THE CLINICIAN'S GUIDE TO
Gastrointestinal Oncology

Michael L. Kochman, MD, FACP

Professor of Medicine
Co-Director, Gastrointestinal Oncology
Gastroenterology Division
University of Pennsylvania
Philadelphia, Pennsylvania

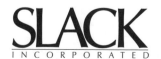

SLACK
INCORPORATED

An innovative information, education, and management company
6900 Grove Road • Thorofare, NJ 08086

Copyright © 2005 by SLACK Incorporated

ISBN-10: 1-55642-682-8
ISBN-13: 978-1-55642-682-7

The procedures and practices described in this book should be implemented in a manner consistent with the professional standards set for the circumstances that apply in each specific situation. Every effort has been made to confirm the accuracy of the information presented and to correctly relate generally accepted practices. The authors, editor, and publisher cannot accept responsibility for errors or exclusions or for the outcome of the material presented herein. There is no expressed or implied warranty of this book or information imparted by it.

Care has been taken to ensure that drug selection and dosages are in accordance with currently accepted/recommended practice. Due to continuing research, changes in government policy and regulations, and various effects of drug reactions and interactions, it is recommended that the reader carefully review all materials and literature provided for each drug, especially those that are new or not frequently used.

Any review or mention of specific companies or products is not intended as an endorsement by the author or publisher.

The work SLACK Incorporated publishes is peer reviewed. Prior to publication, recognized leaders in the field, educators, and clinicians provide important feedback on the concepts and content that we publish. We welcome feedback on this work.

Library of Congress Cataloging-in-Publication Data
The clinician's guide to gastrointestinal oncology / edited by Michael Kochman.
     p. ; cm.
Includes bibliographical references and index.
ISBN-13: 978-1-55642-682-7 (pbk. : alk. paper)
ISBN-10: 1-55642-682-8 (pbk. : alk. paper)
  1. Digestive organs--Cancer.
  [DNLM: 1. Gastrointestinal Neoplasms--diagnosis. 2. Gastrointestinal Neoplasms--therapy. WI 149
C642 2005] I. Kochman, Michael L.
    RC280.D5C58 2005
    616.99'433--dc22
                              2005006970

Printed in the United States of America.

Published by: SLACK Incorporated
                     6900 Grove Road
                     Thorofare, NJ 08086 USA
                     Telephone: 856-848-1000
                     Fax: 856-853-5991
                     www.slackbooks.com

Contact SLACK Incorporated for more information about other books in this field or about the availability of our books from distributors outside the United States.

Last digit is print number: 10   9   8   7   6   5   4   3   2   1

DEDICATION

This book is dedicated to my family: my wife, Mary, and my children Elyse and Sidney, without their indulgence this book would not have been possible.

Over the years a number of key individuals sparked and nurtured my interest in gastrointestinal oncology. Thomas Lad, MD and Jay Goldstein, MD were critical early on in demonstrating to me the need for better diagnostics and additional effective therapies. Tachi Yamada, MD and Chung Owyang, MD had the foresight to allow me the specialized training, which I hope I have put to good use. Drs. Rick Boland, John DelValle, Grace Elta, Robert Hawes, Peter Traber, and Maurits Wiersema were instrumental in helping me acquire and define my skillset and in facilitating my clinical research. My current colleagues at the University of Pennsylvania have been instrumental, with Dan Haller, MD at the forefront.

Clifford Pilz, MD deserves special mention as Chief of Medicine during my medical school, residency, and Chief Residency; he clearly defined the epitome of the all-knowing physician; no question was too small to deserve an answer, no sign or symptom too subtle to be ignored.

CONTENTS

Acknowledgments

I would like to thank the chapter authors who clearly did a phenomenal job conveying their expertise in their respective areas. It is difficult in these times to have genuine experts write chapters due to the complex time demands placed upon them; they are to be congratulated.

The staff at SLACK Incorporated was superb and demonstrated great professionalism; their guidance and expertise shows in the polish of the final product. An individual thanks is due to Carrie Kotlar, without her persistence (and perseverance) this handbook would not have come to fruition.

ABOUT THE EDITOR

Michael L. Kochman, MD, FACP is Professor of Medicine in the Gastroenterology Division at the University of Pennsylvania Medical School and Hospital of the University of Pennsylvania. He is the Endoscopy Training Director and Co-Director of the Gastrointestinal Oncology Program. Dr. Kochman is a graduate of Northwestern University (1982) and the University of Illinois Medical School at Chicago (1986).

At the University of Pennsylvania, he has served on various committees including the Physicians Billing Oversight Committee and Departmental Review Committees. Within the GI division he has served as Fellowship Chairman and has received a number of teaching awards including the Sid Cohen, MD award for the education of fellows. Dr. Kochman has served many local and national societies in a variety of positions. Currently he is President of the Delaware Society for Gastrointestinal Endoscopy and is the Program Chairman for the Pennsylvania State Gastroenterology Society. His major national commitments are to the American Gastroenterological Association (AGA) and the American Society for Gastrointestinal Endoscopy (ASGE). He has served the AGA on the Education Committee and the Program Committee and is currently a member of the Clinical Practice Committee. For the ASGE, Dr. Kochman has served on the Post-Graduate Education Committee, the EUS SIG and is currently a member of the Research Committee and the Program Committee.

Dr. Kochman is the Chairman of the Editorial Board of *Gastrointestinal Endoscopy*, and is coeditor for *Techniques in Gastrointestinal Endoscopy* and the *Yearbook of Gastroenterology*. He also serves on the editorial boards and as a reviewer for a number of journals including *Annals of Internal Medicine* and *Gastroenterology*. Dr. Kochman has published over 120 articles and chapters and a number of videos. He has edited 4 published books and is currently editing 3 books to be published in the near future.

CONTRIBUTING AUTHORS

Jordan Berlin, MD
Vanderbilt University
Nashville, Tennessee

Lynn A. Brody, MD
Memorial Sloan-Kettering Cancer Center
New York, New York

Karen T. Brown, MD
Memorial Sloan-Kettering Cancer Center
New York, New York

Alan L. Buchman, MD, MSPH
Northwestern University Medical School
Chicago, Illinois

Allen W. Burton, MD
UT MD Anderson Cancer Center
Houston, Texas

Navtej Buttar, MD
Mayo Clinic
Jacksonville, Florida

Robert J. Canter, MD
University of Pennsylvania Health System
Philadelphia, Pennsylvania

Bapsi Chak, MD
Vanderbilt University
Nashville, Tennessee

Anne Covey, MD
Memorial Sloan-Kettering Cancer Center
New York, New York

Kristoffel R. Dumon, MD
University of Pennsylvania Health System
Philadelphia, Pennsylvania

Diane Hershock, MD, PhD
University of Pennsylvania Health System
Philadelphia, Pennsylvania

J.J. Karmacharya, FRCS
University of Pennsylvania Health System
Philadelphia, Pennsylvania

John C. Kucharczuk, MD
University of Pennsylvania Health System
Philadelphia, Pennsylvania

Linda S. Lee, MD
Harvard Medical School
Boston, Massachusetts

Paul Limberg, MD, MPH
Mayo Clinic
Jacksonville, Florida

Najjia N. Mahmoud, MD
University of Pennsylvania Health System
Philadelphia, Pennsylvania

Arnold J. Markowitz, MD
Memorial Sloan-Kettering Cancer Center
New York, New York

Patrick M. McQuillan, MD
Penn State College of Medicine
Hershey, Pennsylvania

Carla L. Nash, MD
Memorial Sloan-Kettering Cancer Center
New York, New York

Patrick R. Pfau, MD
University of Wisconsin, Madison
Madison, Wisconsin

Rosemary C. Polomano, PhD, RN, FAAN
University of Pennsylvania School of
Nursing
Philadelphia, Pennsylvania

John M. Poneros, MD
Brigham and Women's Hospital
Boston, Massachusetts

Niraja Rajan, MD
Penn State College of Medicine
Hershey, Pennsylvania

Stephen J. Rulyak, MD, MPH
University of Washington
Harvorview Medical Center
Seattle, Washington

Richard E. Sampliner, MD
University of Arizona Health Sciences
Center
Tucson, Arizona

James S. Scolapio, MD
Mayo Clinic
Jacksonville, Florida

Ilias Scotiniotis, MD
Department of Gastroenterology
Hygeia Hospital
Athens, Greece

Janak N. Shah, MD
San Francisco General Hospital
San Francisco, California

Francis (Frank) Spitz, MD
University of Pennsylvania Health System
Philadelphia, Pennsylvania

Weijing Sun, MD
University of Pennsylvania Health System
Philadelphia, Pennsylvania

Noel N. Williams, MD
University of Pennsylvania Health System
Philadelphia, Pennsylvania

PREFACE

The area of gastrointestinal oncology is an active one. Both clinical research and basic research have come together and changed the diagnostic and treatment protocols for a number of deadly malignancies. A multidisciplinary approach to the diagnosis and treatment appears to be the best paradigm; it allows for each individual medical specialty to apply their knowledge and expertise in an expeditious and effective manner.

Some of the cancers with which we deal are unfortunately all too often ultimately fatal. Our roles are changing; the boundaries between the medical subspecialties are blurring, with progressive leadership we are better able to make the patients feel that their "team" is truly in sync and providing cutting edge therapy. To this end, I have gathered a nationally and internationally recognized group of clinical researchers and clinicians to provide a balanced and multidisciplinary approach to the treatment of the most common of the gastrointestinal malignancies.

It is intended that this book will serve as a resource for trainees and clinicians in the medical and surgical fields. Those that infrequently diagnose or take care of patients with these neoplasms should be able to find enough easily accessible information to be able to converse with their patients and their families, and those who are routinely involved in the care of these patients will gain a better understanding of the capabilities of the other specialties and gain insight into the thought processes behind the often difficult treatment decisions that must be made.

chapter 1

Management of Premalignant Diseases of the Esophagus: Barrett's Esophagus

Richard E. Sampliner, MD

Barrett's esophagus (BE) is the premalignant disease for esophageal adenocarcinoma (EAC), the most rapidly rising incidence cancer in the Western world.[1] Even when BE is not found at endoscopy or at surgical resection in the presence of EAC, it is usually the source. As documented in a study, EAC can overgrow the BE so that the latter is not recognized after chemotherapy. Although pathways of gastroesophageal reflux disease (GERD) progressing to EAC without going through BE have been postulated, such a pathway, if it exists, must be very uncommon.

DEFINITION

The current working definition of BE is based on endoscopic assessment (Table 1-1). The distal esophagus has an abnormal lining—salmon-colored rather than the normal pearl-colored squamous lining. In addition, intestinal metaplasia is present on biopsy. Intestinal metaplasia is a change like the intestine—goblet cells—but in the esophagus. This is the specific epithelium at risk for development of dysplasia and ultimately EAC.

This definition of BE has evolved over the last 3 decades. It is important to differentiate BE from intestinal metaplasia of the gastric cardia. This differentiation requires careful targeting of biopsies by the gastroenterologist and clear communication with the pathologist about the origin of the biopsy. The targeting of biopsies is guided by the recognition of essential endoscopic landmarks (Table 1-2). Missed targeting or mislabeling of the site of biopsy may lead to an incorrect diagnosis. According to one group, BE has a greater concentration of glands than intestinal metaplasia of the gastric cardia and lacks well developed adjacent cardiac mucosa, thus basing the distinction between BE and intestinal metaplasia of the gastric cardia on histologic criteria.

The definition of BE includes patients with intestinal metaplasia of any length in an abnormal distal esophagus. An older definition of BE as columnar lined esophagus greater than 3 cm has led to the current arbitrary classification of short segment BE (<3 cm) and long segment BE (≥3 cm).

Table 1-1

DEFINITION OF BARRETT'S ESOPHAGUS

1. Abnormal appearing distal esophagus mucosa

2. Intestinal metaplasia by biopsy

Table 1-2

ESSENTIAL ENDOSCOPIC LANDMARKS

1. Squamocolumnar junction

2. Esophagogastric junction

3. Diaphragmatic pinch

EPIDEMIOLOGY

The epidemiology of BE is incompletely identified and derived mostly from cohort studies of patients with BE. These studies are retrospective, prospective, and subject to the variability of disease definition, referral bias, and the specifics of the population served at the study site. The mean age of diagnosis is 63 years and the estimated mean age of onset is 40 years.[2] Patients with BE are predominantly male—2:1 male to female ratio.[3] The frequency of BE differs dramatically among ethnic groups. The prevalence of BE in adults undergoing endoscopy ranges from 7.8% of Whites to 4.8% of Hispanic Americans and 1.1% of African Americans. A longer duration of reflux symptoms separates BE from non-Barrett's GERD patients as a group, but there is a great overlap of individual patients. An earlier age of onset of GERD may also be a characteristic of BE.

Reports of families with generations of patients with BE suggest familial aggregation. First-degree relatives of patients with BE and EAC are more likely to have a history of GERD than first-degree relatives of patients with reflux esophagitis.[4] Familial aggregation of BE, EAC and adenocarcinoma of the esophagogastric junction has been demonstrated in White adults.

Hiatal hernia is commonly associated with BE and contributes to the pathophysiology. Ninety-six percent of patients with long segment BE have a hiatal hernia.[5] In fact, a predictive model for the length of BE uses the length of the hiatal hernia and the duration of esophageal acid exposure.[6] On average, patients with BE have greater esophageal acid and bile acid exposure than GERD patients without mucosal disease.

SCREENING FOR BARRETT'S ESOPHAGUS

The rationale for screening for BE is that it is the premalignant lesion for EAC. Recognition of BE allows an opportunity for early recognition of EAC to enable intervention and improvement of outcome. The rising incidence of EAC has been docu-

Table 1-3

HIGH RISK FOR ESOPHAGEAL ADENOCARCINOMA

- Gender: Male
- Ethnicity: White
- Older age
- Chronic GERD
- High body mass index
- Cigarette smoking
- LES relaxing drugs

mented since 1975 and continues to climb. EAC has increased from 5% of esophageal cancers to more than 50% in the last 30 years. Unfortunately, less than 5% of patients with EAC have been previously identified with BE. Only prior detection of BE allows for early intervention.

The annual incidence of EAC in patients with BE has been controversial. A funnel analysis demonstrated publication bias with series with smaller numbers of patients with shorter follow-up having a higher incidence of cancer.[7] This analysis as well as a prospective cohort study suggests the annual incidence to be 0.5%.[8] Even these data are subject to bias from an inadequate length of follow-up. A young patient with BE does not have a greater risk of EAC than an older one just because he has a much longer life expectancy. A more realistic estimate of mortality from EAC can be derived from a population based and a cohort study demonstrating a mortality from EAC in patients with BE of 4.7% and 2.5% respectively.[9,10] The lifetime risk of dying from EAC may be a concept that can be grasped by patients more readily than annual incidence. Patients with BE are usually surprised and reassured that this risk is less than 5%.

The epidemiology of BE and EAC provides information on who is at higher risk for having these diseases (Table 1-3). Who should we screen for BE? Older White males with chronic reflux symptoms will have the highest yield of BE. Evidence-based thresholds for a specific age and years of reflux symptoms are not established. A Veterans Affairs Medical Center study found an age of more than 40 years with heartburn at least weekly to be predictive of BE.[11] There is a 2 phase risk stratification that is necessary: those patients at risk for BE and those with BE at risk for EAC. The risk factors for EAC are similar to those for BE—85% of patients with EAC are White men. Increased frequency, severity, and duration of reflux symptoms are risk factors for EAC. This was documented in a Swedish population-based study. Combining long duration with severity of reflux symptoms has an odds ratio of EAC of 43.5 compared to controls lacking GERD.[12]

Trials of screening a random sample of the population for BE do not exist. BE can even occur in patients lacking evident GERD symptoms. This provides a formidable challenge for screening. In a predominantly male (90%), veteran, and White (73%) group with a mean age of 61 undergoing sigmoidoscopy screening, 7% had long segment BE and 17% short segment.[13] These surprising findings were not substantiated in a larger study of patients with a mean age of 59, 60% male, and 78% White undergoing colonoscopy. Only 0.36% had long segment and 5.2% short segment BE.[14] Long segment BE is uncommon in patients lacking reflux symptoms.

Table 1-4

SUGGESTED SURVEILLANCE FOR BARRETT'S ESOPHAGUS

Dysplasia Grade	Evaluation	Endoscopy Frequency
None	2 endoscopies	3 to 4 years
LGD	Highest grade on second endoscopy	Annual until no dysplasia x 2
HGD	Repeat endoscopy with intensive large forceps biopsy protocol	Mucosal irregularity (EMR)
	Expert pathologist interpretation	Individualize intervention

---

SURVEILLANCE ENDOSCOPY

Once BE is diagnosed, the next step is surveillance in an effort to detect high grade dysplasia (HGD) and EAC for effective intervention. Dysplasia is the currently available clinical biologic marker predicting cancer. Dysplasia is the first step of the neoplastic process. It is characterized by cytologic and architectural changes in intestinal metaplasia that typically involve the surface epithelium. Although a higher grade of dysplasia is associated with a greater risk of EAC, even HGD may apparently regress and may not progress to cancer over even a decade. Progression from HGD to cancer ranges from 59% in 5 years[15] to 16% in 7 years.[16] However, eliminating patients referred for HGD and cancer that develop within the first year of follow-up (prevalence EAC) reduces the higher rate to 24% at 5 years, a still significant risk. All patients with BE and HGD do not inevitably progress to cancer over their lifetime.

The problem with dysplasia as the basis for surveillance is the interobserver variability. Even expert gastrointestinal (GI) pathologists have only a fair agreement in differentiating HGD from intramucosal cancer—kappa value of 0.56.[17] This interobserver variability is not overcome by training. Unfortunately, this basis of clinical decision making is not a clear cut endpoint.

Surveillance endoscopy is intrinsically reasonable and uniformly practiced in the United States,[18] although proof of efficacy is lacking. Retrospective surgical series document a significantly greater survival in patients with cancer found at surveillance endoscopy than patients clinically presenting with EAC (62% to 90% vs 20%). Recent case-control studies also suggest that endoscopy is associated with earlier stage cancer and improved survival.[19,20] The frequency of surveillance endoscopy is based on the grade of dysplasia (Table 1-4).[21] The intervals are derived from prospectively followed patient cohorts and the biopsy protocol is based on modeling studies. With no dysplasia on two consecutive endoscopies, an interval of at least 3 years is recommended. With low grade dysplasia (LGD) after a second endoscopy confirming no higher grade of dysplasia in the esophagus, endoscopy is recommended annually until no dysplasia is detected in 2 consecutive endoscopies. The standard biopsy protocol includes biopsies of any mucosal irregularities and four-quadrant every 2 cm. HGD will be discussed next.

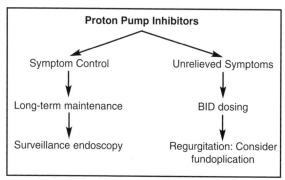

Figure 1-1. Medical management of Barrett's Esophagus.

MEDICAL TREATMENT

The mainstay of medical therapy is proton pump inhibitor therapy. The goal of therapy for patients with BE is control of reflux symptoms and healing of accompanying erosive esophagitis. Symptom control often requires BID dosing (Figure 1-1). Even with appropriate timing prior to meals, esophageal pH is still abnormal in 25% of patients with BE.[22] Patients with postprandial and supine regurgitation may benefit from metoclopramide prior to a late meal. Additionally, intermittent H_2 receptor antagonist use may be of benefit.

Patients with refractory regurgitation and volume reflux, are candidates for surgical fundoplication. Currently, this is performed less invasively and with shorter hospital stay by laparoscopy. Although short term effectiveness is to be expected, a longer term median follow-up of 5 years in 85 BE patients demonstrated recurrent symptoms in 20%.[23] The long term symptomatic durability of surgery is a concern, especially in patients with BE.

Resectional surgery has a definitive role in patients with EAC. It is the only therapy resulting in long-term cancer-free survival. The long-term survival is excellent for early stage disease. TNM staging is utilized (ie, *t*umor, *n*odal involvement, and distant *m*etastases) (see Appendix A). Endosonography provides the most accurate assessment of depth of wall invasion and mediastinal involvement can be directly determined with fine needle aspiration. Intramucosal EAC cancer in the lamina propria and above the muscularis mucosa has less than 5% risk of regional lymph node spread in contrast to submucosal cancer with a 25% risk. With the recognition of the dependence of operative mortality on the institutional volume of esophagectomy, there has been increased motivation to send patients for surgery to high volume centers.[24,25] The role of surgery in the management of HGD will be discussed below.

MANAGEMENT OF HIGH GRADE DYSPLASIA

The management of HGD is complicated by problems including endoscopic sampling, histologic interpretation, variable natural history, coexistence of unrecognized EAC, patient comorbidity, and inconsistent institutional expertise (Figure 1-2). HGD is commonly not visible at endoscopy so that even though a biopsy protocol is systematic, the specific site involved may not be targeted. Therefore, the first step in managing a patient with HGD is to repeat the endoscopy using a therapeutic endoscope and a large

Figure 1-2. Management of HGD.

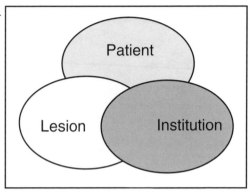

capacity biopsy forceps to obtain larger samples. Four-quadrant biopsies are performed every 1 cm. Biopsies from each level are placed in a separate container to help localize the HGD. Any mucosal irregularity should also be separately biopsied. HGD found in the biopsy of a nodule should be considered a cancer until proven otherwise. This is the ideal setting to apply the new technique of endoscopic mucosal resection. This provides a large sample—usually 1 cm—to more effectively stage the disease for therapeutic decision making. The finding of intramucosal cancer could lead to topical (endoscopic) therapy. Invasion of the muscularis mucosa would lead to an esophageal resection in a patient who is a good surgical candidate because of the risk of regional lymph node spread.

An expert GI pathologist should then confirm the reading of HGD. At this point, it is worthwhile to sit down with the patient and his or her partner to discuss the options—intensive endoscopic surveillance, endoscopic ablation therapy, or esophagectomy. This decision should be individualized based on the patient's age, medical condition, and preferences. A year of surveillance endoscopy every 3 months should not pose a risk of delayed diagnosis in a patient without mucosal irregularities. The finding of cancer at any endoscopy usually simplifies decision making. Factors favoring surgery include younger age, good cardiopulmonary condition, multifocal HGD, recurrently identified HGD, and the availability of a high volume surgical center. Favoring endoscopic surveillance or therapies include an aged patient, major comorbidity, and local endoscopic expertise.

Photodynamic therapy using porfimer sodium as the photosensitizer has been recently approved by the FDA for patients with BE and HGD. A multicenter randomized trial with a 2-year follow-up documented significant improvement in eradication of HGD (77% vs 39% in the nonendoscopically-treated control group) and development of EAC (13% vs 28%).[26] This option offers no procedural mortality and retained esophageal function. One third of patients do develop strictures and patients can still develop EAC. Endoscopic therapy may include a combination of endoscopic mucosal resection of mucosal irregularities and photodynamic therapy of the entire segment of BE.

The patient has to weigh the risk of operative mortality and morbidity against the opportunity for cancer-free survival. In contrast, the patient choosing endoscopic therapy balances the avoidance of procedural mortality and maintenance of esophageal function for the continuing risk of developing EAC and the need to maintain endoscopic surveillance. The risk of developing EAC after endoscopic therapy has been documented to continue for as long as 6 years.

CANCER PREVENTION OPPORTUNITIES

Biologic markers of progression from BE to EAC have been pursued as the holy grail of risk stratification over the last decades. Despite the evaluation of scores of markers ranging from indicators of proliferation, differentiation, growth factors, enzymes, and gene mutations, only 2 have been assessed in a prospectively followed cohort of BE patients. The baseline histology and marker status were determined and the clear endpoint of EAC utilized. Flow cytometric abnormalities were found to be predictive of EAC—aneuploidy (abnormal cellular DNA content) and increased 4N fractions.[15] Perhaps the most pragmatic finding was that none of 215 patients with no or LGD lacking flow cytometric abnormalities progressed to cancer over 5 years (95% confidence interval 0 to 4.7%). The same group found the baseline 17p (p53) loss of heterozygosity (a tumor suppressor gene) predicted progression to EAC, relative risk 16.[27] Clinical application of these markers awaits their validation in multicenter cohorts of patients with BE. Surveillance endoscopy could then be focused on the highest risk group likely to progress to EAC.

Preliminary reports have highlighted new concepts in the molecular biology of BE. Methylation of the adenomatous polyposis coli (APC) gene was expressed in 92% of EAC and 25% of these patients' plasma.[28] This approach could result in a blood test to screen for EAC. Using microarray technology and a verified complementary DNA library containing 8064 clones, BE was separated from EAC. Over- and underexpressed genes in BE and EAC were identified for further study of neoplastic progression.[29]

The optical detection of dysplasia during endoscopy offers the potential for real time recognition of HGD and treatment. Many technologies are in the developmental stage and have preliminary data. Fluorescence spectroscopy takes advantage of fluorescent molecules within tissue re-emitting absorbed light at differing wavelengths that are then analyzed. Laser-induced fluorescence can recognize HGD.[30] Tissue fluorescence can be examined after administration of exogenous fluorescent agents such as 5-aminolevular acid at a lower dose than used for photodynamic therapy.[31] Light scattering spectroscopy utilizes reflected light to determine the size distribution of nuclei in the mucosa. Analysis of enlarged nuclei and nuclear crowding can detect both low and HGD with excellent sensitivity and specificity.[32] Raman spectroscopy provides detailed biochemical information about tissue from a small fraction of scattered light undergoing shifts in wavelength—this can be analyzed by algorithms to detect dysplasia.[33] Optical coherence tomography provides cross-sectional tissue images with high spatial resolution by detecting light reflected back from mucosal structures and thereby can identify dysplasia.[34] Magnification endoscopy with or without chromoendoscopy can identify fine mucosal detail suggestive of dysplasia. These techniques could potentially replace endoscopic biopsy or at least guide the targeting of biopsies for a higher yield of neoplasia. Which techniques will emerge and be clinically validated remains to be seen.

The only therapies that can prevent the development of cancer are resectional surgery and photodynamic therapy. The hope for the future is the prevention of carcinogenesis—chemoprevention. Understanding the molecular biology, the cytokines and growth factors, and microenvironment factors would allow for precise targeting of pathways. A current example of such potential targeting is cyclooxygenase-2 (COX-2). COX-2 expression can be induced by cytokines, growth factors, and tumor promoters. It can be upregulated *ex vivo* by acid and bile. COX-2 expression increases during progression of intestinal metaplasia to dysplasia and subsequently EAC.[35] Selective COX-2 inhibition decreases proliferation in cell cultures. Both nonselective and selective COX-2 inhibition significantly reduce the development of EAC in an esophagojejunostomy anastomosis rat model of BE.[36] In humans, a meta-analysis of epidemiologic case-control studies documents a significant reduction of EAC with aspirin and other NSAIDs.[37] The above data have led to the initiation of a large randomized prospective trial of aspirin to test the chemopreventive impact on the development of EAC in patients with BE.

There has been an expansion of information and literature about BE. The definition has evolved. Screening and surveillance are still based on preliminary information lacking an evidence basis. Surveillance intervals are based on the relatively crude marker of dysplasia. Yet advances in therapy include endoscopic technology development and improved surgical outcomes. Breakthroughs in the understanding of molecular biology, development of optical techniques, and progress in chemoprevention should highlight the future.

REFERENCES

1. Brown LM, Devesa SS. Epidemiologic trends in esophageal and gastric cancer in the United States. *Surg Oncol Clin N Am.* 2002;11:235-256.

2. Cameron AJ, Lomboy CT. Barrett's esophagus: age, prevalence and extent of columnar epithelium. *Gastroenterology.* 1992;103:1241-1245.

3. O'Connor JB, Falk GW, Richter JE. The incidence of adenocarcinoma and dysplasia in Barrett's esophagus. *Am J Gastroenterol.* 1999;94(8):2037-2042.

4. Romero Y, Cameron AJ, Locke GR, et al. Familial aggregation of gastroesophageal reflux in patients with Barrett's esophagus and esophageal adenocarcinoma. *Gastroenterology.* 1997;113:1449-1456.

5. Cameron AJ. Barrett's esophagus: prevalence and size of hiatal hernia. *Am J Gastroenterol.* 1999;94(8):2054-2059.

6. Wakelin DE, Al-Mutawa TS, Wendel CS, et al. A predictive model for length of Barrett's esophagus with hiatal hernia length and duration of esophageal acid exposure. *Gastrointest Endosc.* 2003;58:350-355.

7. Shaheen NJ, Crosby MA, Bozymski EM. Is there publication bias in the reporting of cancer risk of Barrett's esophagus? *Gastroenterology.* 2000;119:333-338.

8. Drewitz DJ, Sampliner RE, Garewal HS. The incidence of adenocarcinoma in Barrett's esophagus—a prospective study of 170 patients followed 4.8 years. *Am J Gastroenterol.* 1997;92(2):212-215.

9. Anderson LA, Murray LJ, Murphy SJ, et al. Mortality in Barrett's esophagus: results from a population based study. *Gut.* 2003;52:1081-84.

10. VanDerBurgh A, Doos J, Hop WJC, VanBlankenstein M. Esophageal cancer is an uncommon cause of death in patients with Barrett's oesophagus. *Gut.* 1996;39:5-8.

11. Eloubeide MA, Provenzale D. Clinical and demographic predictors of Barrett's esophagus among patients with gastroesophageal reflux disease. *J Clin Gastroenterol.* 2001; 33(4):306-309.

12. Lagergren J, Bergstrom R, Lindgren A, Nyren O. Symptomatic gastroesophageal reflux as a risk factor for esophageal adenocarcinoma. *N Engl J Med.* 1999;340(11):825-831.

13. Gerson LB, Sheltler K, Triadafilopoloulos G. Prevalence of Barrett's esophagus in asymptomatic individuals. *Gastroenterology.* 2002;123:461-467.

14. Rex DK, Cummings OW, Shaw M, et al. Screening for Barrett's esophagus in colonoscopy patients with and without heartburn. *Gastroenterology.* 2003;125:1670-1677.

15. Reid B, Levine D, Longton G, Blount P, Rabinovitch P. Predictors of progression to cancer in Barrett's esophagus: baseline histology and flow cytometry identify low and high risk patient subsets. *Am J Gastroenterol.* 2000;95:1669-1676.

16. Schnell TG, Sontag SJ, Chejfec G, et al. Long-term nonsurgical management of Barrett's esophagus with high-grade dysplasia. *Gastroenterology.* 2001;120:1607-1619.

17. Ormsby AH, Petras RE, Henricks WH, et al. Interobserver variation in the diagnosis of superficial oesophageal adenocarcinoma. *Gut.* 2002;51:671-676.

18. Falk GW, Ours TM, Richter J. Practice patterns for surveillance of Barrett's esophagus in the United States. *Gastrointest Endosc.* 2000;52:197-203.

19. Corley DA, Levin TR, Habel LA, Weiss NS, Buffler PA. Surveillance and survival in Barrett's adenocarcinomas: a population-based study. *Gastroenterology.* 2002;122:633-640.

20. Cooper GS. Endoscopic screening and surveillance for Barrett's esophagus: can claims data determine its effectiveness? *Gastrointest Endosc.* 2003;57(7):914-915.

21. Sampliner RE, Practice Parameters Committee ACG. Updated guidelines for the diagnosis, surveillance, and therapy of Barrett's esophagus. *Am J Gastroenterol.* 2002; 97:1888-1895.

22. Fass R, Sampliner RE, Malagon IB, et al. Failure of oesophageal acid control in candidates for Barrett's oesophagus reversal on a very high dose of proton pump inhibitor. *Aliment Pharmacol.* 2000;14:597-602.

23. Hofstetter WL, Peters JH, DeMeester T, et al. Long-term outcome of antireflux surgery in patients with Barrett's esophagus. *Ann Surg.* 2001;234(532-9).

24. Begg CB, Cramer LD, Hoskins WJ, Brennan MF. Impact of hospital volume on operative mortality for major cancer surgery. *JAMA.* 1998;280:1747-1751.

25. Birkmeyer JD, Siewers AE, Finlayson EVA, et al. Hospital volume and surgical mortality in the United States. *N Engl J Med.* 2002;346:1128-1137.

26. Overholt B, Lightdale C, Wang K, et al. International, multicenter, partially blinded, randomized study of the efficacy of photodynamic therapy (PDT) using porfimer sodium (POR) for the ablation of high-grade dysplasia (HGD) in Barrett's esophagus (BE): results of 24-month follow-up. *Gastroenterology.* 2003;124:A20.

27. Reid B, Prevo L, Galipeau P, et al. Predictors of progression in Barrett's esophagus II: baseline 17p (p53) loss of heterozygosity identifies a patient subset at increased risk for neoplastic progression. *Am J Gastroenterol.* 2001;96:2839-2848.

28. Kawakami K, Brabender J, Lord RV, et al. Hypermethylated APC DNA in plasma and prognosis of patients with esophageal adenocarcinoma. *J Natl Cancer Inst.* 2000; 92:1805-11.

29. Xu Y, Selaru FM, Yin J, et al. Artificial neural networks and gene filtering distinguish between global gene expression profiles of Barrett's esophagus and esophageal cancer. *Cancer Research.* 2002;62:3943-97.

30. Panjehpour M, Overholt BF, Vo-Dinh TH, et al. Endoscopic fluorescence detection of high grade dysplasia in Barrett's esophagus. *Gastroenterology.* 1996;111:93-101.

31. Endlicher E, Knuechel R, Hauser T, Szeimies RM, Scholmerich J, Messmann H. Endoscopic fluorescence detection of low and high grade dysplasia in Barrett's oesophagus using systemic or local 5-aminolaevulinic acid sensitization. *Gut.* 2001;48:314-319.

32. Wallace MB, Perelman LT, Backman V, et al. Endoscopic detection of dysplasia in patients with Barrett's esophagus using light-scattering spectroscopy. *Gastroenterology.* 2000;119:677-682.

33. Kendall C, Stone N, Shepherd NA, et al. Raman spectroscopy, a potential tool for the objective identification and classification of neoplasia in Barrett's oesophagus. *J Pathol.* 2003;200:602-609.

34. Poneros JM, Nishioka NS. Diagnosis of Barrett's esophagus using optical coherence tomography. *Gastrointest Endosc Clin N Am.* 2003;13:309-323.

35. Shirvani VN, Ouatu-Lascar R, Kaur B, Omary B, Triadafilopoloulos G. Cyclooxygenase 2 expression in Barrett's esophagus and adenocarcinoma: ex vivo induction by bile salts and acid exposure. *Gastroenterology.* 2000;118:487-496.

36. Buttar NS, Wang KK, Leontovich O, et al. Chemoprevention of esophageal adenocarcinoma by COX-2 inhibitors in an animal model of Barrett's esophagus. *Gastroenterology.* 2002;122:1101-1112.

37. Corley DA, Kerlikowske K, Verma R, Buffler PA. Protective association of aspirin/NSAIDs and esophageal cancer: a systematic review and meta-analysis. *Gastroenterology.* 2003;124:47-56.

chapter 2

Surgical Approaches to Esophageal Neoplasms

John C. Kucharczuk, MD

INTRODUCTION

Several important factors influence the surgical approach to an esophageal neoplasm. These include the nature of the neoplasm (benign vs malignant), the overall health of the patient, and the expertise of the surgeon. The intent of this chapter is to familiarize the reader with the different approaches available for resection of esophageal neoplasms. Special emphasis will be placed on the expected benefits as well as potential risk of each operative approach to aide in the dialogue between the gastroenterologist and surgeon. This dialogue is vital in providing an individual patient with the surgical approach that is most likely to be safe and effective.

BENIGN ESOPHAGEAL NEOPLASM

ESOPHAGEAL LEIOMYOMA

Esophageal leiomyoma is the most common benign esophageal neoplasm. These lesions are most frequently found in the middle and lower thirds of the esophagus.[1] Indications for surgical resection are 1) dysphagia, 2) size over 3 cm, 3) progressive increase in size, 4) mucosal ulceration, and 5) to obtain definitive tissue diagnosis.[2,3]

We recently published an extensive review on the management of esophageal leiomyoma.[4] The surgical approach to these lesions depends on the size, location, and character of the leiomyoma. Leiomyoma less than 8 cm without annular characteristics (Figure 2-1) are best treated by surgical extramucosal enucleation. Those greater than 8 cm or annular in character usually require esophageal resection (Figure 2-2).

The surgical approach to extramucosal enucleation is dictated by anatomic location of the lesion. Leiomyoma in the middle third of the esophagus are approached through the right chest. Those occurring in the distal third of the esophagus are approached via the left chest. On occasion, lesions occurring in the very distal esophagus just above the gastroesophageal junction can be approached via the upper abdomen.

Figure 2-1. Endoscopic view of small midesophageal leiomyoma. (Photo courtesy of Michael Kochman, MD, University of Pennsylvania Medical Center.) *For a full-color version, see page CA-I of the Color Atlas.*

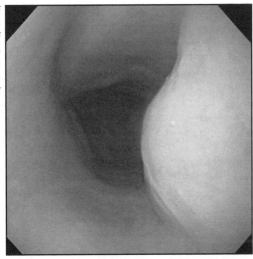

Figure 2-2A. Coronal MRI image of a massive esophageal leiomyoma in a symptomatic 15-year-old girl.

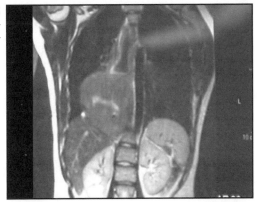

Figure 2-2B. Corresponding CT scan axial image.

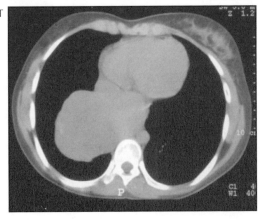

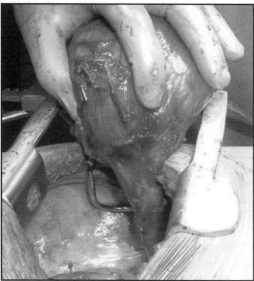

Figure 2-2C. Intraoperative photo through right thoracotomy showing massive leiomyoma and resected esophagus. This patient required a complete esophagectomy via right thoracotomy, upper midline abdominal incision, and left neck incision. Continuity was restored by creation of a gastric tube with cervical anastomosis. (Photo from author's personal collection.) *For a full-color version, see page CA-II of the Color Atlas.*

Traditionally, enucleation of leiomyomata has been performed in an "open" fashion either by thoracotomy or laparotomy. More recently, minimally invasive approaches utilizing thoracoscopy and laparoscopy have been introduced for selected patients.

The principles and technique of extramucosal enucleation, whether performed open or with minimally invasive techniques, is similar. The open technique is illustrated in Figures 2-3A to D. This involves mobilizing the esophagus above and below the lesion. Once the esophagus is mobilized, a longitudinal myotomy is performed (Figure 2-3B). The cut muscle edges are slowly elevated and easily dissect away from the leiomyoma; an avascular, encapsulated mass (Figure 2-3C). Dissection is facilitated by placement of a silk suture through the lesion or use of a ringed forceps for retraction. Care is taken to avoid mucosal injury which results in a postoperative intrathoracic esophageal leak, a potentially devastating complication. Once the enucleation is completed, the myotomy is reapproximated to avoid later mucosal bulging and formation of a symptomatic pseudodiverticulum (Figure 2-3D). Prior to completing the procedure, the chest is flooded with sterile saline, the esophagus distal to the enucleation site is manually occluded, and air is insufflated into the proximal esophagus either by a nasogastric tube or esophagoscope. The absence of an air leak insures mucosal integrity. Following this a chest tube is place and the incisions are closed.

The expected mortality rate following thoracotomy for the extramucosal resection is less than 1%. Complications are infrequent but can include esophageal leak, cardiopulmonary complications, chyle leak, and chronic thoracotomy pain. The long-term outcomes are outstanding with more than 90% of patients remaining symptom free at 5 years following operation.[5] Recurrence is rare with only 2 cases reported in the literature.[6] A thoracoscopic approach also appears appropriate in selected patients with anatomically favorable locations and smaller size (<5 cm).[7] Proponents have argued that a thoracoscopic approach results in less pain, shorter hospitalization, and better cosmetic outcome. At present the role of thoracoscopic resection is evolving.

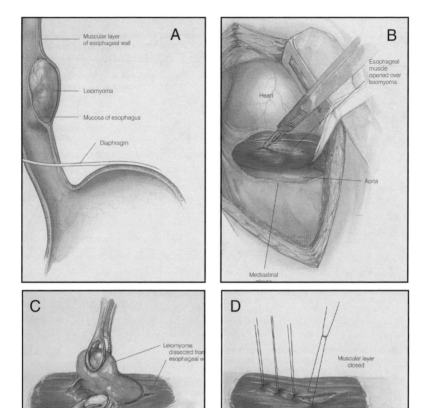

Figure 2-3. (A) Typical small esophageal leiomyoma appropriate for extramucosal enucleation. (B) A longitudinal myotomy is performed exposing the leiomyoma. C) The leiomyoma is gently dissected away from the esophageal mucosa. (D) The myotomy is closed to prevent pseudodiverticulum formation. (Reprinted from *Atlas of Surgery*, 2e, Cameron JL, pp 73-75, Copyright 1994 with permission from Elsevier.) *For full color version, see pages CA-II and CA-III of the Color Atlas.*

OTHER UNCOMMON BENIGN ESOPHAGEAL NEOPLASMS

As mentioned above, leiomyomata of the esophagus are uncommon but they represent the most frequently occurring benign esophageal neoplasm. A number of other benign esophageal neoplasms have been reported but are distinctly unusual. Included in this group are adenomatous polyp, lipoma, fibroma, neurofibroma, hemangioma, and papilloma. The surgical treatment for these benign lesions is resection. Endoscopic removal is appropriate in selected patients; however, particular attention must be given to large lesions located in cervical esophagus. Endoscopic snare removal can result in uncontrollable bleeding, and very large cervical esophageal lesions should usually be approached via a left cervical esophagotomy.[8]

MALIGNANT ESOPHAGEAL NEOPLASM

Malignant esophageal neoplasms include adenocarcinoma, squamous cell carcinoma, small cell carcinoma, leiomyosarcoma, rhabdomyosarcoma, fibrosarcoma, liposarcoma, lymphomas, and metastatic lesions to the esophagus from distant primary sites. Clearly adenocarcinoma and squamous cell carcinoma are the most frequently encountered and many surgeons complete entire careers without seeing the less common types of malignant esophageal neoplasms.

The goal of esophageal resection, whether as primary treatment or as part of a multimodality plan, is cure. Palliative esophagectomy is associated with mortality rates in excess of 20%, morbidity rates as high as 50%, and should be avoided.[9] Very effective palliation can be obtained with chemotherapy, radiation therapy, and endoscopic interventions.

There are several surgical approaches to esophagectomy. These include the transhiatal approach (Orringer),[10] the transabdominal transthoracic approach (Ivor-Lewis),[11] the "Three Stage" approach (McKeown),[12] the thoracoabdominal approach, and the "minimally invasive" approach. Each approach has its own set of risks and benefits as well as outspoken opponents and proponents. Selection of the appropriate approach for an individual patient requires experienced surgical judgment. Despite the rhetoric, several studies have shown equivalent outcomes among the multiple approaches. It appears that the experience of the surgeon[13] and the volume of like cases performed at a particular institution are the most important factors determining outcome.[14] A recent high volume single institution review showed that technical complications following esophagectomy were associated with increased length of hospital stay and increased in hospital mortality and was predictive of a poorer overall long-term survival.[15]

TRANSHIATAL APPROACH TO ESOPHAGECTOMY

The transhiatal approach to esophagectomy was popularized by Orringer in 1978. Today, the transhiatal approach is preferred by many surgeons, nevertheless, debate continues over whether this approach really has lower morbidity and mortality than other approaches involving thoracotomy and whether it provides an adequate cancer operation. Proponents argue that this approach results in less surgical trauma by avoiding thoracotomy and thus less postoperative morbidity, especially pulmonary complication. Furthermore, by placing the anastomosis in the neck, a leak—should it occur—can be treated by simple cervical drainage. In contrast, a leak in the chest can result in mediastinitis and be life threatening.

This procedure is performed with the patient is in a supine position with the neck extended and turned toward the right (Figure 2-4). The transhiatal approach is begun with an upper midline laparotomy. After exploration of the peritoneal cavity to rule out disseminated disease, the stomach is mobilized for creation of a gastric tube. Due to its robust blood supply, ease of mobilization, and its ability to reach the neck, the gastric tube is the conduit of choice. The use of colon is more complex and has an increased morbidity when compared to gastric transposition.[16] I reserve the use of colon or jejunum for patients with an unusable stomach due to previous surgery, tumor extension, or other technical considerations. The right gastroepiploic artery is preserved and

Figure 2-4. Typical cervical and abdominal incision placement for transhiatal esophagectomy. (Reprinted from *Atlas of General Thoracic Surgery*, Kaiser LR, Copyright 1997, with permission from Elsevier.)

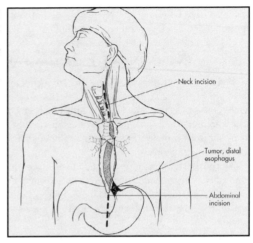

Neck incision

Tumor, distal esophagus

Abdominal incision

protected throughout the dissection as this will become the major blood supply to the gastric tube. As dissection is continued along the greater curvature of the stomach, the short gastric vessels are individually identified and ligated. If there are dense adhesions in the left upper quadrant, the spleen is at risk for injury and bleeding. On rare occasion, a splenectomy is required. On the lesser curvature side, the left gastric artery is identified, ligated, and divided. Lymph nodes around the celiac axis are dissected away and brought up with the mobilized stomach. A "Kocher maneuver" is performed to mobilize the duodenum, providing more mobility to the gastric remnant. At this point the transhiatal dissection is begun.

The hiatus is opened and a Penrose drain is passed around the distal esophagus for retraction. Although some have referred to this operation as a "blind esophagectomy," this is a misnomer. The transhiatal dissection is actually performed under direct vision by placing Deaver retractors in the hiatus (Figure 2-5). The first move is to identify the right and left vagus nerves running along the distal esophagus and to divide them. This move provides a significant amount of esophageal mobility. Next, the posterior dissection along the spine is performed. All attachments are dissected, clipped, and divided. Care is taken with the lateral attachments containing the blood supply to the esophagus directly from the thoracic aorta. Avulsion of branches coming directly from the aorta can lead to significant bleeding and must be avoided. Often, the patient will experience hypotension during dissection due to compression of the heart by anteriorly directed hiatal retraction. In these circumstances, close communication between the surgeon and the anesthesiologist is vital as simple intermittent relaxation of retraction allows for recovery of blood pressure. Often the dissection is completed with multiple short episodes or retraction followed by recovery to minimize the effects of prolonged hypotension. Finally, the anterior portion of the dissection is performed. In moving more proximally on the anterior surface of the esophagus, special care must be taken to avoid injury to the membranous portions of the airway, especially the left mainstem bronchus. One also needs to be aware of potential disruption of the azygous vein as the dissection proceeds higher on the right side. Both injuries can be life threatening and require conversion to a right thoracotomy for repair (note that for the thoracic surgeon,

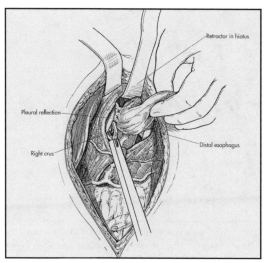

Figure 2-5. Transhiatal disection. (Reprinted from *Atlas of General Thoracic Surgery*, Kaiser LR, Copyright 1997, with permission from Elsevier.)

the proximal left mainstem bronchus is approached from the right chest; approaching through the left chest obstructs access).

Next, a cervical incision is made along the border of the left sternocleidomastoid muscle. The platysma is divided, the sternocleidomastoid is retracted, and the omohyoid muscle is identified. The omohyoid is divided and dissection is carried down directly onto the prevertebral fascia, which is incised; at this point, a dissecting finger can easily palpate the posterior cervical esophagus. The esophagus is gently mobilized (Figure 2-6). No deep retractors are placed in the incision to avoid damage to the recurrent laryngeal nerve. The recurrent nerve is identified in the tracheal esophageal groove and protected throughout the dissection. A Penrose drain is placed around the cervical esophagus and used for retraction. The esophagus is mobilized from above to meet the mobilization already completed through the hiatus. Once mobilized, the esophagus is divided in the neck and the distal esophagus is brought down through the hiatus. The gastric tube creation is completed in the abdomen with multiple firings of a stapling device. The resected specimen is oriented and forwarded to pathology. A pyloromyotomy or pyloroplasty is performed to aid in gastric tube emptying since the vagus nerves have been divided. Finally, the gastric tube is delivered into the neck in an oriented fashion through the bed of the resected esophagus (Figure 2-7). Multiple techniques have been described for the cervical esophagogastric tube anastomosis. At present, the modified stapled anastomosis[17] appears to have the lowest leak rate, about 2% as compared to sutured techniques, which are as high as 15%. The final reconstruction is shown in Figure 2-8.

The transhiatal approach can be utilized in the majority of patients with very good results. The reported hospital mortality rates are under 5% and major morbidity, including hemorrhage, recurrent nerve damage, chylothorax, and tracheal laceration, is less than 1%.[18] Despite concerns regarding the lack of a complete lymph node dissection with the transhiatal approach, review of the published English literature revealed no difference in the 3 or 5 year survival when comparing transthoracic versus the transhiatal

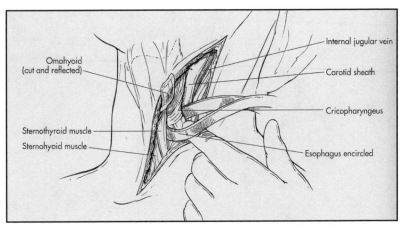

Figure 2-6. View through the hiatus after the stomach has been mobilized. Retractors are placed in the hiatus which has been enlarged. This allows for direct visualization of the lateral attachments that contain the blood supply to the esophagus. A small clip applier is used to control the vessels prior to division. (Reprinted from *Atlas of General Thoracic Surgery*, Kaiser LR, Copyright 1997, with permission from Elsevier.)

Figure 2-7. The gastric tube has been completed and is supplied by the gastroepiploic artery. It is pulled up orthotopically through the mediastinum and delivered into the cervical incision for completion of the cervical esophagogastric anastomosis. (Reproduced with permission from Skinner DB. *Atlas of Esophageal Surgery*. New York: Churchill Livingstone; 1991.)

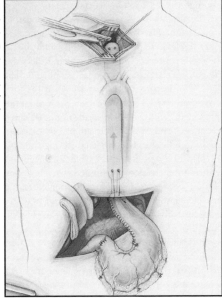

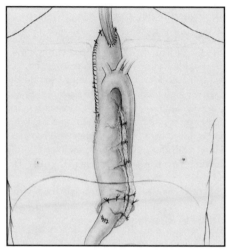

Figure 2-8. The completed transhiatal esophagectomy with gastric interposition. (Reproduced with permission from Skinner DB. *Atlas of Esophageal Surgery*. New York: Churchill Livingstone; 1991.)

approach; however, the early pulmonary complications appear higher in the transthoracic approach.[19]

TRANSTHORACIC TRANSABDOMINAL APPROACH TO ESOPHAGECTOMY

The transabdominal transthoracic approach was initially described by Ivor-Lewis and is often referred to as the "Ivor-Lewis esophagectomy." This approach includes an upper midline laparotomy for mobilization of the stomach with creation of a gastric tube in the same manner employed for the transhiatal esophagectomy and described above. Once the stomach has been mobilized, the hiatus is opened and the gastroesophageal junction and distal esophagus are mobilized. At this point the abdomen is closed, the patient is repositioned in the left lateral decubitus position, and a right fifth intercostal space thoracotomy is performed. The intrathoracic esophagus is mobilized under direct vision up to the level of the azygous vein, which is the level at which the intrathoracic esophagogastric anastomosis is performed. The azygous vein is usually divided to provide additional mobilization. The proximal esophagus is divided with a GI stapler and the gastric remnant is pulled into the right chest. The esophagogastric anastomosis is performed in either a hand sewn fashion or in a modified stapled fashion as described above for the transhiatal technique.

The advantage of this approach is that the intrathoracic esophagus is mobilized directly with full exposure of the mediastinum. This may be of value in avoiding injury to the airway or other mediastinal structures with bulky tumors in the middle third of the esophagus. Unfortunately, these patients are subject to increased early postoperative pulmonary complications due to the thoracotomy incision. In addition, placing the anastomosis in the chest can lead to life threatening mediastinitis should an anastomotic leak occur.

TRANSABDOMINAL TRANSTHORACIC TRANSCERVICAL ESOPHAGECTOMY

This approach is often referred to as the "Three Hole" or "Three Stage" McKeown esophagectomy. The operation begins with the patient in a left lateral decubitus position for a right thoracotomy to mobilize the intrathoracic esophagus. Following this, the patient is moved to a supine position with the neck extended and turned toward the right. An upper midline laparotomy is used for mobilization of the stomach in the same way as in the transhiatal and Ivor Lewis approach. Once this has been completed, a left neck incision is made and the cervical esophagus is mobilized. The esophagus is divided in the neck and the portion to be resected is pulled back into the abdomen. The resected specimen is removed from the operative field; the gastric tube is completed in the abdomen and directed through the mediastinum in an oriented fashion to the neck. The anastomosis is performed in the neck.

Proponents of this approach fall into 2 categories. The first group utilizes this approach to selectively resect large intrathoracic lesions of the mid esophagus. Clearly exposure, especially at the level of the carina and left mainstem bronchus, is superior as compared to the transhiatal approach. Since the visualization is improved, the injury rate to nearby structures, especially the airway and azygous vein is lower. The second group utilizes this approach to perform a complete "two" or "three" field lymph node dissection suggesting that this approach provides a better operation from an oncologic viewpoint and thus improved long term survival.[20] It is interesting that this approach had acceptable morbidity and mortality; however, it was reported out of a single US center. On the other hand, a large randomized Dutch trial comparing transhiatal resection with extended transthoracic resection showed that the transhiatal approach was associated with a lower morbidity and no statistically different overall, disease-free, and quality-adjusted survival.[21]

MINIMALLY INVASIVE ESOPHAGECTOMY

Numerous "minimally invasive" techniques to esophagectomy have been described including laparoscopic, hand-assisted, thoracoscopic, and robotic-assisted. The hope of these procedures is that minimizing the incision size will decrease the morbidity of the operation at the same time providing adequate resection. The largest study included 222 patients from the University of Pittsburgh.[22] Initially, they performed transhiatal dissection via laparoscopy (n=7), however, later refined the approach to include thoracoscopy, laparoscopy, and a left neck incision (n=217). They observed equivalent results as compared to open techniques and suggest development of a multicenter trial to determine the role of minimally invasive esophagectomy. At present, the usefulness of this approach remains undefined.

REFERENCES

1. Seremetis MG, Lyons WS, deGuzman VC, Peabody JW Jr. Leiomyomata of the esophagus. An analysis of 838 cases. *Cancer.* 1976;38:2166-2177.
2. Hatch GF 3rd, Wertheimer-Hatch L, Hatch KF, et al. Tumors of the esophagus. *World J Surg.* 2000;24:401-411.
3. Zuccaro G Jr, Rice TW. Tumors of the esophagus. In: Brandt LJ, ed. *Clinical Practice of Gastroenterology.* Philadelphia: Churchill Livingstone; 1999:131-134.

4. Lee LS, Singhal S, Brinster CJ, et al. Current management of esophageal leiomyoma. *J Am Coll Surg.* 2004;198:136-146.

5. Bonavina L, Segalin A, Rosati R, et al. Surgical therapy of esophageal leiomyoma. *J Am Coll Surg.* 1995;181:257-262.

6. Hatch GF III, Wertheimer-Hatch L, Hatch KF, et al. Tumors of the esophagus. *World J Surg.* 2000;24:401-411.

7. Bardini R, Segalin A, Ruol A, et al. Videothoracoscopic enucleation of esophageal leiomyoma. *Ann Thorac Surg.* 1992;54:576-577.

8. Eberlin TJ, et al. Benign schwannoma of the esophagus presenting as a giant fibrovascular polyp. *Ann Thorac Surg.* 1992;53:343.

9. Orringer MB. Substernal gastric bypass of the excluded esophagus—results of an ill-advised operation. *Surgery.* 1984;96:467.

10. Orringer MB, Sloan H. Esophagectomy without thoracotomy. *J Thorac Cardiovasc Surg.* 1978;76:643-654.

11. Lewis I. The surgical treatment of carcinoma of the esophagus with special reference to a new operation for growths of the middle third. *Br J Surg.* 1946;34:18.

12. McKeown KC. Total three-stage oesphagectomy for cancer of the esophagus. *Br J Surg.* 1976;51:259.

13. Bolten JS. Teng S. Transthoracic or transhiatal esophagectomy for cancer of the esophagus—does it matter. *Surg Oncol Clin N Am.* 2002; 11(2)365-375.

14. Dimick JB, Pronovost PJ, Cowan JA, Lipsett PA. Surgical volume and quality of care for esophageal resection: do high-volume hospitalshavehospitals have fewer complications? *Ann Thor Surg.* 2003;75(2):337-341.

15. Rizk NP, Bach PB, Schrag D, et al. The impact of complications on outcomes after resection for esophageal and gastroesophageal junction carcinoma. *J Am Coll Surg.* 2004; 42-50.

16. Davis PA, Law S, Wong J. Colonic Interposition after esophagectomy for cancer. *Arch Surg.* 2003;138(3):303-8.

17. Orringer MB, Marshall B, Iannettoni MD. Eliminating the cervical esophagogastric anastomotic leak with a side-to-side stapled anastomosis. *J Thorac Cardiovasc Surg.* 2000;119(2);277-285.

18. Orringer MB, Marshall B, Iannettoni MD. Transhiatal esophagectomy: clinical experience and refinements. *Ann Surg.* 1999;230(3):392-400.

19. Hulscher JB, Tijissen JG, Obertop H, van Lanschot JJ. Transthoracic versus transhiatal resection for carcinoma of the esophagus: a meta-analysis. *Ann Thorac Surg.* 2001; 72(1):306-313.

20. Altorki N, Kent M, Ferrara C, Port J. Three-field lymph node dissection for squamous cell and adenocarcinoma of the esophagus. *Ann Surg.* 2002;236:177-183.

21. Hulscher JB, van Sandick JW, de Boer AG, et al. Extended transthoracic resection compared with limited transhiatal resection for adenocarcinoma of the esophagus. *NEJM.* 2002;374(21):1662-1669.

22. Luketich JD, Alvelo-Rivera M, Buenaventura PO, Christie NA, McCaughan JS, Little VR, Schauer PR, Close JM, Fernando HC. Minimally invasive esophagectomy: outcomes in 222 patients. *Ann Surg.* 2003:238(4):486-494.

chapter 3

Approach to Chemotherapy and Radiation for Gastric and Esophageal Cancer

Diane Hershock, MD, PhD

INTRODUCTION

Both gastric and esophageal cancers remain amongst the 10 most common cancers in the world with variations in incidence and survival based on geographic sites. Gastric cancer is the second most common tumor worldwide with 60% of cases in developing countries.[1] It appears gastric cancer worldwide is second to lung cancer with a reported 798, 300 new cases in 1990 and is more common than breast and colorectal cancers in other areas of the world. The highest incidences are in Japanese men; rates are also increased in Eastern Europe, South America, and Eastern Asia, but lower in the United States, North Africa, and Australia.[1] Esophageal cancer is the seventh leading cause of death in men in the United States and unfortunately 90% of patients diagnosed with this cancer will die from their disease.[2] Metastatic disease is seen in approximately 50% of patients at the time of diagnosis. The effectiveness of surgery, chemotherapy, radiation therapy, or the combination of the above modalities has been investigated for decades with varied results. This chapter will discuss the strategies and dilemmas in treating both gastric and esophageal cancers, which are often included together in many clinical trials. The reasons for this are similar clinical behavior, histology, and responses to various chemotherapeutic agents. Additionally, eligibility criteria for clinical trials, particularly in this country, typically include both cancers.

GASTRIC CANCER

INCIDENCE/EPIDEMIOLOGY

The pattern of occurrence of gastric cancer has changed over the years with population migration. Although it remains the second most common tumor in the world, the incidence of gastric cancer has declined dramatically since 1930 in developed countries, particularly the United States.[3] This decline may be attributed to reclassification of adenocarcinoma of the gastric cardia and the lower third of the esophagus as gastroesophageal junction cancers since both behave in a similar biologic and clinical fashion. Additionally, there has been a decline in the well-differentiated adenocarcinomas of the fundus and antrum.[4]

PATHOGENESIS AND ETIOLOGY

Neither the pathogenesis of gastric or esophageal cancers has been well established. It has been postulated that p53 mutations, the adenomatous polyposis coli (APC) gene, K-*ras* alterations, loss of heterozygosity of the deleted-in-colorectal-cancer gene (DCC), and translocated promoter region-MET (TPR-MET) rearrangement may play a role in gastric cancer development.[5-7] It is unclear whether there is a sequenced order of progression from an adenoma, as in colon cancer. However, it has been suggested by one study that TPR-MET activation may play an early role in gastric cancer development; K-*ras* may predict further progression.[7,8] Variations in p53 mutations may explain differences in Asian and European cases. [9] G:C→A:T transitions are seen more commonly in Europeans whereas A:T→G:C transitions/transversion are seen in Asians.[9] Food associations and other risk factors may also be more closely linked to p53 differences in the pathogenesis of Western vs Asian gastric cancers.[10] Microsatellite instability (MSI) and loss of heterozygosity (LOH) are purported to cause progression of gastric cancers.[11-14]

Familial aggregates of gastric cancer have also been observed and may account for a substantial number of cases. Carriers of mismatch repair gene mutations like hMSH2 responsible of hereditary nonpolyposis colorectal carcinoma syndrome (HNPCC) have a significant risk (approximately 19 times) of developing gastric cancer as well.[15-17] Again, MSI and LOH may be due to other genes responsible for DNA replication fidelity.[18-19] Additionally, those with familial adenomatous polyposis (FAP) are at increased risk of gastric cancer as well, though secondary to mutations at exon 10 to 15H.[20] Those with Li-Fraumeni syndrome infrequently develop gastric cancer, suggesting that risk may not be increased by a p53 mutation.[21-23]

CLASSIFICATION/PROGNOSTIC INDICATORS

Suspected causative agents in gastric cancer include dietary factors such as poor nutrition, salted and smoked foods, alcohol, decreased intake of fruits/vegetables, and nitrates.[24,25] Lifestyle issues such as smoking and low socioeconomic status have been noted. Vitamin E, vitamin C, beta-carotene, selenium, and other micronutrients have been reported to be protective but data are relatively inconsistent.[26,27]

Gastroesophageal junction tumors (GEJ) appear to differ significantly in their etiology as compared to gastric cancers. GEJ tumors arise from GERD resulting in esophagitis, gastric metaplasia and BE. It appears also that obese people are at increased risk of GERD.[28] It may be related to increased intra-abdominal pressure from an increased body mass index. Tobacco, alcohol, and low socioeconomic status may also be risk factors for GES tumors.[29,30]

Helicobacter pylori (*H. Pylori*) has been investigated as an etiological agent in non-GEJ gastric cancer. *Helicobacter* has been listed as a known carcinogen and has been postulated initially as inducing an inflammatory response that leads to the release of pro-inflammatory cytokines, many of which cause a reactive oxygen species, leading to oxidative stress and a milieu conducive to carcinogen development.[31-33] Controversy remains, however, and it may be the cytotoxin, CagA, causing an increased risk. Those individuals positive for both CagA and *Helicobacter* appear to have an increased risk of developing gastric cancer.[34-36]

Histologically, gastric cancers are classified as diffuse or intestinal. Diffuse gastric cells are small cells that grow diffusely into the surrounding gastric tissue; intestinal type is more glandular in appearance and is delimited. Linitis plastica is an antomicpathological entity due to diffuse infiltration by the small, diffuse type which appears rigid and tubular. The diffuse type appears to have an overall worse prognosis even after TMN staging is considered. WHO classifies gastric cancer cells histologically into mucinous, tubular, signet ring, and papillary.[37]

Immunohistochemistry and molecular prognostic indicators are now coming into investigation. p53 has been evaluated to the greatest extent. One study reported an inverse relationship between p53 protein overexpression and survival, but a multivariate analysis was not performed and only 120/427 patients were evaluable.[38-40] Serum antibodies to p53 were measured in 501 patients with gastric cancer and were associated with a poor prognosis, lymph node metastasis, and poorly differentiated nuclear grade.[41] Other prognostic markers include Bcl-2, c-met, c-erb, vascular endothelial growth factor (VEGF), urokinase plasminogen activator, DNA ploidy, CD44 expression, and nm23.[42-50] Large trials investigating their utility in predicting outcome have not been done.

In general, gastric cancers have a poor outcome and thus prognosis. The overall survival rate, particularly in the United States, has been reported to be 37%, 18%, 11% and 5% for Stage II, IIIA, IIIB, and IV diseases.[51] The survival rates are thought to be so poor in this country due to late detection. However, rates are similar to European data. In Japan, Stage IA and IB cancers are more frequently found due to screening programs and thus the five year survival is reported to be 75%.[52-53]

Until the last decade, the management of gastric cancer for curative intent was with surgery; chemotherapy and radiotherapy were generally used for palliation. With newer chemotherapy and radiotherapy techniques, multimodality approaches are now coming into existence, with newer data suggesting curative benefit. These therapies will be discussed subsequently.

SURGICAL MANAGEMENT

Surgery has been the mainstay of treatment of gastric cancers for curative intent for the past century. Debate now exists as to the optimum surgical technique in terms of total vs subtotal gastrectomy, the extensive lymph node dissection done by Japanese surgeons, and the approach to early gastric cancers.

Two randomized trials in Western Europe were designed to address the question of total vs subtotal gastrectomy. The French Association for Surgical Research randomized 169 patients with adenocarcinoma to total or subtotal gastrectomy.[54] The 5-year survival rate in both groups was the same at 48% with a higher surgical mortality in the subtotal group. A second study conducted by the Italian Gastrointestinal Tumor Study Group randomized 624 patients with gastric cancer in the distal half of the stomach to subtotal or total gastrectomy.[55] Again, 5-year survival rates were similar at 65% and 62% respectively, but those with subtotal gastrectomy and lymphadenectomy of compartments one and two had a better quality of life and nutritional status.

Lymph node metastasis clearly affects prognosis in gastric cancer. The issue of performing extensive lymph node dissection when performing a gastrectomy has been a huge debate over the past 30 years.[56-59] Removal of the perigastric lymph nodes only is called D1 resection. D2 lymphadenectomy adds removal of the lymphatic chains along the celiac axis, the common hepatic and splenic artery, and at the splenic hilum. The Japanese Society for Research in Gastric Cancer attempted to standardize this procedure by classifying 16 lymph node stations or 4 levels. The D2 procedure is done to achieve accurate staging and regional lymph node disease control, is safe if done by a skilled surgeon, avoids pancreatic and splenic resections, and benefits a group with occult disease in D2 nodes.

Eight prospective randomized trials demonstrated a significant survival advantage for D2 over D1 resections especially in patients with stage II or IIIA disease. A small trial from South Africa looked at 43 patients who were randomized to D1 or D2 resections that showed no survival advantage in the D2 arm with increased surgical morbidity and prolonged hospital courses.[60] Another trial from Hong Kong in which 55 patients either underwent D1 or D3 resections showed an overall survival advantage in the D1 group again with increased surgical morbidity and mortality in the D3 group.[61] Two major randomized trials from the UK and Dutch Gastric Cancer Group have been reported.[62-65] Seven hundred eleven and 400 patients, respectively, either underwent D1 or D2 resections. Again, the complication rates were higher in the D2 resection, even in the Dutch trial in which supervision in the operating room by Japanese surgeons was made available. Neither trial showed a survival advantage with D2 resection although the 5-year survival rate was slightly better in the Dutch study which was attributed to a lower number of patients with T4 disease. The morbidity associated with D2 resections is postulated due to lesions to the pancreatic tail or because the pancreas needs to be resected to achieve complete removal of the lymph nodes at the splenic hilum. Splenectomy was also included in the D2 resection and it is also thought that T-cell immunosuppression from splenectomy may contribute to surgical mortality. It is now recommended that splenectomy is an adverse prognostic factor and should only be performed in locally advanced tumor in the upper third of the stomach, greater curvature, gastric cardia, or macroscopic disease to the splenic hilum.[66]

In Japan, early gastric cancer represents 50% of newly diagnosed cases. The 10-year survival rate in Japan is between 80% and 95%.[67] Submucosal invasion has been noted in 20% of cases which can be associated with lymph node involvement, thus suggesting a poorer prognosis.[68-70] Thus, detection of early lymph node involvement is controversial and an ongoing debate in terms of accuracy of staging endoscopy/endoscopic ultrasound.[71-73] It has been suggested that size and submucosal invasion should determine the extent of surgical resection.[74,75]

Surgery, therefore, remains an intricate part of curative management of resectable gastric cancer. Debate continues as to the extent of resection and thus, adding other effective modalities of treatment may be important, particularly in the adjuvant setting. The next sections will review the current literature on chemotherapy and radiation in this setting.

Systemic Chemotherapy

In order to understand the current literature in the neoadjuvant and adjuvant settings, a review of chemotherapy agents in the metastatic disease will be discussed. As with many cancers, gastric cancer was thought to be relatively insensitive to chemotherapy. Most agents used in gastric cancer did not induce a complete response as is the norm in most cancers. Responses in general were poor, and time to progression was short. Table 3-1 contains a list of single agent drugs with some activity in gastric cancer.

Table 3-1

ACCUARY OF SINGLE CHEMOTHERAPEUTIC AGENTS[76]

Drug	Patients Studied (First Line/Second Line)	Responses (%)
5-Fluorouracil	392	21
Mitomycin C	211	30
Cisplatin	14/115	36/20
Etoposide	14	21
Doxorubicin	124/78	17/17
Methotrexate	28	11
Carboplatin	29	7
BCNU	55	20

Adapted from Roth AD. Curative treatment of gastric cancer: towards a multidisciplinary approach? *Critical Rev in Oncology Hematology.* 2003;46:59-100.

The standard first line salvage regimen through the 1980s was FAM for 5-fluorouracil (5-FU), adriamycin and mitomycin C with an initial reported response rate of 50%.[77] This combination, though, was subsequently evaluated by multiple investigators with less convincing response rates.[78-81] Randomized trials subsequently followed, the largest from the European Organization for Research and Treatment of Cancer (EORTC). Response rates were reported at 9% with a median survival of 6.5 months.[82] In the United States, 252 patients were evaluated comparing 5-FU to FAM as well as other combinations such as CCNU with FAM and low dose cisplatin with 5-FU and adriamycin.[83] None of these combination agents had any advantage.

Attempts to evaluate more aggressive multiple drug combinations were then pursued. FAMTX or the addition of high dose methotrexate to the standard FAM with leucovorin rescue (LV) was compared to FAM alone.[82,84,85] FAM again demonstrated a 9% response compared to 42% with FAMTX; additionally, a median survival of 29 vs 42 weeks with FAMTX was reported. Thus, FAMTX became the standard of care in metastatic gastric cancer.

Cisplatin (CDDP) in single agent trials had a mediocre response and thus was subsequently studied. Synergy was known to exist between 5-FU and cisplatin and thus trials were designed to exploit this. Regimens such as FUP (5-FU/CDDP), FLP (5-FU/LV/CDDP), PELF (CDDP/Epirubicin/LV/5-FU), and ELF (Etoposide/LV/5-FU) had responses ranging from 37% to 72% with duration of response reported between 4 and 7 months (see Table 3-2).[86-91]

Phase III trials compared the above regimens to each other. FAM vs 5-FU vs FUP, which is 5-FU/CDDP, suggested responses of 25%, 51%, and 26% in 166 patients with measurable disease.[93] Time to progression was 21 weeks in the FUP arm compared to 12 weeks for either 5-FU or FAM; however, no statistical significance was found. FAM was compared to PELF with PELF nonstatistically superior in terms of median time to

Table 3-2

RESPONSES TO CHEMOTHERAPY REGIMENS

Combination	Patients	Response Rate (RR%)	Survival (Months)
FAMTX	317	25	6 to 10[84-85,92]
FUP/FLP	226	44	8 to 11[89,93]
PELF	85	43	8[91]
ELF	63	49	7 to 11[88]

progression.[91] FAMTX was compared to etoposide, adriamycin, and CDDP (EAP) but suspended due to unacceptable toxicities.[92] The EORTC did a multicenter trial comparing FAMTX, FUP and ELF with responses of 12%, 20%, and 9% respectively with median survivals of 6.7 to 7.2 months.[94] Thus, other drugs found their way into therapy in the metastatic setting.

Continuous infusion 5-FU was investigated based on new knowledge of the pharmacokinetics of the drug and method of administration. Bolus 5-FU appears to favor binding of the drug into RNA, leading to disruption of maturation of nuclear RNA. Infusional 5-FU on the other hand favors inhibition of thymidylate synthetase (TS) after its conversion to 5-fluoro-2'-deoxy-5' monophosphate (FdUMP) and thus DNA synthesis. Based on data derived from colon cancer, response rates with the infusional form were noted to be 32% vs 7% for the bolus arm with no survival advantage to either arm.[95] This led to the evolution of ECF or 5-FU continuous infusion with epirubicin and CDDP with responses of 71%.[96-98] Responses compared to FAMTX were 45% vs 21% with a superior median time to progression of 7.4 vs 3.4 months and a significant survival advantage (8.9 vs 5.7 months).[99]

Many of the above regimens have been given on the every 3 to 4 week cycling due to various toxicities. High dose weekly regimens have been investigated such as EPFL or epirubicin, CDDP, 5-FU, and LV with 62% response rates but unacceptable neutropenia.[100] Another study looked at an additional drug, etoposide with the EPFL regimen with responses of 71% again with considerable toxicity.[101]

Other active agents have now been looked at in the past 5 to 10 years, including the taxanes-paclitaxel or docetaxel as well as irinotecan (CPT11) as single agents and in combination. Other newer agents include Oxaliplatin and Xeloda or oral 5-FU.

Paclitaxel or Taxol (Bristol-Myers Squibb, New York, NY) is an antimitotic agent that binds microtubules that promote microtubular assembly and stabilize microtubules.[102] Taxol as a single agent in gastric cancer has reported response rates of 5 to 17%, as well as 20%.[103-105] Taxol in combination with 5-FU, or CDDP, or both have reported responses of 32% to 64% with time to progression of 4 to 8 months and overall median survival from 6 to 11 months.[106-109] Paclitaxel with CDDP and etoposide was evaluated in 25 chemotherapy naïve patients with locally advanced, unresectable, or metastatic gastric and esophageal cancer with a high response rate; both adenocarcinoma and squamous cell were included and thus differences may have been due to histology as well as the inclusion of locally advanced but nonmetastatic patients.[110]

Docetaxel or Taxotere (Aventis, Bridgewater, NJ) is reported to be twice as potent as paclitaxel-inhibiting microtubule depolymerization. Using docetaxel as a single agent, three phase II trials report responses ranging from 17% to 24% in gastric cancer.[111-113] Phase I studies combining CDDP with docetaxel revealed dose-limiting myelosuppression.[114] Lower doses appeared tolerable and the Europeans reported combinations of CDDP with docetaxel as well as continuous infusion 5-FU with docetaxel and CDDP.[115,116] The first study evaluated 47 patients with every 3 week CDDP at 75 mg/m^2 and docetaxel at 85 mg/m^2. Responses were reported at 56% with median time to progression of 6.6 months and overall survival of 9 months. Toxicity profile was acceptable. The second trial involving this regimen with continuous infusion 5-FU was then pursued. Fifty percent of patients (52 patients) responded with an overall survival rate of 9.3 months. Further investigations and randomized studies are underway in the first line metastatic setting.

In those patients in which docetaxel was used as second line therapy, studies have demonstrated 20% responses as a single agent and 21% responses in combination with epirubicin.[117,118]

Irinotecan or CPT11 is a DNA topoisomerase I inhibitor converted to its active metabolite SN38 by hepatic carboxyesterase. It has been shown to have first line activity as a single agent of 18 to 23%.[119-120] Studies incorporating CDDP have been done in both gastric and esophageal cancer with reported responses of 42% to 58% in chemotherapy naïve patients.

Oxaliplatin is a third-generation cisplatin analog with a 1.2-diaminocyclohexane carrier ligand. It forms diaminocyclohexane-platinum adducts with DNA. It appears to have activity in tumors marginally sensitive to other platinum agents and is neither nephrotoxic or ototoxic. Its main side effect is cold neuropathy, which can be exacerbated by cold exposure. Oxaliplatin has been demonstrated to have additive or synergistic activity with 5-FU, especially in 5-FU resistant, as well as CDDP resistant, tumor cell lines.[124] A recent Phase II study in which bolus 5-FU at 400 mg/m^2 with oxaliplatin at 85mg/m^2 followed by infusional 5-FU over 48 hours reported response rates of 26% with median time to progression of 4.3 months.[125] Toxicity profiles were tolerable. Thus, this is yet another chemotherapeutic agent with promise.

Matrix metalloproteinases (MMP) agents are zinc-containing enzymes responsible for degradation of various proteins in the extracellular matrix. These may be important in invasion and metastatic spread of tumors. A study done in patients with gastric cancer who failed other chemotherapies looked at oral Marimastat for 18 months; median survival was more than 5 months.[126] Many other agents are currently under investigation.

In conclusion, the ECF or epirubicin, CDDP, and 5-FU regimen is standard in Europe and is being investigated in the United States since data suggest superiority to FAMTX. Other agents such as taxanes, CPT11, and Oxaliplatin are encouraging in Phase II trials and warrant further investigation.

ADJUVANT CHEMOTHERAPY

It is well known that despite complete resections for curative intent, locoregional failures have been noted in gastric cancers. Patients can subsequently present with local disease, peritoneal carcinomatosis, or distant disease. Over the years, various neoadjuvant and adjuvant strategies have been investigated with the intent of treating microscopic residual disease postsurgery. Meta analysis have suggested benefit to adjuvant chemotherapy but more recently, the Intergroup 0116 Study reported information with improved disease-free and overall survival with combination chemoradiotherapy, which will be discussed in detail subsquently.[127]

Initial adjuvant chemotherapy trials revealed less than encouraging data. The Gastrointestinal Tumor Study Group published a positive trial looking at methyl-CCNU with 5-FU.[128] The median survival was reported at 33 months in those who did not receive postoperative chemotherapy; the median survival in the chemotherapy arm was more than 4 years. Unfortunately, these results were not confirmed in a larger trial setting. Mitomycin C was used by the Japanese Surgical Adjuvant Chemotherapy Group with various dosing schedules; all trials but one were negative.[129]

Multiple adjuvant trials have been conducted in Japan; unfortunately, few had surgery alone as a control arm and many of these trials merely compared chemotherapy regimens. Several studies in the United States and Europe looked at regimens such as FAM and did compare surgery alone as the control; most were negative trials with sufficient numbers of patients enrolled.

Several meta-analyses have attempted to prove or disprove the use of adjuvant chemotherapy by creating larger sample sizes. One study published by the Dutch, based on 14 randomized trials including 2096 patients, did not suggest a survival advantage from adjuvant chemotherapy.[130] Another meta-analysis in 1999 analyzed 13 trials demonstrating a small but significant survival benefit for patients receiving postoperative chemotherapy.[131] There was an absolute risk reduction from 65 to 61% in relapse-free survival after postoperative chemotherapy. A third meta-analysis based on 20 trials was published by the Gruppo Italiano per lo Studio dei Carcinomi dell'Apparato Digerente (GISCAD). Patients received either 5-FU alone or in combination with adriamycin-based chemotherapy with a reduced risk of death of 18% in the chemotherapy arm.[132] This translated to an overall absolute risk reduction of about 4% in 5-year survival.

Thus, from the above trials and published meta-analyses, many negative trials appear to exist in the adjuvant setting, none of which were powered to show a 5-year survival advantage. The few positive trials published were too small in sample size to suggest validity. The effectiveness of adjuvant chemotherapy alone remains controversial at best; if a benefit exists in terms of survival, it needs to be evaluated in terms of acceptable toxicity and quality of life.

RADIOTHERAPY

The rationale for adjuvant radiation therapy is similar to chemotherapy; it is used to decrease the locoregional relapse rate observed after surgery. Based on tissue tolerance/toxicity to the local area, such as spinal cord, pancreas, small bowel, liver, and kidneys, the dose of external beam is limited to 45 Gy.[133-134]

Many of the radiation studies published in the literature were retrospective in nature and had methods, issues making evaluation and interpretation difficulty. Issues include underpowered studies, variations in doses of radiation, no control arm (no treatment), or inadequate randomization. Only one study using chemotherapy in one arm, radiation in another arm, and surgery alone suggested a benefit from radiation.[135] In general, none of the studies suggested a true survival benefit to radiation alone in the adjuvant setting.

Intraoperative radiation therapy (IORT) is another modality in which a single dose of radiation is given directly into the operative field at the time of surgery. The initial theory is based on immediate local treatment of any residual microscopic disease that may remain in that operative bed, sparing normal tissue from field effects. There are technical difficulties associated with this type of treatment in that a radiation setup must be available in the sterile arena of the operative suite, which is not necessarily practical.

The Japanese have conducted several nonrandomized trials in which single doses of 30 to 35 Gy were given to the local area, particularly lymph nodes less than 3 cm; if no nodes were noted, 28 Gy was given to the operative bed alone.[136,137] Further data suggested that doses of 30 to 40 Gy decreased primary tumor size but was insufficient to eradicate all disease.[138] Many of the above studies were feasibility studies; little has been determined regarding improvement in overall survival. Patterns of local recurrence after this type of radiation were assessed and felt to be of little to no benefit if surgical margins were positive.[139]

Two randomized trials in the United States have been published with varied results. One study conducted at the National Cancer Institute (NCI) compared surgery alone in Stage I/II disease vs single dose 50 Gy/surgery in those with Stage III/IV disease.[140] Forty-one patients were evaluable; locoregional failure occurred in 44% of IORT patients and 92% of surgery alone patients. No difference in median survival was documented. The second study reviewed 211 patients with no comment on staging or type of surgical resection performed; patients were randomized at the time of the procedure.[141] This report suggested a significant survival benefit but again, major flaws appear to exist based on the information published.

Based on local and regional recurrence rates at the tumor bed, the anastomosis site or regional lymph nodes 40% to 65% of the time in those undergoing surgery for curative resection and the unsatisfying data from adjuvant chemotherapy and radiation trials alone, the SWOG/ECOG/RTOG/CALGB/NCCTG cooperative groups designed the landmark Intergroup 0116 trial.[127] This study demonstrated that adjuvant chemoradiotherapy after surgical resection of high-risk localized gastric cancer resulted in an improved relapse-free survival from 31% to 48% at 3 years. Overall survival at 3 years was 52% vs 41%. The treatment arm consisted of the Mayo Clinic method of administration of one cycle of 5-FU/LV (425 mg/m² plus 20 mg/m² LV daily times 5 days) followed 1 month later by combined 5-FU/LV days 1 to 4 as above with 180 cGy/day of external beam radiation and the same chemotherapy again in the last week of radiation for 3 days. The total fraction of radiation was 4500 Gy. Two subsequent cycles of adjuvant chemotherapy alone at the above doses were given thereafter. There was a 44% relative improvement in relapse-free survival and a 28% relative improvement in survival with median survival of 42 and 27 months, respectively. Radiotherapy techniques were closely monitored due to variations in target volume. Flaws in this study included the initial requirement that all patients have D2 resections; 54% of the patients ultimately only received a D1 resection, which is less than standard. Thus, the issue of benefit from chemoradiation may have been because of inadequate surgery.

NEOADJUVANT CHEMOTHERAPY

The rationale for preoperative neoadjuvant chemotherapy is based on treating an intact vascular tumor with no reason for treatment-induced resistance for a better response rate de novo. There have always been arguments that responses are improved with the fibrotic remodeling of the tumor bed following surgical removal. Additionally, surgery may be less invasive if an adequate response occurs prior to that procedure and thus issues of organ preservation are considered.

There have been extensive debates in the literature as to the utility of neoadjuvant chemotherapy in the treatment of any cancer. In locoregionally advanced rectal cancers, neoadjuvant radiotherapy has been considered superior to surgery alone or followed by adjuvant radiotherapy in terms of risk of locoregional relapse.[142,143] Neoadjuvant chemotherapy is also used in inflammatory breast cancer as well as osteosarcoma.[144,145] Arguments exist about its use in esophageal cancer which will be discussed later in this chapter.

There are several issues as to the use of neoadjuvant chemotherapy in gastric cancer. The decision for adjuvant treatment is often made based on the final pathological diagnosis and features postoperatively; the decision to perform or not perform a preoperative intervention relies on clinical staging, which is not as accurately known without the benefit of surgery. The primary tumor extension is not necessarily obvious on routine CT scans or MRIs and the invaded lymph nodes may not be detectable on conventional scans. Endoscopic ultrasonography is the only option for estimating the T and N stage with a known diagnostic accuracy of 70%.[146] Peritoneal carcinomatosis is also difficult to determine without surgical exploration and thus many trials investigating neoadjuvant therapy have suggested laparoscopic staging.

Few randomized studies have been done comparing neoadjuvant chemotherapy followed by surgery vs surgery alone. One study looked at 107 patients after receiving 2 to 3 cycles of CDDP/VP16/5-FU with surgery vs surgery alone.[147] A higher curative resection rate was noted in the investigative arm, with evidence of downstaging after chemotherapy. As with many studies, though, no survival advantage was reported. Another randomized trial looked at 2 to 4 cycles of FAMTX/surgery vs surgery alone.[148] Fifty-nine patients were studied and the study was ultimately suspended due to toxicity and poor accrual.

Two randomized trials with neoadjuvant radiation have been published as well. Three hundred seventeen patients with adenocarcinoma of the cardia were randomized to radiation therapy/surgery vs surgery alone.[149] Forty Gy were administered as 2 Gy/day; surgery was done 2 to 4 weeks later. The reported 5-year survival was 30% vs 20% in the XRT/surgery arm vs surgery. Issues with this study include inadequate staging and the variation in the radiation fields. Another randomized study investigated XRT/surgery, XRT/local hyperthermia followed by surgery vs surgery alone.[150] Again, 20 Gy were given. The 5-year survival rates were 45%, 52%, and 30%, respectively.

The MRC Adjuvant Gastric Infusional Chemotherapy (MAGIC) trial, a UK-driven trial, is investigating the role of pre- and postoperative epirubicin, CDDP and 5-FU chemotherapy in combination with surgery compared with surgery alone; results are pending. The EORTC is comparing neoadjuvant systemic therapy with surgery vs surgery alone using weekly CDDP and high dose 5-FU/LV. The French have a similar trial to the EORTC using infusional 5-FU/CDDP every 3 to 4 weeks. Taxotere with 5-FU/CDDP is currently in trial in Italy with 4 neoadjuvant cycles followed by surgery.

MULTIMODALITY THERAPY

The treatment of gastric cancer with potential curative resection has become a question of multidisciplinary management. The roles of surgery, radiation, and chemotherapy and their sequence in treatment are still evolving. New treatment regimens based on novel cytotoxic agents such as docetaxel, paclitaxel, irinotecan, and biologic agents such as epidermal growth factor receptor inhibitors and antiangiogenesis may find a role in the management of gastric cancer, either in the neoadjuvant, adjuvant, or combined modality setting. The limited benefit from adjuvant therapy in many trials to date might be due to residual tumor burden after surgery, delay in the administration of chemotherapy, insufficient activity of current chemotherapy, inadequate sample sizes of treatable patients, or the need for better local therapies with combination radiation/chemotherapy. Optimal surgical intervention needs to be better defined as well. Thus, much work remains in determining the best strategies for the treatment of gastric cancer.

ESOPHAGEAL CANCER

INCIDENCE/EPIDEMIOLOGY

Carcinoma of the esophagus, including the gastroesophageal junction, remains relatively uncommon in the United States, with approximately 13,000 new cases and almost an equal number of deaths in 2003.[151] As with gastric cancer, surgery has generally been considered the standard of care for local regionally confined esophageal cancer; the survival, though, has remained poor, with 6% to 24% of patients in the Western world alive at 5 years.[152] The Japanese report 5-year survival rates around 24% as well.[153] The lifetime risk of developing this cancer is 0.8% for men and 0.3% for women with risk increasing with age.[154-155] In the United States, Black men are more affected than White males and is the seventh leading cause of cancer death; it is the sixth leading cause worldwide.[156]

PATHOGENESIS

There are 2 major histological classifications of esophageal cancer; 90% are either squamous cell or adenocarcinomas.[155] Less than 10% are of other subtypes such as GI stromal tumors, lymphomas, carcinoids, or melanoma. Squamous cell carcinomas are generally noted in the middle to lower third of the esophagus whereas adenocarcinomas are located predominantly in the distal esophagus.[155,157] The cervical esophagus generally involves squamous cell histology and is usually treated in a similar fashion to those of the head/neck region.

The pathogenesis remains uncertain, and epidemiologic studies have investigated potential causes for the rise in esophageal cancer. Data suggest risk factors such as smoking, oxidants, reflux (which causes inflammation), and esophagitis. This will be discussed subsequently. More than 50% of patients at the time of diagnosis have locally advanced unresectable disease or distant metastatic disease. Fourteen percent to 21% of T1b or submucosal lesions and 38% to 60% of T2 lesions metastasize to regional lymph nodes.

Smoking remains a significant risk factor for both squamous cell carcenoma and adenocarcinoma. The inhalation and ingestion of tobacco carcinogens, particularly nitrosamines, from direct contact with the mucosa of the esophagus and risk correlates with the number and duration of cigarettes smoked.[158,159] Both subtypes can be seen in patients with prior cancers treated with radiation such as those with a history of primary breast, non-Hodgkin's and Hodgkin's lymphoma and lung cancers. These generally occur more than 10 years from primary radiotherapy.[160]

The initial cause of SC carcinoma may be related to chronic surface irritation and inflammation. Leading agents of causality include alcohol, tobacco, and the incidences with the combination of alcohol/tobacco. Ninety percent of cases worldwide are associated with alcohol and/or tobacco etiologies.[159] This is the same association as with head and neck cancers. In fact 1% to 2% of those with esophageal cancer have head and neck cancer as well.[161] Additionally, other irritants can include esophageal diverticuli with retained bacterial decomposition, which release local chemical irritants, and achalasia.[162] Caustic fluids and lye can initiate this cancer as can the chronic consumption of very hot beverages.[163,164] Generally, squamous cell histology is linked to a lower socioeconomic status.[159] Nutritional deficiencies were linked to this cancer in the past but diseases such as Plummer-Vinson syndrome, characterized by dysphagia, iron-deficiency anemia, and esophageal webs, is now rare worldwide. There is only one recognized familial syndrome that predisposes patients to squamous cell esophageal cancer—nonepidermolytic palmoplantar keratoderma (tylosis).[165] This is a rare autosomal dominant disorder defined by a genetic abnormality at chromosome 17q25. It is diagnosed in those with hyperkeratosis of the palms and soles and thickening of the oral mucosa. Lifetime risk of developing this disease in those affected is 95% by age 70.[166]

There are several risk factors associated with the development of adenocarcinoma, which has increased in incidence to almost epidemic numbers in the United States. In fact, during the 1990s, this had become the predominant histology for esophageal cancer in this country.[167] The reason for this may be related to chronic reflux (GERD), a cause of BE. Those people with recurrent symptoms of reflux appear to have an 8-fold increase in risk of esophageal cancer.[168] Other factors which suggest risk include hiatal hernia; ulcers; frequent use of H_2 blockers and drugs that relax the gastroesophageal sphincter, such as anticholingergics, aminophylline, and beta blockers.[169-170]

There is ongoing debate as to the role of *H. pylori* in the development of esophageal cancer. Certain strains of *H. pylori*, in particular those that are positive for the CagA protein, may decrease the risk of severe GERD and thus be protective against esophageal cancer development.[171-173] The literature suggests that *H. pylori* infection leads to atrophic gastritis and reduced gastric acidity and a decline in infection by this bacteria may actually lead to increased GERD, BE, and esophageal cancer.[174]

Another risk factor for adenocarcinoma of the esophagus is obesity.[158,170] The basis for this is increased intra-abdominal pressure leading to chronic GERD. Again, there is little data to support this etiology but there is literature suggesting this mechanism as a viable agent in women.[175,176]

BE has been found in 5 to 8% of people with GERD.[177] Changes in the epithelium have been histologically documented with replacement of stratified squamous cell epithelium with specialized columnar epithelium similar to that in the intestine/stomach areas. Mutations may develop within this tissue, leading to dysplasia. The risk of neoplastic transformation in patients with BE has been reported at 0.5%.[178] Frequent chromosomal aberrations have been noted although not distinguished as definitive causes of transformation to esophageal cancer in those with BE. Cancers that have arisen from BE have chromosomal losses in 4q, 5q, 9p, and 18q and gains in 8q, 17q, and 20q.[179-181] The gene products that may be involved in the development of this cancer include COX-2, Bcl-2, p53, p16, p27, cyclin D1, retinoblastoma protein, epidermal growth factor and receptor, erb-b2, E-cadherin, α catenin, and ß catenin.[181-188]

Prevention/Surveillance/Prognostic Indicators

Tobacco and alcohol use are major risk factors in the development of squamous cell esophageal cancers; cessation of tobacco and alcohol do significantly decrease risk of this cancer.[189] This, however, does not apply to adenocarcinoma development. Fresh fruit and vegetable intake as opposed to foods high in nitrosamines or contaminated with bacterial or fungal toxins may decrease risk by approximately 50%.[190]

Screening has not been found cost-effective or indicated since this is a relatively low-incidence form of cancer with no definable hereditary link and few symptoms at early onset. Those patients diagnosed with BE are generally followed endoscopically due to the incidence of both LGD and HGD.[191-193] It has been recommended that an endoscopic procedure be performed every 3 to 5 years in the absence of dysplasia and more frequently if LGD is found.[193] The management of HGD, conversely, is greatly debated in terms of prophylactic esophagectomy since occult invasive cancer has frequently been identified at the time of resection.[194] It has been reported that over half of patients identified with HGD will develop esophageal cancer within 3 to 5 years without treatment.[195] Use of proton pumps can lead to healing of erosive gastritis and remains unclear if this treatment reduces the risk of esophageal cancer.[196]

The prognosis for esophageal cancer treated with standard approaches such as surgery and/or radiation are poor. Large retrospective studies of patients treated with either radiotherapy alone or surgery alone have noted 5-year survival rates of 6% for radiotherapy and 11% for surgery.[197,198] This has prompted studies involving the use of preoperative chemotherapy followed by surgery, combined preoperative chemoradiotherapy followed by surgery, or definitive chemoradiotherapy alone without surgery.

SURGICAL MANAGEMENT

Localized esophageal cancer is resected and is covered in more surgical detail in Chapter 2. The right transthoracic approach combines a laparotomy and right-sided thoracotomy leading to an esophagogastric anastomosis either in the upper chest (the Ivor-Lewis) or in the neck (the three-field technique). A laparotomy with blunt dissection of the thoracic esophagus and anastomosis in the neck is the transhiatal approach. Greater morbidity and mortality exists when using the transthoracic approach due to cardiopulmonary complications. However, the tumor is better visualized and the lymphatics are more thoroughly dissected. The Ivor-Lewis technique places the patient at an even higher risk of anastomotic leak into the chest. Although no trial has demonstrated a significant difference in overall survival, the transhiatal approach has a lower rate of perioperative complications and lower incidence of a thoracic duct leak.[199-201] Patients undergoing surgery as the only method of treatment independent of stage had a median survival rate of 13 to 19 months, a 2-year survival rate of 35% to 42%, and a 5-year survival rate of 15% to 24%.[202]

RADIOTHERAPY

The use of radiotherapy as an alternative to surgery was evaluated in patients found to be poor surgical risks. A review of noncontrolled patients treated with radiotherapy alone to doses of 5000 to 6800 cGy demonstrated survival data similar to that with surgery alone.[203] There appears to be less perioperative morbidity but the effectiveness of this modality is questionable. Primary radiotherapy alone does not appear to be a successful mode for palliation as compared to surgery. It does not provide significant relief of dysphagia/odynophagia and has a real risk of local complications independent of recurrence such as esophagotracheal fistula development.

Radiation, whether given either preoperatively or postoperatively has, to date, not demonstrated a survival advantage. Six randomized trials involving more than 100 patients have been reported comparing preoperative radiotherapy followed by immediate surgery. Patients received probably inadequate dosing ranging from 2000 to 4000 cGy and the predominant histology reported was squamous cell; no survival advantage was noted.[204] Adjuvant or postoperative radiotherapy has also failed to improve survival. Detrimental effects on survival have been noted except in the setting of recurrence rates for node-negative patients.[205,206] RTOG 8501, in which radiation was given in combination with chemotherapy, was reported to have a significant advantage over radiation alone.[207] Thus, chemotherapy may play a role in management of esophageal cancer and will be discussed subsequently.

SYSTEMIC CHEMOTHERAPY

Currently available chemotherapy agents have modest activity in esophageal cancer. The traditional active agents have included CDDP, 5-FU, and mitomycin with response rates of 15% to 28% as single agents. Initial combination agents in the metastatic setting included CDDP, bleomycin and vindesine with reported responses of 33% and 29% in two respective studies.[208-209] The most commonly used combination regimen has included 5-FU and CDDP with reported responses of 50% to 60% with a toxicity profile including myelosuppression and mucositis.[210-212] This combination is considered "standard" based on common practice in the community, synergism between the 2 agents, and radio-sensitizing properties.[213-215] Only one trial has compared single agent CDDP to CDDP/5-FU in a phase II setting with a higher response rate in the combined arm of 35% and median survival of 33 weeks.[216] The CDDP arm reported responses of 19% with a median survival of 28 weeks which was not statistically different. Patients included in this trial were those with esophageal, GEJ, and gastric cancer of either adenocarcinoma or squamous cell histology. In GEJ and gastric adenocarcinoma, a trial was published included epirubicin (E) combined with a protracted, 6-week infusion of 5-FU/CDDP known as the ECF regimen and compared to 5-FU/doxorubicin and methotrexate (FAMTX).[217] The median survival in the ECF arm was 8.9 months compared to 5.7 months for FAMTX with a response rate of 45% vs 21% and less toxicity. As described previously, another trial in GEJ/gastric cancer compared CDDP with 5-day infusional 5-FU to FAMTX or etoposide, leucovorin, and 5-FU (ELF) with responses of 10% to 20% and a median survival of less than 8 months.[94] Thus, controversy remains as to the benefit of CDDP/5-FU or in combination with other agents.

Thus, newer agents such as paclitaxel and irinotecan (CPT11) have been used in combination with CDDP or 5-FU or as single agents in the metastatic setting. Responses of 15 to 30% have been noted with either 5-FU or CDDP.[218-225] In general as previously explained, chemotherapy is essentially used for palliation of symptoms with responses to chemotherapy lasting several months, with little influence on overall survival. Thus, the therapeutic benefit of combination chemotherapy with its associated toxicity must be weighed against single agent regimens.

Paclitaxel is a very active agent, alone and in combinations, for esophageal cancer. Initially, paclitaxel was given as a 24-hour infusion at a dose of 250 mg/m^2 every 3 weeks with granulocyte support; response rates were reported at 32% in either squamous or adenocarcinoma.[226] Three hour infusional paclitaxel, which is the standard method of administration, has not been tested as a single agent in this cancer. Weekly paclitaxel has been demonstrated in a multicenter national trial to have a 17% response rate in chemotherapy naïve patients.[227] Docetaxel as mentioned in the gastric cancer section has been used as a single agent every 3 weeks in gastric cancer; 8 patients on that study had esophageal cancer with a response rate of 25%.[228]

Paclitaxel has also been investigated in combination trials. In a phase II, multicenter trial, paclitaxel was given over 3 hours with infusional 5-FU over 96 hours and CDDP every 28 days in patients with either squamous or adenocarcinoma of the esophagus with a reported 48% response rate.[229] Significant toxicity was reported. Twenty-four hour infusional paclitaxel was evaluated with CDDP and no 5-FU with less toxicity and an overall response rate of 44%.[230] Biweekly scheduling of paclitaxel and CDDP has been reported from Europe where 3 hour paclitaxel is given with CDDP every 14 days.[231] Forty percent responses were noted with less myelosuppression and neurotoxicity. Increased doses of paclitaxel to 200mg/m^2 biweekly with CDDP rendered a 52% objective response rate.[232] Carboplatin (AUC5) with 3-hour infusional paclitaxel (200 mg/m^2) every 3 weeks has been reported with an approximate 40% response rate.[233]

Another active drug is the topoisomerase II inhibitor, irinotecan or CPT-11. Single agent use on a weekly schedule has reported response rates of 15%.[234,235] A recently published phase II trial from New York with CDDP 30 mg/m^2 and CPT-11 65 mg/m^2 weekly for 4 weeks demonstrated a 57% response rate with myelosuppression as the rate limiting factor.[236] Patients' quality of life appeared improved, with less dysphagia reported. Studies are ongoing looking at alterations in the dosing schedule to weekly for 2 weeks vs 4 weekly therapies. CPT-11 has been used with mitomycin C and also in a randomized phase II trial comparing it to infusional 5-FU/CPT-11 with CDDP/CPT-11.[237,238] The CDDP/CPT-11 combination is now being investigated in the combined modality setting with radiation.

Other active drugs in metastatic esophageal cancer include the vinca alkaloid, vinorelbine, and a new platinum agent, nedaplatin. Vinorelbine as a single agent at 25 mg/m^2 weekly has reported response rates of 20%.[239] Nedaplatin is being investigated in Japan in those with metastatic squamous cell with reported single agent responses of 52% but dose limited by thrombocytopenia.[240] Gemcitabine and oxaliplatin are also being investigated in this disease as with gastric cancer.[241-245]

NEOADJUVANT CHEMOTHERAPY

The role of preoperative chemotherapy alone has been investigated in 2 multicenter trials.[246,247] Both studies used CDDP/5-FU as the chemotherapy regimen. The first study conducted in North America showed no benefit, with 35% of patients alive at 2 years who received chemotherapy/surgery compared to 37% of patients who underwent surgery alone. A similar British study revealed a 34% response rate for surgery alone compared to 43% in the chemotherapy/surgery arm. The differences in these studies include more intensive chemotherapy in the American arm, delaying surgery as well as staging prechemotherapy CT scans.

COMBINED PREOPERATIVE CHEMOTHERAPY/RADIOTHERAPY

There have been at least 8 trials addressing the issue of concurrent chemoradiation in the preoperative setting. Table 3-3 is a summary of those studies/results.

Of the above trials, one published by Walsh et al demonstrated a benefit to chemotherapy in those with adenocarcinoma who either had immediate surgery or received CDDP/5-FU with 4000 cGy radiation preoperatively.[248] There appeared to be a trend to a significant 3-year survival advantage, but this study was limited by a small number of patients, brief follow up, and poor outcome in the surgery arm. Only 6% of patients in the surgery arm were alive at 3 years compared to 26% estimated survival

Table 3-3

PREOPERATIVE CHEMOTHERAPY AND RADIOTHERAPY WITH SURGERY VS SURGERY ALONE IN PATIENTS WITH LOCALIZED ESOPHAGEAL CANCER

Study	N	Diagnosis	Chemo (cGy)	Radiation	Months	3 Year Survival (%)
Nygaard, et al[249]						
S	41	SCC	CDDP/	3500	—	9
CRS	47		Bleomycin		—	17
LePrise, et al[250]						
S	41	SCC	CDDP/5-FU	2000	10	14
CRS	41				10	19
Apinop, et al[251]						
S	34	SCC	CDDP/5-FU	4000	7	20
CRS	35				10	26
Walsh, et al[248]						
S	55	A	CDDP/5-FU	4000	11	6*
CRS	58				16	32
Bosset, et al[252]						
S	139	SCC	CDDP	3700	19	3
CRC	143				19	39
Law, et al[253]						
S	30	SCC	CDDP/5-FU	4000	27	—
CRS	30				26	—
Urba, et al[254]						
S	50	SCC/A	CDDP/5-FU/	4500	18	16
CRS	50		Vinblastine		17	30
Burmeister, et al[255]						
S	128	SCC/A	CDDP/5-FU	3500	22	—
CRS	128				19	—

N=number of patients, SCC=squamous, A=adenocarcinoma, S=surgery, CRS=chemoradiation/surgery
*Significant difference

from historical controls. Thus, 6 of the above trials were negative; one was questionably positive.[248-255] The Nygaard trial used one chemotherapy agent other than 5-FU (bleomycin) with no significant difference in either arm.[249] Squamous cell histology alone was looked at in the trial by Bosset, et al with CDDP at 80 mg/m^2 given 2 days prior to the initiation of radiotherapy; median follow-up of 55 months revealed no survival differences.[252] Urba et al employed three chemotherapy drugs, CDDP/5-FU and vinblastine days 1 to 21 with hyperfractionated radiotherapy at 150 cGy/day for a total dose of 4500 cGy followed by a transhiatal esophagectomy on day 42.[254] Three-year survival was reported at 30% in the chemotherapy/XRT/surgery arm vs 16% in the surgery alone but this was statistically significant based on the small number of patients. Thus, no conclusions have been made as to the benefit of chemoradiation in the neoadjuvant setting despite significant use of these regimens.

POSTOPERATIVE CHEMOTHERAPY/RADIATION THERAPY

Postoperative chemotherapy given concurrently with radiation has been given to patients with approaching positive surgical margins but without any documentation as to benefit in the absence of residual disease.

COMBINED MODALITY THERAPY IN UNRESECTABLE DISEASE

RTOG 8501 addressed the question of radiotherapy alone in unresectable esophageal cancer compared to chemoradiation.[256-258] In this phase III prospective trial involving 123 patients, 4 courses of combined 5-FU (1000 mg/m²/4 days) with CDDP (75 mg/m² Day 1) with 50 Gy of radiation were compared to 64 Gy of radiation. Surgery was not an option in this study. Patients with either squamous cell or adenocarcinoma confined to the esophagus with no mediastinal/supraclavicular nodal involvement were allowed to enroll. The chemoradiation arm had a 12 and 24 month survival rate of 50% and 38% with a 3-year survival rate of 35%. A 5-year follow-up has now been reported at 26% compared to 0% in the radiotherapy group alone. More intensive regimens with or without neoadjuvant chemotherapy or brachytherapy have shown no survival benefit.

TARGETED THERAPIES

Because of the significant challenge of treating esophageal cancer and the less than satisfying outcomes to chemotherapy, radiation, surgery, or the combination, novel molecular targets may play a greater role in treatment. Additionally, markers assessing chemo- or radiotherapy resistance may help tailor treatment.

As mentioned in the section on gastric cancer, growth factor pathway inhibitors, inhibitors of tyrosine kinase involved in signaling and antiangiogenesis inhibitors may take on a greater role in this cancer as well. The monoclonal antibody, C225, which is an EGF-R inhibitor, has synergy with both chemotherapy and radiotherapy in phase I and II trials in head/neck squamous cell cancer and colon cancer and may have a role in esophageal cancer as well.[259,260] OSI 774 and ZD 1839 with activity in both lung and head/neck cancer is being investigated in esophageal cancer.

Markers of resistance to chemotherapy are also under investigation. One potential marker of response to chemotherapy is the degree of expression of the target enzyme for 5-FU, thymidylate synthase. There may be some correlation between response to 5-FU in gastric cancer based on thymidylate synthase expression.[261] The DNA excision repair gene, ERCC-1, may be a marker of response to CDDP.[261]

CONCLUSIONS

Both gastric and esophageal cancers remain a challenge in terms of surgical, radiotherapy, chemotherapy or combined modality therapy. Progress with newer chemotherapy agents and optimal radiotherapy techniques may improve responses to combined modality treatment with more limited toxicities. The advent of molecular targets may also play a key role in therapeutic options. Quality of life indices now need to be considered, especially in patients with such a short median life expectancy. Potential markers of response or resistance may come into play as well that may aid in developing targeted therapies to improve patient response.

REFERENCES

1. Parkin DM. Epidemiology of cancer global patterns and trends. *Toxicol Lett.* 1998;102-103:227-234.
2. Ilson DH. Oesophageal cancer: new developments in systemic therapy. *Cancer Treatment Reviews.* 2003;29:525-532.
3. Howson CP, Hiyama T, Wynder EL. The decline in gastric cancer epidemiology of an unplanned triumph. *Epidemiol Rev.* 1986;8:1-27.
4. Correa P. The epidemiology of gastric cancer. *World J Surg.* 1991;15;228-234.
5. Dijkhuizen SM, et al. Multiple hyperplastic polyps in the stomach: evidence for clonality and neoplastic potential. *Gastroenterology.* 1997;112:561-562.
6. Shiao YH, et al. Implications of p53 mutation spectrum for cancer etiology in gastric cancers of various histologic types from a high-risk area of central Italy. *Carcinogenesis.* 1998;10:2145-2149.
7. Correa P, Shiao YH. Phenotypic and genotypic events in gastric carcinogenesis. *Cancer Res.* 1994;54:1941s-1943s.
8. Gong C, et al. KRAS mutations predict progression of preneoplastic gastric lesions. *Cancer Epidemiol Biomarkers Prev.* 1999;8:167-171.
9. Hongyo T, et al. Mutations of the K-ras and p53 genes in gastric adenocarcinomas from a high-incidence region around Florence, Italy. *Cancer Res.* 1995;55:2665-2672.
10. Fedriga R, et al. Relation between food habits and p53 mutational spectrum in gastric cancer patients. *Int J Oncol.* 2000;17:127-133.
11. Strickler JG, et al. P53 mutations and microsatellite instability in sporadic gastric cancer: when guardians fail. *Cancer Res.* 1994;54:4750-4755.
12. Chong JM, et al. Microsatellite instability in the progression of gastric carcinoma. *Cancer Res.* 1994;54:4595-4597.
13. Kobayashi K, et al. Genetic instability in intestinal metaplasia is a frequent event leading to well-differentiated early adenocarcinoma of the stomach. *Eur J Cancer.* 2000;36:1113-1119.
14. Palli D, et al. Red meat, family history, and increased risk of gastric cancer with microsatellite instability. *Cancer Res.* 2001;61:5415-5419.
15. Lin KM, et al. Cumulative incidence of colorectal and extracolonic cancers in MLH1 and MSH2 mutation carriers of hereditary nonpolyposis colorectal cancer. *J Gastrointest Surg.* 1998;2:67-71.
16. Vasen HF, et al. Cancer risk in families with hereditary nonpolyposis colorectal cancer diagnosed by mutation analysis. *Gastroenterology.* 1996;110:1020-1027.
17. Akiyama Y, et al. Frequent microsatellite instabilities and analyses of the related genes in familial gastric cancers. *Jpn J Cancer Res.* 1996;87:595-601.
18. Yanagisawa Y, et al. Methylation of the hMLH1 promoter in familial gastric cancer with microsatellite instability. *Int J Cancer.* 2000;85:50-53.

19. Keller G, et al. Microsatellite instability and loss of heterozygosity in gastric carcinoma in comparison to family history. *Am J Pathol.* 1998;152:1281-1289.

20. Enomoto M, et al. The relationship between frequencies of extracolonic manifestations and the position of APC germline mutation in patients with familial adenomatous polyposis. *Jpn J Clin Oncol.* 2000;30:82-88.

21. Shinmura K, et al. Familial gastric cancer: clinicopathological characteristics, RER phenotype and germline p53 and E-cadherin mutation. *Carcinogenesis.* 199;20:1127-1131.

22. Varley JM, et al. An extended Li-Fraumeni kindred with gastric carcinoma and a codon 175 mutation in PT53. *J Med Genet.* 1995;32:942-945.

23. Sugano K, et al. Germline p53 mutation in a case of Li-Fraumeni syndrome presenting as gastric cancer. *Jpn J Clin Oncol.* 1999;29:513-516.

24. Neugut AI, Hayek M, Howe G. Epidemiology of gastric cancer. *Semin Oncol.* 1996;23:281-291.

25. Chyou PH, et al. A case-cohort study of diet and stomach cancer. *Cancer Res.* 1990;50:7501-7504.

26. Blot WJ, et al. Nutrition intervention trials in Linxian, China: supplementation with specific vitamin/mineral combinations, cancer incidence, and disease-specific mortality in the general population. *J Natl Cancer Institute.* 1993;85:1483-1492.

27. Benner SE, Hong WK. Clinical chemoprevention: developing a cancer prevention strategy. *J Natl Cancer Inst.* 1993;85:1446-1447.

28. Chow WH, et al. Body mass index and risk of adenocarcinomas of the esophagus and gastric cardia. *J Natl Cancer Inst.* 1998;90:150-155.

29. Gammon MD, et al. Tobacco, alcohol, and socioeconomic status and adenocarcinomas of the esophagus and gastric cardia. *J Natl Cancer Inst.* 1997;89:1277-1284.

30. Zhang ZF, Kurtz RC, Marshall JR. Cigarette smoking and esophageal and gastric cardia adenocarcinoma. *J Natl Cancer Inst.* 1997;89:1247-1249.

31. Ernst P. Review article: the role of inflammation in the pathogenesis of gastric cancer. *Aliment Pharmacol Ther.* 1999;13:13-18.

32. Graham DY. *Helicobacter pylori* infection in the pathogenesis of duodenal ulcer and gastric cancer: a model. *Gastroenterology.* 1997;113:1983-1991.

33. Danesh J. *Helicobacter pylori* and gastric cancer: time for mega-trials? *Br J Cancer.* 1999;80:927-929.

34. Parsonnet J, et al. Risk for gastric cancer in people with CagA positive or CagA negative Helicobacter pylori infection. *Gut.* 1997;40:297-301.

35. Blaser MJ, et al. Infection with *Helicobacter pylori* strains possessing cagA is associated with an increased risk of developing adenocarcinoma of the stomach. *Cancer Res.* 1995;55:2111-2115.

36. Deguchi R, et al. Association between CagA + *Helicobacter pylori* infection and p53, bax and transforming growth factor-beta-RII gene mutations in gastric cancer patients. *Int J Cancer.* 2001;91:481-485.

37. Oota K, Sobin LH. *Histological typing of gastric and oesophageal tumors in international histological classification of tumors.* Geneva:WHO; 1977.

38. Maehara Y, et al. Prognostic value of p53 expression for patients with gastric cancer—a multivariate analysis. *Br J Cancer.* 1999;79:1255-1261.

39. Fonseca L, et al. P53 detection as a prognostic factor in early gastric cancer. *Oncology.* 1994;51:485-490.

40. Aizawa K, et al. Apoptosis and bcl-2 expression in gastric carcinomas: correlation with clinicopathological variables, p53 expression, cell proliferation and prognosis. *Int J Oncol.* 1999;14:85-91.

41. Wu CW et al. Serum anti-p53 antibodies in gastric adenocarcinoma patients are associated with poor prognosis lymph node metastasis and poorly differentiated nuclear grade. *Br J Cancer.* 1999;79:1255-1261.

42. Maeda K, et al. Expression of p53 and vascular endothelial growth factor associated with tumor angiogenesis and prognosis in gastric cancer. *Oncology.* 1998;55:594-599.

43. Martin HM, et al. p53 expression and prognosis in gastric carcinoma. *Int J Cancer.* 1992;50:859-862.

44. Polkowski W, et al. Prognostic value of Lauren classification and c-erbB-2 oncogene overexpression in adenocarcinoma of the esophagus and gastroesophageal junction. *Ann Surg Oncol.* 1999;6:290-297.

45. Nakajtma M, et al. The prognostic significance of amplification and overexpression of c-met and c-erb B-2 in human gastric carcinomas. *Cancer.* 2000;85:1894-1902.

46. Heiss MM, et al. Tumor-associated proteolysis and prognosis: new functional risk factors in gastric cancer defined by the urokinase-type plasminogen activator system. *J Clin Oncol.* 1995;13:2084-2093.

47. Heiss MM, et al. Individual development and uPA-receptor expression of disseminated tumour cells in bone marrow: a reference to early systemic disease in solid cancer. *Nat Med.* 1995;1:1035-1039.

48. Yonemura Y, et al. Prediction of lymph node metastasis and prognosis from the assay of the expression of proliferating cell nuclear antigen and DNA ploidy in gastric cancer. *Oncology.* 1994;51:251-257.

49. Muller W, et al. Expression and prognostic value of the CD44 splicing variants v5 and v6 in gastric cancer. *J Pathol.* 1997;183:222-227.

50. Yoo CH, et al. Prognostic significance of CD44 and nm23 expression in patients with stage II and stage IIIA gastric carcinoma. *J Surg Oncol.* 1999;71:22-28.

51. Hundahl SA, et al. The National Cancer Data Base report on gastric carcinoma. *Cancer.* 1997;80:2233-2241.

52. Nakamura K, et al. Pathology and prognosis of gastric carcinoma. Findings in 10000 patients who underwent primary gastrectomy. *Cancer.* 1992;70:1030-1037.

53. Fuchs CS, Mayer RJ. Gastric carcinoma. *New Engl J Med.* 1995;333:32-41.

54. Gouzi JL, et al. Total vs subtotal gastrectomy for adenocarcinoma of the gastric antrum. A French prospective controlled study. *Ann Surg.* 1989;209:162-166.

55. Italian Gastrointestinal Tumor Study Group, Bozzetti F, et al. Subtotal vs total gastrectomy for gastric cancer five-year survival rates in a multicenter randomized Italian trial. *Ann Surg.* 2000;230:170-178.

56. Roukos DH, Kappas AM, Encke A. Extensive lymph-node dissection in gastric cancer is it of therapeutic value. *Cancer Treat Rev.* 1996;22:247-252.

57. Roukos DH. Extended lymphadenectomy in gastric cancer when, for whom and why. *Ann R Coll Surg Engl.* 1998;80:16-24.

58. Jessup JM. Is bigger better. *J Clin Oncol.* 1995;13:5-7.

59. Lawrence W, Jr, Horsley JS. Extended lymph node dissections for gastric cancer—is better? (editorial). *J Surg Oncol.* 1996;61:85-89.

60. Dent DM, Madden MV, Price SK. Randomized comparison of R1 and R2 gastrectomy for gastric carcinoma. *Br J Surg.* 1988;75:110-112.

61. Robertson CS, et al. A prospective randomized trial comparing P1 subtotal gastrectomy with R3 total gastrectomy for antral cancer (see comments). *Ann Surg.* 1994;220:176-182.

62. Dutch Gastric Cancer Group, Bonenkamp JJ, et al. Extended lymph-node dissection for gastric cancer. *New Engl J Med.* 1999;340:908-914.

63. Bonenkamp JJ, et al. Randomised comparison of morbidity after D1 and D2 dissection for gastric cancer in 996 Dutch patients. *Lancet.* 1995;345:745-748.

64. Surgical Cooperative Group, Cuchieri A, et al. Patient survival after D1 and D2 resections for gastric cancer: long-term results of the MRC randomized surgical trial. *Br J Cancer.* 1999;79:1522-1530.

65. The Surgical Cooperative Group, Cuchieri A, et al. Post-operative morbidity and mortality after D1 and D2 resections for gastric cancer preliminary results of the RMC randomised controlled surgical trial. *Lancet.* 1996;347:995-999.

66. Maruyama K, et al. Pancreas-preserving total gastrectomy for proximal gastric cancer. *World J Surg.* 1995;19:532-536.

67. Jentschura D, et al. Surgery for early gastric cancer, a European one-center experience. *World J Surg.* 1997;21:845-848.

68. Iriyama K et al. Is extensive lymphadenectomy necessary for surgical treatment of intramucosal carcinoma of the stomach. *Arch Surg.* 1989;124:309-311.

69. Hanazaki K, et al. Clinicopathologic features of submucosal carcinoma of the stomach. *J Clin Gastroenterol.* 1997;24:150-155.

70. Hanazaki K, et al. Surgical outcome in early gastric cancer with lymph node metastasis. *Hepatogastroenterology.* 1997;44:907-911.

71. Yanai H, et al. Diagnostic utility of 20-megahertz linear endoscopic ultrasonography in early gastric cancer. *Gastrointest Endosc.* 1996;44:29-33.

72. Akahoshi K, et al. Pre-operative TN staging of gastric cancer using a 15 MHz ultrasound miniprobe. *Br J Radiol.* 1997;70:703-707.

73. Akahoshi K, et al. Endoscopic ultrasonography: a promising method for assessing the prospects of endoscopic mucosal resection in early gastric cancer. *Endoscopy.* 1997;29:614-619.

74. Takeshita K, et al. Rational lymphadenectomy for early gastric cancer with submucosal invasion: a clinicopathological study. *Surg Today.* 1998;28:580-586.

75. Sano T, Kobori O, Muto T. Lymph node metastasis from early gastric cancer: endoscopic resection of tumour. *Br J Surg.* 1992;79:241-244.

76. Roth AD. Curative treatment of gastric cancer: towards a multidisciplinary approach? *Critical Rev in Oncology Hematology.* 2003;46:59-100.

77. Macdonald JS, et al. 5-fluorouracil, adriamycin and mitomycin-C (FAM) combination chemotherapy in treatment of advanced gastric cancer. *Cancer.* 1979;44:42-47.

78. Cunningham D, et al. Advanced gastric cancer experience in Scotland using 5-fluorouracil adriamycin and mitomycin-C. *Br J Surg.* 1984;71:673-676.

79. Haim N, et al. Treatment of advanced gastric carcinoma with 5-fluorouracil adriamycin and mitomycin C (FAM). *Cancer Chemother Pharmacol.* 1982;8:277-280.

80. Haim N, et al. Further studies on the treatment of advanced gastric cancer by 5-fluorouracil, Adriamycin (doxorubicin) and mitomycin C (modified FAM). *Cancer.* 1984;54:1999-2002.

81. Macdonald JS, Gohmann JJ. Chemotherapy of advanced gastric cancer: present status, future prospects. *Semin Oncol.* 1988;15:42-49.

82. Wils JA, et al. Sequential high-dose methotrexate and fluorouracil combined with doxorubicin-A step ahead in the treatment of advanced gastric cancer. A trial of the European Organization for Research and Treatment of Cancer Gastrointestinal Tract Cooperative Group. *J Clin Oncol.* 1991;9:827-831.

83. North Central Cancer Treatment Group, Cullinan SA, et al. Controlled evaluation of three drug combination regimens vs fluorouracil alone for the therapy of advanced gastric cancer. *J Clin Oncol.* 1994;12:412-416.

84. Wils J, et al. An EORTC Gastrointestinal Group evaluation of the combination of sequential methotrexate and 5-fluorouracil, combined with adriamycin in advanced measurable gastric cancer. *J Clin Oncol.* 1986;4:1799-1803.

85. Murad Am, et al. Modified therapy with 5-fluorouracil, doxorubicin and methotrexate in advanced gastric cancer. *Cancer.* 1993;72:37-41.

86. Leichman L, Berry BT. Cisplatin therapy for adenocarcinoma of the stomach. *Semin Oncol.* 1991;18 (Suppl3):25-33.

87. Wilke H, et al/ Preoperative chemotherapy in locally advanced and nonresectable gastric cancer: a phase II study with etoposide, doxorubicin and cisplatin. *J Clin Oncol.* 1989;7:1318-1326.

88. Wilke H, et al. Etoposide, folinic acid and 5-fluorouracil in carboplatin-pretreated patients with advanced gastric cancer. *Cancer Chemother Pharmacol.* 1991;29:83-84.

89. Ychou M, et al. A phase II study of 5-fluorouracil, leucovorin and cisplatin (FLP) for metastatic gastric cancer. *Eur J Cancer.* 1996;32A:1933-1937.

90. Preusser P, Wilke H, Achterrath W. Phase II study with the combination etoposide, doxorubicin and cisplatin in advanced measurable gastric carcinoma. *J Clin Oncol.* 1989;7:1310-1317.

91. Cocconi G, et al. Fluorouracil, doxorubicin and mitomycin combination vs PELF chemotherapy in advanced gastric cancer: a prospective randomized trial of the Italian Oncology Group for Clinical Research. *J Clin Oncol.* 1994;12;2687-2693.

92. Kim NK, et al. A phase III randomized study of 5-fluorouracil and cisplatin vs 5-fluorouracil, doxorubicin and mitomycin C vs 5-fluorouracil alone in the treatment of advanced gastric cancer. *Cancer.* 1993;71:3813-3818.

93. Kelsen D, et al. FAMTX vs etoposide, doxorubicin and cisplatin: a random assignment trial in gastric cancer. *J Clin Oncol.* 1992;10:541-548.

94. Vanhoefer U et al. Final results of a randomized phase III trial of sequential high-dose methotrexate, fluorouracil and doxorubicin vs etoposide, leucovorin and fluorouracil vs infusional fluorouracil and cisplatin in advanced gastric cancer: a trial of the European Organization for Research and Treatment of Cancer Gastrointestinal Tract Cancer Cooperative Group. *J Clin Oncol.* 2000;11:301-306.

95. Lokich JJ, et al. A prospective randomized comparison of continuous infusion fluorouracil with a conventional bolus schedule in metastatic colorectal carcinoma: a Mid-Atlantic Oncology Program Study. *J Clin Oncol.* 1989;7:425-432.

96. Findlay M, et al. A phase II study in advanced gastroesophageal cancer using epirubicin and cisplatin combination with continuous infusion 5-fluorouracil (ECF). *Ann Oncol.* 1994;5: 6609-6616.

97. Bamias A, et al. Epirubicin, cisplatin, and protracted venous infusion of 5-fluorouracil for esophagogastric adenocarcinoma: response, toxicity, quality of life and survival. *Cancer.* 1996; 77:1978-1985.

98. Zaniboni A, et al. Epirubicin, cisplatin and continuous infusion 5-fluorouracil is an active and safe regimen for patients with advanced gastric cancer. An Italian Group for the Study of Digestive Tract Cancer (GISCAD) report. *Cancer.* 1995;76:1694-1699.

99. Webb A, et al. Randomized trial comparing epirubicin, cisplatin, and fluorouracil vs fluorouracil, doxorubicin and methotrexate in advanced esophagogastric cancer. *J Clin Oncol.* 1997;15:261-267.

100. Cascinu S, et al. Intensive weekly chemotherapy for advanced gastric cancer using fluorouracil, cisplatin, epi-doxorubicin, 6S-leucovorin, glutathione and filgrastim: A report from the Italian Group for the Study of Digestive Tract Cancer. *J Clin Oncol.* 1997;15:3313-3319.

101. Chi KH, et al. Weekly etoposide, epirubicin, cisplatin 5-fluorouracil and leucovorin: an effective chemotherapy in advanced gastric cancer. *Br J Cancer.* 1998;77:1984-1988.

102. Schiff PB, Horwitz SB. Taol assembles tubulin in the absence of exogenous guanosine 5'triphosphate or microtubule-associated proteins. *Biochemistry.* 1981;20:3247-3252.

103. Einzig AI, et al. Phase II trial of Taxol in patients with adenocarcinoma of the upper gastrointestinal tract (UGIT). The Eastern Cooperative Oncology group (ECOG) results. *Invest New Drugs.* 1995;13:223-227.

104. Ajani JA, et al. Phase II study of Taxol in patients with advanced gastric carcinoma. *Cancer J Sci Am.* 1998;4:269-275.

105. Ohtsu A, et al. An early phase II study of a 3 h infusion of paclitaxel for advanced gastric cancer. *Am J Clin Oncol.* 1998;21:416-419.

106. Cascinu S, et al. A phase I study of paclitaxel and 5-fluorouracil in advanced gastric cancer. *Eur J Cancer.* 1997;33:1699-1702.

107. Bokemeyer C, et al. A phase II trial of paclitaxel and weekly 24 h infusion of 5-fluorouracil/folinic acid in patients with advanced gastric cancer. *Anticancer Drugs.* 1997;8:396-399.

108. Chun H, et al. Chemotherapy (CT) with cisplatin, fluorouracil (FU) and paclitaxel for adenocarcinoma (AC) of the stomach and gastroesophageal junction (GEJ). *ASCO Proc.* 1999; 18:280a.

109. Kim YH, et al. Paclitaxel, 5-fluorouracil and cisplatin combination chemotherapy for the treatment of advanced gastric carcinoma. *Cancer.* 1999;85:295-301.

110. Lokich JJ, et al. Combined paclitaxel, cisplatin and etoposide for patients with previously untreated esophageal and gastroesophageal carcinomas. *Cancer.* 1999;85:2347-2351.

111. Einzig AI, et al. Phase II trial of docetaxel (Taxotere) in patients with adenocarcinoma of the upper gastrointestinal tract previously untreated with cytotoxic chemotherapy: the Eastern Cooperative Oncology Group (ECOG) results of protocol E1293. *Med Oncol.* 1996;13:87-93.

112. EORTC Early Clinical Trials Group, Sulkes A, et al. Docetaxel (Taxotere) in advanced gastric cancer, results of a Phase II clinical trial. *Br J Cancer.* 1994;70:380-383.

113. Mai M, et al. A late phase II clinical study of RP56976 (docetaxel) in patients with advanced or recurrent gastric cancer; a cooperative study group trial (group B). *Gan To Kagaku Ryoho.* 1999;26:487-496.

114. Verweij J, Clavel M, Chevalier B. Paclitaxel(Taxol) and docetaxel (Taxotere): not simply two of a kind. *Ann Oncol.* 1994;5:495-505.

115. Roth AD, et al. Docetaxel (taxotere)-cisplatin (TC): an effective drug combination in gastric carcinoma. Swiss Group for Clinical Cancer Research (SAKK) and the European Institute of Oncology (EIO). *Ann Oncol.* 2000;11:301-306.

116. Roth AD, et al. 5-FU as protracted continuous IV infusion (5-FUpiv) can be added to full dose taxotere-cisplatin (TC) in advanced gastric carcinoma (AGO). *Eur J Cancer.* 1999;35:S130-139.

117. Vanhoefer U, et al. Phase II study of docetaxel as second line chemotherapy (CT) in metastatic gastric cancer. *ASCO Proc.* 1999;18:303a.

118. Andre T, et al. Docetaxel-epirubicin as second-line treatment for patients with advanced gastric cancer. *ASCO Proc.* 1999;18:277a.

119. CPT-11 Gastrointestinal Cancer Study Group, Futatsuki K, et al. Late phase II study of irinotecan hydrochloride (CPT-11) in advanced gastric cancer. *Gan To Kagaku Ryoho.* 1994; 21:1033-1038.

120. Kohne CH, et al. Final results of a phase II trial of CPT-1 in patients with advanced gastric cancer. *ASCO Proc.* 1999;18:258a.

121. Shirao K, et al. Phase I-II study of irinotecan hydrochloride combined with cisplatin in patients with advanced gastric cancer. *J Clin Oncol.* 1997;15:921-927.

122. Boku N, et al. Phase II study of a combination of irinotecan and cisplatin against metastatic gastric cancer. *J Clin Oncol.* 1999;17:319-323.

123. Ajani JA, et al. Irinotecan plus cisplatin in advanced gastric or gastroesophageal junction carcinoma. *Oncology.* 2001;15:52-54.

124. Raymond E, Chaney SG, Taamma A, et al. Oxaliplatin: a review of preclinical and clinical studies. *Ann Oncol.* 1998;9:1053-1071.

125. Kim DY, Kim JH, Lee SH, et al. Phase II study of oxaliplatin, 5-fluorouracil and leucovorin in previously platinum-treated patients with advanced gastric cancer. *Ann Oncol.* 2003;14: 383-387.

126. Murray GI, et al. Matrix metalloproteinases and their inhibitors in gastric cancer. *Gut.* 1998; 43:791-797.

127. Macdonald JS, Smalley SR, Benedetti J, et al. Chemoradiotherapy after surgery compared with surgery alone for adenocarcinoma of the stomach or gastroesophageal junction. *N Engl J Med.* 2001;345:725-730.

128. The Gastrointestinal Tumor Study Group. Controlled trial of adjuvant chemotherapy following curative resection for gastric cancer. *Cancer.* 1982;49:1116-1122.

129. Imanaga H, Nakazato H. Results of surgery for gastric cancer and effect of adjuvant mitomycin C on cancer recurrence. *World J Surg.* 1977;2:213-221.

130. Hermans J, et al. Adjuvant therapy after curative resection for gastric caner: meta-analysis of randomized trials. *J Clin Oncol.* 1993;11:1441-1447.

131. Pignon JP, Ducreux M, Rougier P. Meta-analysis of adjuvant chemotherapy in gastric cancer: a critical reappraisal. *J Clin Oncol.* 1994;12:877-878.

132. Mari E, et al. Efficacy of adjuvant chemotherapy after curative resection for gastric cancer: a meta-analysis of published randomised trials. A study of the GISCAD (Gruppo Italiano per lo Studio dei Carcinomi dell'Apparato Digerente). *Ann Oncol.* 2000;11:837-843.

133. Minsky BD. The role of radiation therapy in gastric cancer. *Semin Oncol.* 1996;23:390-396.

134. Budach VG. The role of radiation therapy in the management of gastric cancer. *Ann Oncol.* 1994;5:37-48.

135. Hallissey MT, et al. The second British Stomach Cancer Group trial of adjuvant radiotherapy or chemotherapy in resectable gastric cancer: a 5 year follow-up. *Lancet.* 1994;343:1309-1312.

136. Abe M et al. Clinical experiences with intraoperative radiotherapy of locally advanced cancers. *Cancer.* 1980;45:40-48.

137. Abe M, et al. Japan gastric trials in intraoperative radiation therapy. *Int J Radiat Oncol Biol Phys.* 1988;15:1431-1433.

138. Abe M, et al. Intraoperative radiotherapy of gastric cancer. *Cancer.* 1974;34:2034-2041.

139. Pelton JJ, et al. The influence of surgical margins on advanced cancer treated with intraoperative radiation therapy (IORT) and surgical resection. *J Surg Oncol.* 1993;53:30-35.

140. Sindelar WF, et al. Randomized trial of intraoperative radiotherapy in carcinoma of the stomach. *Am J Surg.* 1993;165:178-186.

141. Abe M et al. Intraoperative radiotherapy in carcinoma of the stomach and pancreas. *World J Surg.* 1987;11:459-464.

142. Frykholm GJ, Glimelius B, Pahlman L. Preoperative or postoperative irradiation in adenocarcinoma of the rectum: final treatment results of a randomized trial and an evaluation of late secondary effects. *Dis Colon Rectum.* 1993;36:564-572.

143. Swedish Rectal Cancer Trial. Improved survival with preoperative radiotherapy in resectable rectal cancer. *New Engl J Med.* 1997;336:980-987.

144. Singletary SE. Current treatment options for inflammatory breast cancer. *Ann Surg Oncol.* 1999;6:228-229.

145. Provisor AJ, et al. Treatment of nonmetastatic osteosarcoma of the extremity with preoperative and postoperative chemotherapy: a report from the Children's Cancer Group. *J Clin Oncol.* 1997;15:76-84.

146. Martinez-Monge R, et al. Patterns of failure and long-term results in high-risk resected gastric cancer treated with post-operative radiotherapy with or without intraoperative electron boost. *J Surg Oncol.* 1997;66:24-29.

147. Kang YK, et al. A phase III randomized comparison of neoadjuvant chemotherapy followed by surgery vs surgery for locally advanced stomach cancer. *ASCO Proc.* 1996;15:210-215.

148. The Dutch Gastric Cancer Group (DGCD), Songun I et al. Chemotherapy for operable gastric cancer: results of the Dutch randomised FAMTX trial. *Eur J Cancer.* 1999;35:558-562.

149. Zhang ZX, et al. Randomized clinical trial on the combination of preoperative irradiation and surgery in the treatment of adenocarcinoma of gastric cardia (AGC): report on 370 patients. *Int J Radiat Oncol Biol Phys.* 1998;42:929-934.

150. Shchepotin IB et al. Intensive preoperative radiotherapy with local hyperthermia for the treatment of gastric carcinoma. *Surg Oncol.* 1994;3:37-44.

151. Jemal A, Murray T, Samuels A, et al. Cancer statistics. *CA Cancer J Clin.* 2003;53:5-16.

152. Roth JA, Putnam JB Jr. Surgery of cancer of the esophagus. *Semin Oncol.* 1994;21:453-461.

153. Japanese Committee for Registration of Esophageal Carcinoma Cases. Parameters linked to 10 year survival in Japan of resected esophageal carcinoma. *Chest.* 1989;96:1005-1011.

154. Ries LAG, Eisner MP, Kosary C, et al. *SEER cancer statistics review, 1973-1999.* Bethesda, Md: National Cancer Institute; 2002.

155. Daly JM, Fry WA, Little AG, et al. Esophageal cancer: results of an American College of Surgeons patient care evaluation study. *J Am Coll Surg.* 2000;190:562-567.

156. Pisani P, Parkin DM, Bray F, Ferlay J. Estimates of the worldwide mortality from 25 cancers in 1990. *Int J Cancer.* 1999;83:18-29.

157. Siewert JR, Stein HJ, Feith M, et al. Histologic tumor type is an independent prognostic parameter in esophageal cancer: lessons from more than 1000 consecutive resections at a single center in the Western world. *Ann Surg.* 2001;234:360-367.

158. Wu AH, Wan P, Bernstein L. A multiethnic population-based study of smoking, alcohol, and body size and risk of adenocarcinoma of the stomach and esophagus (United States). *Cancer Causes Control.* 2001;12:721-732.

159. Brown LM, Hoover R, Silverman D, et al. Excess incidence of squamous cell esophageal cancer among US black men: role of social class and other risk factors. *Am J Epidemiol.* 2001;153: 114-122.

160. Ahsan H, Neugut A. Radiation therapy for breast cancer and increased risk for esophageal carcinoma. *Ann Intern Med.* 1998;128:114-117.

161. Erkal HS, Mendenhall WM, Amdur RJ, Villaret DB, et al. Synchronous and metachronous squamous cell carcinomas of the head and neck mucosal sites. *J Clin Oncol.* 2001;19:1358-1362.

162. Sandler RS, Nyren O, Ekbom A, et al. The risk of esophageal cancer in patients with achalasia: a population-based study. *JAMA.* 1995;274:1359-1362.

163. Csikos M, Horvath O, Petri A, et al. Late malignant transformation of chronic corrosive oesophageal strictures. *Langenbecks Arch Chir.* 1985;365:231-238.

164. Avisar E, Luketich J. Adenocarcinoma in a mid-esophageal diverticulum. *Ann Thorac Surg.* 2000;69:288-289.

165. Risk JM, Mills HS, Garde J, et al. The tylosis esophageal cancer (TOC) locus: more than just a familial cancer gene. *Dis Esophagus.* 1999;12:173-176.

166. Ellis A, Field JK, Field EA, et al. Tylosis associated with carcinoma of the oesophagus and oral leukoplakia in a large Liverpool family—a review of six generations. *Eur J Cancer B Oral Oncol.* 1994;30B:102-112.

167. Devesa SS, Blot WJ, Fraumeni JF Jr. Changing patterns of incidence of oesophageal and gastric carcinoma in the United States. *Cancer.* 1998;83:2049-2053.

168. Lagergren J, Bergstrom R, Lindgren A, Nyren O. Symptomatic gastroesophageal reflux as a risk factor for esophageal adenocarcinoma. *N Engl J Med.* 1999;340:825-831.

169. Farrow DC, Vaughan TL, Sweeney C, et al. Gastroesophageal reflux disease, use of H_2 receptor antagonists and risk of esophageal and gastric cancer. *Cancer Causes Control.* 2000;11: 231-238.

170. Vaughan TL, Farrow DC, Hansten PD, et al. Risk of esophageal and gastric adenocarcinomas in relation to use of calcium channel blockers, asthma drugs and other medications that promote gastroesophageal reflux. *Cancer Epidemiol Biomarkers Prev.* 1998;7:749-756.

171. Vicari JJ, Peek RM, Falk GW, et al. The seroprevalence of cagA-positive *Helicobacter pylori* strains in the spectrum of gastroesophageal reflux disease. *Gastroenterology.* 1998;115:50-57.

172. Warburton-Timms VJ, Charlett A, Valori RM, et al. The significance of cagA (+) *Helicobacter pylori* in reflux oesophagitis. *Gut.* 2001;49:341-346.

173. Chow WH, Blaser MJ, Blot WJ, et al. An inverse relation between cagA_strains of *Helicobacter pylori* infection and risk of esophageal and gastric cardia adenocarcinoma. *Cancer Res.* 1998;58:588-590.

174. Roth JA, Putnam JB, Rich TA, et al. Cancer of the esophagus. In: Devita VT, et al, eds. *Cancer: Principles and Practice of Oncology.* 5th ed. Philadelphia: Lippincott-Raven; 1997: 980-1021.

175. Lagergren J, Bergstrom R, Nyren O. No relation between body-mass and gastroesophageal reflux symptoms in a Swedish population based study. *Gut.* 2000;47:26-29.

176. Nilsson M, Lundegardh G, Carling L, et al. Body mass and reflux oesophagitis: an oestrogen-dependent association? *Scand J Gastroenterol.* 2002;37:626-630.

177. Romeo Y, Cameron AJ, Schaid DJ, et al. Barrett's esophagus: prevalence in symptomatic relatives. *Am J Gastroenterol.* 2002;97:1127-1132.

178. Shaheen N, Ransohoff DF. Gastroesophageal reflux, Barrett's esophagus, and esophageal cancer: scientific review. *JAMA.* 2002;287:1972-1981.

179. Walch AK, Zitzelsberger HF, Bruch J, et al. Chromosomal imbalances in Barrett's adenocarcinoma and the metaplasia-dysplasia-carcinoma sequence. *Am J Pathol.* 2000;156:555-556.

180. Varis A, Puolakkainen P, Savolainen H, et al. DNA copy number profiling in esophageal Barrett adenocarcinoma: comparison with gastric adenocarcinoma and esophageal squamous cell carcinoma. *Cancer Genet Cytogenet.* 2001;127:53-58.

181. Wijnhoven BP, Tilanus HW, Dinjens WN. Molecular biology of Barrett's adenocarcinoma. *Ann Surg.* 2001;233:322-337.

182. Singh SP, Lipman J, Goldman H, et al. Loss or altered subcellular localization of p27 in Barrett's associated adenocarcinoma. *Cancer Res.* 1998;58:1730-1735.

183. Shirvani VN, Ouatu-Lascar R, Laur BS, et al. Cyclooxygenase 2 expression in Barrett's esophagus and adenocarcinoma: ex vivo induction by bile salts and acid exposure. *Gastroenterology.* 2000;118:487-496.

184. Katada N, Hinder RA, Smyrk TC, et al. Apoptosis is inhibited early in the dysplasia-carcinoma sequence of Barrett's esophagus. *Arch Surg.* 1997;132:728-733.

185. Arber N, Lightdale C, Rotterdam H, et al. Increased expression of the cyclin D1 gene in Barrett's esophagus. *Cancer Epidemiol Biomarkers Prev.* 1996;5:457-459.

186. Yacoub L, Goldman H, Odze RD. Transforming growth factor-alpha, epidermal growth factor receptor, and MiB-1 expression in Barrett's associated neoplasia; correlation with prognosis. *Mod Pathol.* 1997;10:105-112.

187. Polkowski W, van Sandick JW, Offerhaus GJ, et al. Prognostic value of Lauren classification and c-erbB-2 oncogene overexpression in adenocarcinoma of the esophagus and gastroesophageal junction. *Ann Surg Oncol.* 1999;6:290-297.

188. Krishnadath KK, Tilanus HW, van Blankenstein M, et al. Reduced expression of the cadherin-catenin complex in oesophageal adenocarcinoma correlates with poor prognosis. *J Pathol.* 1997;182:2049-2053.

189. Blot WJ, McLaughlin JK. The changing epidemiology of esophageal cancer. *Semin Oncol.* 1999;26S15:2-8.

190. Terry P, Lagergren J, Hansen H, et al. Fruit and vegetable consumption in the prevention of oesophageal and cardia cancers. *Eur J Cancer Prev.* 2001;10:365-369.

191. Katz D, Rothstein R, Schned A, et al. The development of dysplasia and adenocarcinoma during endoscopic surveillance of Barrett's esophagus. *Am J Gastroenterol.* 1998;93:536-541.

192. O'Connor JB, Falk GW, Richter JE. The incidence of adenocarcinoma and dysplasia in Barrett's esophagus: report on the Cleveland Clinic Barrett's Esophagus Registry. *Am J Gastroenterol.* 1999;94:2037-2042.

193. Spechler SJ. Barrett's esophagus. *N Engl J Med.* 2002;346:836-842.

194. Falk GW, Rice TW, Goldblum JR, Richter EJ. Jumbo biopsy forceps protocol still misses unsuspected cancer in Barrett's esophagus with high-grade dysplasia. *Gastrointest Endosc.* 1999;49:170-176.

195. Buttar NS, Wang KK Sebo TJ, et al. Extent of high-grade dysplasia in Barrett's esophagus correlates with risk of adenocarcinoma. *Gastroenterology.* 2001;120:1630-1639.

196. Morales TG, Sampliner RE. Barrett's esophagus: update on screening, surveillance and treatment. *Arch Intern Med.* 1999;159:1411-1416.

197. Earlam R, Cunha-Melo JR. Oesophageal squamous cell carcinoma: II. A critical view of radiotherapy. *Br J Surg.* 1980;67:457-461.

198. Muller JM, Erasmi H, Stelzner M, et al. Surgical therapy of oesophageal carcinoma. *Br J Surg.* 1990;77:845-857.

199. Pommier RF, Bveto JT, Ferris BL, et al. Relationships between operative approaches and outcomes in esophageal cancer. *Am J Surg.* 1998;175:422-425.

200. Goldminc M, Maddern G, Le Prise E, et al. Oesophagectomy by a transhiatal approach or thoracotomy: a prospective randomized trial. *Br J Surg.* 1993;80:367-370.

201. Hulscher JBF, van Sandick JW, et al. Extended transthoracic resection compared with limited transhiatal resection for adenocarcinoma of the esophagus. *N Engl J Med.* 2002;47:1662-1669.

202. Kelsen DP, Ginsberg R, Pajak TF, et al. Chemotherapy followed by surgery compared with surgery alone for localized esophageal cancer. *N Engl J Med.* 1998;339:1979-1984.

203. Earlam R, Cunha-Melo JR. Oesophageal squamous cell carcinoma. II. A critical review of radiotherapy. *Br J Surg.* 1980;339:1979-1984.

204. Arnott SJ, Duncan W, et al. Preoperative radiotherapy in esophageal carcinoma: a meta-analysis using individual patient data (Oesophageal Cancer Collaborative Group). *Int J Radiat Oncol Biol Phys.* 1998;41:579-583.

205. Fok M, Sham JST, et al. Postoperative radiotherapy for carcinoma of the esophagus: a prospective randomised controlled trial. *Surgery.* 1993;113;138-147.

206. Teniere P, Hay JM, Fingerhut A, et la. Postoperative radiation therapy does not increase survival after curative resection for squamous cell carcinoma of the middle and lower esophagus as shown by a multicenter controlled trial. *Surg Gynecol Obstet.* 1991;173:123-130.

207. Cooper JS, Guo MD, Herskovic A, et al. Chemoradiotherapy of locally advanced esophageal cancer: long-term follow-up of a prospective randomised trial (RTOG 8501). *JAMA.* 1999; 281:1623-1627.

208. Kelsen D, Hilaris B, Coonley C, et al. Cisplatin, vindesine and bleomycin chemotherapy of local-regional and advanced esophageal carcinoma: Eastern cooperative oncology group experience. *Am J Med.* 1983;75:645-652.

209. Dinwoodie WR, Bartorucci AA, Lyman GH, et al. Phase II evaluation of cisplatin, bleomycin and vindesine in advanced squamous cell carcinoma of the esophagus: a Southeastern Cancer Study Group trial. *Cancer Treat Rep.* 1986;70:267-270.

210. Hilgenberg AD, Carey RW, Wilkins EW, et al. Preoperative chemotherapy, surgical resection and selective postoperative therapy for squamous cell carcinoma of the esophagus. *Ann Thorac Surg.* 1988;45:357-363.

211. Ajani JA, Ryan B, Rich TA, et al. Prolonged chemotherapy for localized squamous cell carcinoma of the esophagus. *Eur J Cancer.* 1992;28A:880-884.

212. Mercke C Albertsson M, Hambraeus G, et al. Cisplatin and 5-FU combined with radiotherapy and surgery in the treatment of squamous cell carcinoma of the esophagus. *Acta Oncologica.* 1991;30:617-622.

213. Scanlon KJ, Newman YL, Priest DG. Biochemical basis for cisplatin and 5-fluorouracil synergism in human ovarian carcinoma cell lines. *Proc Natl Acad Sci USA.* 1986;83:8923-8925.

214. Byfield JE. Combined modality infusional chemotherapy with radiation. In: Lokich JJ, ed. *Cancer Chemotherapy by Infusion.* 2nd ed. Chicago, Ill: Percepta Press; 1990:521-551.

215. Double EB, Richmond RC. A review of interactions between platinum coordination complexes and ionizing radiation: implication for cancer therapy. In: Prestayko AW, Croke ST, Karter SK, eds. *Cisplatin: Current Status and New Developments.* Orlando, Fla: Academic Press; 1980:125-157.

216. Bleiberg H, Conroy T, et al. Randomized phase II study of cisplatin and 5-FU vs cisplatin alone in advanced squamous cell oesophageal cancer. *Eur J Cancer.* 1997;33:1216-1220.

217. Webb A, Cunningham D, et al. A randomised trial comparing ECF with FAMTX in advanced oesophago-gastric cancer. *J Clin Oncol.* 1997;15:61-67.

218. Enzinger PC, Ilson DH, Kelsen DP. Chemotherapy in esophageal cancer. *Semin Oncol.* 1999; 26(Supp 15):12-20.

219. Enzinger PC, Kulke MH, Clark JW, et al. Phase II trial of CPT-11 in previously untreated patients with advanced adenocarcinoma of the esophagus and stomach. *Prog Proc Am Soc Clin Oncol.* 2000;19:315a.

220. De Besi P, Silen VC, Salvagno L, et al. Phase II study of cisplatin, 5-FU, and allopurinol in advanced esophageal cancer. *Cancer Treat Rep.* 1986;70:909-910.

221. Ilson DH, Forastiere A, Arquette M, et al. A phase II trial of paclitaxel and cisplatin in patients with advanced carcinoma of the esophagus. *Cancer.* 2000;6:316-323.

222. Ilson DH, Saltz L, Enzinger P, et al. Phase II trial of weekly irinotecan plus cisplatin in advanced esophageal cancer. *J Clin Oncol.* 1999;17:3270-3275.

223. Bleiberg H, Conroy T, Paillot B, et al. Randomised phase II study of cisplatin and 5-fluorouracil (5-FU) vs cisplatin alone in advanced squamous cell oesophageal cancer. *Eur J Cancer.* 1997;33:1216-1220.

224. Webb A, Cunningham D, Scarffe JH, et al. Randomized trial comparing epirubicin, cisplatin, and fluorouracil vs fluorouracil, doxorubicin and methotrexate in advanced esophagogastric cancer. *J Clin Oncol.* 1997;15:261-267.

225. Ross P, Nicholson D, Cunningham D, et al. Prospective randomized trial comparing mitomycin, cisplatin, and protracted venous-infusion fluorouracil (PVI 5-FU) with epirubicin, cisplatin, and PVI 5-FU in advanced esophagogastric cancer. *J Clin Oncol.* 2002;20:1996-2004.

226. Ajani J, Ilson D, Daugherty K, et al. Activity of taxol in patients with squamous cell carcinoma and adenocarcinoma of the oesophagus. *J Natl Cancer Inst.* 1994;86:1086-1091.

227. Kelsen DP, Ilson D, Wadleigh R, et al. A phase II multi-center trial of paclitaxel as a weekly one-hour infusion in advanced oesophageal cancer. *Proc ASCO.* 2000;19:1266.

228. Einzig AI, Neuberg D, et al. Phase II trial of docetaxel (Taxotere) in patients with adenocarcinoma of the upper gastrointestinal tract previously untreated with cytotoxic chemotherapy: the Eastern Cooperative Oncology Group (ECOG) results of protocol E1293. *Med Oncol.* 1996;13:87-93.

229. Ilson DH, Ajani J, Bhalla K, et al. Phase II trial of paclitaxel, fluorouracil, and cisplatin in patients with advanced carcinoma of the oesophagus. *J Clin Oncol.* 1998;16:1826-1834.

230. Garcia-Alfonso P, Guevara S, et al. Taxol and cisplatin and 5-fluorouracil sequential in advanced oesophageal cancer. *Pro ASCO.* 1998;17:998.

231. Petrasch S, Welt A, et al. Chemotherapy with cisplatin and paclitaxel in patients with locally advanced recurrent or metastatic oesophageal cancer. *Br J Cancer.* 1998;78:511-514.

232. Van der Gaast A, kok TC, et al. Phase I study of a biweekly schedule of a fixed dose of cisplatin with increasing doses of paclitaxel in patients with advanced oesophageal cancer. *Br J Cancer.* 1999;80:1052-1057.

233. Philip PS, Gadgeel M, Hussain M, et al. Phase II study of paclitaxel and carboplatin in patients with advanced gastric and esophageal cancers. *Proc ASCO.* 1998;17:1001.

234. Enzinger PC, Kulke MH, et al. Phase II trial of CPT-11 in previously untreated patients with advanced adenocarcinoma of the oesophagus and stomach. *Proc ASCO.* 2000;19:1243.

235. Lin L, Hecht JR. A phase II trial of irinotecan in patients with advanced adenocarcinoma of the gastrooesophageal (GE) junction. *Proc ASCO.* 2000;19:1130.

236. Ilson D, Saltz L, Enzinger P, et al. A phase II trial of weekly irinotecan plus cisplatin in advanced oesophageal cancer. *J Clin Oncol.* 1999;17:3270-3275.

237. Gold PJH, Carter G, Livingston R. Phase II trial of irinotecan and mitomycin C in the treatment of metastatic oesophageal and gastric cancers. *Proc ASCO.* 2001;20:644.

238. Pozzo C, Bugat R, et al. Irinotecan in combination with CDDP of 5-FU and folinic acid is active in patients with advanced gastric or gastrooesophageal junction adenocarcinoma: final results of a randomised phase II study. *Proc ASCO.* 2001;20:531.

239. Conroy T, Etienne PL, et al. Phase II trial of vinorelbine in metastatic squamous cell esophageal carcinoma. *J Clin Oncol.* 1996;14:164-170.

240. Taguchi T, Wakui A, Nabeya K, et al. A phase II study of cis-diammine glycolate platinum, 254-S for gastrointestinal cancers. *Jpn J Cancer Chemother.* 1992;19:483-488.

241. Burris HA, Moore MJ, et al. Improvements in survival and clinical benefit with gemcitabine as first-line therapy for patients with advanced pancreatic cancer: a randomized trial. *J Clin Oncol.* 1997;15:2403-2413.

242. Shirao K, Shimada Y, et al. Phase I-II study of irinotecan hydrochloride combined with cisplatin in patients with advanced gastric cancer. *J Clin Oncol.* 1997;15:921-927.

243. Boku N, Ohtsu A, et al. Phase II study of a combination of CDDP and CPT-11 in metastatic gastric cancer: CPT-11 study group for gastric cancer. *Proc Am Soc Clin Oncol.* 1997;16: 264.

244. Becouam Y, Ychou M, et al. Oxaliplatin (L-OHP) as first-line chemotherapy in metastatic colorectal cancer (MCRC) patients: preliminary activity/toxicity report. *Proc Am Soc Clin Oncol.* 1997;16:2291.

245. Giacchetti S, Zidani R, et al. Phase III trial of 5-flourouracil (5-FU) folinic acid (FA) with or without oxaliplatin (OXA) in patients (pts) with metastatic colorectal cancer (MCC). *Proc Am Soc Clin Oncol.* 1997;16:264.

246. Kelsen DP, Ginsberg R, et al. Chemotherapy followed by surgery compared with surgery alone for localized esophageal cancer. *N Engl J Med.* 1998;339:1979-1984.

247. Medical Research Council Oesophageal Cancer Working Group. Surgical resection with or without postoperative chemotherapy in oesophageal cancer: a randomised controlled trial. *Lancet.* 2002;359:1727-1733.

248. Walsh T, Noonan N, et al. A comparison of multimodal therapy and surgery for esophageal adenocarcinoma. *N Engl J Med.* 1999;341:384.

249. Nygaard K, Hagen S, et al. Pre-operative radiotherapy prolongs survival in operable esophageal carcinoma: a randomized multicenter study of preoperative radiotherapy and chemotherapy: the second Scandinavian trial in esophageal carcinoma. *World J Surg.* 1992;16:1104-1110.

250. LePrise E, Etieene PL, et al. A randomized study of chemotherapy, radiation therapy and surgery vs surgery for localized squamous cell carcinoma of the esophagus. *Cancer.* 1994;73: 1179-1184.

251. Apinop C, Puttsiak P, et al. A prospective study of combined therapy in esophageal cancer. *Hepatogastroenterology.* 1994;41:391-393.

252. Bosset J-F, Gignoux M, et al. Chemoradiotherapy followed by surgery compared with surgery alone in squamous-cell cancer of the esophagus. *N Engl J Med.* 1997;337:161-167.

253. Law S, Kwong D, et al. Preoperative chemoradiation for squamous cell esophageal cancer: a prospective randomized trial. *Can J Gastroenterol.* 1998;12:56B.

254. Urba SG, Orringer MB, Turrisi, et al. Randomized trial of preoperative chemoradiation vs surgery alone in patients with locoregional esophageal carcinoma. *J Clin Oncol.* 2001;19: 305-313.

255. Burmeister BH, Smithers BM, et al. A randomized phase III trial of preoperative chemoradiation followed by surgery (CR-S) vs surgery alone (S) for localized resectable cancer of the esophagus. *Prog Proc Am Soc Clin Oncol.* 2002;21:130a.

256. Herskovic A, Martz K, Al-Sarraf M, et al. Combined chemotherapy and radiotherapy compared with radiotherapy alone in patients with cancer of the esophagus. *N Engl J Med.* 1992; 326:1593-1598.

257. Al-Sarraf M, Martz K, Herskovic A, et al. Progress report of combined chemoradiotherapy vs radiotherapy alone in patients with esophageal cancer: an intergroup study. *J Clin Oncol.* 1997;15:866.

258. Cooper JS, Guo MD et al. Chemoradiotherapy of locally advanced esophageal cancer: long-term follow up of a prospective randomized trial (RTOG 85-01). *JAMA.* 1999;281:1623-1627.

259. Raben D, Helfrich B, et al. Anti-EGFR antibody potentiates radiation (RT) and chemotherapy (CT) cytotoxicity in human non-small cell lung cancer (NSCLC) cells in vitro and in vivo. *Proc ASCO.* 2001;20:1026.

260. Saltz L, Rubin M, et al. Cetuximab plus irinotecan is active in CPT-11 refractory colorectal cancer that expresses epidermal growth factor receptor. *Proc ASCO.* 2001;20:7.

261. Metzger R, Leichman CG, et al. ERCC1 mRNA levels complement thymidylate synthase mRNA levels in predicting response and survival for gastric cancer patients receiving combination cisplatin and fluorouracil chemotherapy. *J Clin Oncol.* 1998;16:309-316.

chapter 4

Surgical Approach to Gastric and Gastroesophageal Neoplasms

Francis (Frank) Spitz, MD

Cancers of the esophagus and stomach are relatively uncommon neoplasms, together accounting for an estimated 3% of newly diagnosed cancers in the United States in 2003.[1] While the incidence of gastric cancer has seen a decline over the past several decades, esophageal adenocarcinoma, now the most common type of esophageal cancer, has increased over the past 3 decades. Both cancers, particularly in advanced stages, have a generally dismal prognosis and 5-year survival, although several advancements have been made in recent years toward treatment of these diseases. Surgical resection has historically been a critical component of therapy for localized gastroesophageal neoplasms, and while it remains integral for curative treatment, it finds itself increasingly in the evolving context of a multimodal approach with adjuvant or neoadjuvant chemoradiation. This chapter aims to review esophageal and gastric cancer adenocarcinomas separately, outlining the epidemiology, risk factors, and diagnostic and preoperative evaluation of these entities, with particular attention to their management and surgical treatment.

CANCERS OF THE ESOPHAGUS

EPIDEMIOLOGY

Nearly 14,000 new cases of esophageal cancer were estimated in the United States in 2003 and 13,000 esophageal cancer related deaths, making it responsible for an estimated 2% of all cancer deaths.[1] The mean age of diagnosis is 67.3 years,[2] and while relatively uncommon in patients under 40 years of age, increases in occurrence in an age-related manner. Squamous cell carcinoma of the esophagus accounted for the majority of esophageal cancers, but has been supplanted over the past couple of decades by adenocarcinoma. The lifetime risk for esophageal cancer is approximately 2- to 3-fold higher in males than in females, and this risk is nearly doubled when one considers esophageal adenocarcinomas separately. Esophageal cancer is the seventh most common cause of cancer death in United States men, accounting for an estimated 4% of all cancer deaths in this population.[1] With regard to race, esophageal squamous cell cancers are more common (approximately 5-fold) in Blacks in the United States whereas adenocarcinoma occurs more frequently in Whites. Other malignancies of the esophagus include leiomyosarcoma, lymphoma, small cell cancer, melanoma, and others, although combined these are responsible for less than 10% of all esophageal malignancies.

RISK FACTORS AND PATHOGENESIS

The majority (75% to 90%) of adenocarcinomas occur in the distal esophagus where the squamous cell epithelium can frequently undergo metaplastic change to columnar epithelium. Both environmental and genetic factors seem to be involved in the pathogenesis of these adenocarcinomas. BE appears to most strikingly increase the risk of occurrence (over 100-fold)[2,3] of esophageal adenocarcinoma, with obesity, persistent reflux disease, and tobacco use also serving as environmental factors which lead to an increased risk. Several genes (including bcl-2, P53, cyclin D1, p16, APC, ß-catenin, BRCA2 and others)[3-5] have been postulated to be implicated in the pathogenesis of esophageal adenocarcinoma with some understanding of the pathogenesis pathway, although the precise genetic mechanisms responsible for the transformation to malignancy are still not clearly delineated.

CLINICAL PRESENTATION, DIAGNOSIS, PREOPERATIVE EVALUATION, AND STAGING

The majority of patients with esophageal cancer (>70%) will present with symptoms of dysphagia.[2] Less commonly, patients will complain of other symptoms including weight loss, odynophagia, hematemesis, or Horner's syndrome if the sympathetic chain is involved. Preoperative assessment usually includes plain chest x-rays, CT scan of the chest and abdomen, and, if neurological symptoms are present, an enhanced CT scan of the head or brain MRI. While an esophagogram may be useful in localizing the lesion and assessing the extent of luminal stenosis, upper endoscopy with ultrasound is more commonly used and provides the added benefit of potentially providing a tissue diagnosis. Bronchoscopy is integral for excluding invasion of airway structures particularly for more proximal esophageal cancers.

The staging of esophageal cancers criteria is most commonly done according to the American Joint Committee on Cancer (AJCC) (2002) TNM classification, which considers the extent of the primary tumor, the involvement of regional nodes, and the presence or absence of metastatic disease. The current AJCC TNM staging of esophageal cancer is depicted in Appendix A. It should be noted that most patients present with Stage III or IV disease (ie, with regional node involvement or metastatic disease, and approximately 50% of patients are considered unresectable at the time of diagnosis).

Resectability can be assessed by a variety of noninvasive and invasive modalities. CT scan can reliably predict the T stage of the tumor in approximately 50% of cases[6,7] and the nodal involvement generally in a slightly smaller percentage of patients. MRI generally does not provide increased yield over CT scan in accurately staging patients. Endoscopic ultrasound (EUS) is an immensely important tool for esophageal cancer staging, providing accurate tumor depth data (T stage) in over 80% of patients,[8] and sensitivity for nodal involvement as high as 89%.[9] EUS also provides information on the extent of local invasion and with ultrasound-guided fine-needle aspiration (FNA), can provide tissue diagnosis. Minimally invasive techniques including laparoscopy, laparo-scopic ultrasound, and thoracoscopy have increased the accurate staging of esophageal cancer to greater than 95%.[10] The role of positron-emission tomography (PET) with flu-deoxyglucose 18, whose sensitivity in detecting metastatic disease may be quite high and may identify metastases in as many as 14% of patients[11] otherwise thought to have localized disease by conventional imaging techniques is expanding. In our practice, endoscopy/endoscopic ultrasound with CT scan of the chest, abdomen and pelvis are routinely obtained for diagnosis and determining surgical resectability.

SURGICAL APPROACH TO ESOPHAGEAL CANCER

Surgery has traditionally been considered integral in the management of esophageal cancer and has generally been thought of as the only modality to provide a definitive cure for localized disease. Despite this, the 5-year survival rates with surgery alone are generally reported to be less than 25%[24,25] with a median survival time of 1 to 2 years. Complete response data from chemoradiation studies approach these numbers and may therefore be redefining the role of surgical intervention.

Resection of esophageal lesions can be achieved either with (transthoracic approach) or without a thoracotomy incision (transhiatal approach). For the transthoracic approach (TTE), either 1) a right thoracotomy can be made to dissect out the esopha-gus (this is more common), along with either a midline or transverse upper abdominal incision to mobilize the stomach; or 2) a left thoracotomy or thoracoabdominal approach can also be used to resect distal esophageal neoplasms or lesions of the gastric cardia, although this approach is generally less favored because of decreased accessibility of the esophagus. A three-field technique involves a laparotomy incision for stomach mobilization, a thoracotomy for esophageal and nodal dissection and a cervical incision for esophagogastric anastomosis in the neck versus in the thorax.

The transhiatal esophagectomy (THE) entails a laparotomy incision only with blunt dissection of the esophagus from the esophageal hiatus superiorly with an anastomosis in the neck. For both TTE and THE, generally the stomach is mobilized for the anas-tomosis to restore GI continuity, taking care to preserve the right gastroepiploic artery. Kocherization of the duodenum assists in providing the necessary length for the esoph-agogastric anastomosis. Since the vagus is usually divided with esophageal resection, a pyloromyotomy or pyloroplasty is generally performed. In some cases, other conduits are used for anastomosis with the remnant esophagus, the next most common being colon, although jejunum is also used. For very distal esophageal lesions, subtotal esophagectomy can be performed with an intrathoracic anastomosis, although, complete resection is required for proximal surgical margins positive for malignancy. The esopha-gogastric anastomosis can be performed either hand sewn or by use of a stapling device. These 2 methods carry about the same risk of anastomotic leak, and which method is used is generally based upon surgical preference, although the stapling method may have an increased rate of stricture formation.[22]

A significant amount of debate exists concerning which surgical approach for esophagectomy is the preferred method. Proponents of TTE argue that it provides bet-ter visualization of the dissection, thereby reducing the incidence of injury to intratho-racic structures (such as the azygous vein, recurrent laryngeal nerve, or thoracic duct) caused by blunt blind dissection while offering the opportunity for a more extensive lymph node dissection. Opponents of TTE defend the transhiatal approach as a satis-factory means of safely performing a thorough resection while avoiding the perioperative pulmonary and other complications associated with a thoracotomy incision. They also point to the generally shorter intraoperative time of THE and the potentially devastating consequences of a leak from an intrathoracic anastomosis whose mortality can be as high as 50%.

Several randomized prospective studies and retrospective meta-analyses to date have shown no significant differences in 5-year survival rates between the transhiatal and transthoracic approaches to esophagectomy.[25] One larger randomized trial with 220 patients with esophageal adenocarcinoma[12] demonstrated a statistically significant increase in the number of postoperative pulmonary complications associated with TTE (50%) as compared to THE (25%), but again no statistical difference in median or 5-year survival.

The same randomized trial demonstrated a statistically significant difference between the 2 surgical approaches in terms of the number of lymph nodes resected with the esophagectomy specimen, with almost twice as many obtained from the TTE approach as compared to THE. The clinical significance of this result is unclear however. While the incidence of positive lymph nodes in the neck may be as high as 30%[13] for mid- and distal esophageal neoplasms, which would support the extended lymphadenectomy approach (entailing resection of celiac, superior mediastinal, and cervical lymph nodes), the finding of similar 5-year survival rates between THE and TTE despite their difference in lymph node dissection suggests there may not be increased benefit from more radical resections.

The operative mortality of patients undergoing esophagectomy can range from less than 5% to over 25% in some reports (recent Phase III trials report mortality rates of 0 to 9%).[14,15] While variability in patient selection may play a role in these differences, there seems to be a clear decrease in mortality rates in high volume centers where the surgical and intensive care staff have frequent exposure to and experience with these patients.

With relatively low 5-year survival rates (25%) in patients undergoing THE and TTE, there is impetus for the development of less invasive and potentially less morbid operative methods. The use of laparoscopy, hand-assisted laparoscopy, and/or video-assisted thoracoscopy for various portions of the operation from gastric to esophageal mobilization has been successfully employed in several centers. The most frequent combination is the use of video-assisted thoracoscopy for esophageal dissection with an open incision for gastric mobilization and cervical anastomosis. Theoretically, these minimally invasive approaches could combine the benefits (and reduce the risks) of THE and TTE by allowing good visualization of intrathoracic structures and for extensive lymphadenectomy while at the same time reducing the potential complications of a large thoracotomy incision. Indeed, the extent of lymphadenectomy by thoracoscopic methods (as measured by lymph nodes resected) has been found to be similar to that achieved by TTE. Despite this, there has been no established significant difference found in morbidity and mortality between thoracoscopic and open methods, although some reports indicate a small benefit in postoperative pulmonary function and decreased pulmonary morbidity. Other considerations with minimally invasive techniques include the learning curve and training required for time-efficient performance of the surgery and operative costs. A multi-institutional trial would help sort out these various issues and critically examine any benefits that may exist with these methods.

Nonsurgical Treatments of Esophageal Cancer

Various studies have compared the use of radiation, chemotherapy, and their combination in the treatment of esophageal cancer with or without surgical intervention. The use of adjuvant chemotherapy or radiation therapy has largely been disappointing in the absence of known residual disease. Many studies have thus recently focused on neoadjuvant therapy.

No statistically significant benefit in survival has been demonstrated in pre-operative radiotherapy vs surgery alone through a number of randomized trials (most having histology of squamous cell CA) with radiation doses ranging from 20 to 45 Gy over a period of 8 days to 4 weeks. Whether there is truly any survival benefit to preoperative chemotherapy vs surgery alone is less clear. A large prospective randomized trial with 440 patients in the North America demonstrated no difference in 2-year survival rates between patients with esophageal cancer receiving preoperative chemotherapy with cisplatin and fluorouracil (35%) vs those undergoing esophagectomy alone (37%).[16] A trial in Great Britain with 802 patients, however, found an almost 10% (43% vs 34%) 2-year survival benefit.[17] Differences between the trials included different requirements of pre-operative staging and a longer chemotherapy treatment course (3 cycles vs 2 cycles) in the North American trial. Neither study nor the results of three other randomized trials demonstrated a statistically significant difference in median survival time between patients receiving pre-operative chemotherapy vs surgery alone.

Several randomized trials have compared the use of preoperative chemotherapy and radiotherapy vs surgery alone. Only one prospective randomized study published in 1996[18] with relatively few patients having esophageal adenocarcinoma demonstrated any significant survival benefit between combined neoadjuvant therapy vs esophagectomy alone. This study estimated a 3-year survival benefit for combined therapy, but was limited by its unstringent requirements of preoperative staging and its relatively poor survival outcomes of patients undergoing surgery alone as compared to other studies. A meta-analysis[19] of 9 randomized control trials with 1116 patients also concluded a 3-year survival benefit to combined neoadjuvant radiochemotherapy performed concurrently, thought to be achieved through an increase in locoregional control of disease (a nonsignificant trend was noted to treatment mortality with combined treatment). The rate of esophageal resection was lower in the group receiving combined adjuvant therapy, although the rate of complete (R0) resections was higher. Despite the negative results of the other multiple randomized control trials, the practice of treatment of patients with esophageal cancer has generally trended toward the use of combined chemoradiation therapy. Clearly, a large multi-institutional randomized trial is needed to sort out the exact benefit of this multimodality therapy.

A recent randomized trial[20] comparing chemoradiation with fluorouracil and cisplatin versus radiation alone demonstrated a significant survival benefit of the former with 5-year survival percentage (26%). Increasing the level of radiation in the combination chemoradiotherapy (64.8 Gy vs 50.4 Gy of radiation) does not seem to provide any significant benefit with local control or survival.[21] The use of other chemotherapeutic agents in the combination therapy may improve upon these results and/or decrease toxicity associated with the treatments. Investigations are currently underway with irinotecan/cisplatin and paclitaxel/cisplatin chemotherapy regimens.

While much has been learned in the management of patients with esophageal cancer, continued relatively poor 5-year survival statistics for this disease entity indicate that there is still much to be discovered. A better understanding of the tumor biology at the molecular level can help guide more effective treatment strategies whose true benefit can be assessed by large multi-institutional trials.

CANCERS OF THE STOMACH

EPIDEMIOLOGY

Approximately 22,400 new cases of gastric cancer were estimated for 2003 with an estimated 12,100 deaths for that year.[1] The overwhelming majority of these malignancies (>95%) are adenocarcinomas, followed by lymphoma. Gastric sarcomas, of which leiomyosarcoma is the most common, account for 1% to 3% and occur most frequently in the proximal portion of the stomach. Interestingly, the incidence of gastric cancer related deaths has steadily decreased in the United States in both males and females since the 1930s. The reasons for this are not entirely clear although dietary and other environmental influences may be involved. The incidence of gastric cancer is higher in males than females (1.5:1), and the peak age incidence is in the seventh and eighth decades of life, with a median age of 65 years.[29] There is considerable geographic variation in the incidence (and survival statistics) of gastric cancer, suggesting environmental and/or genetic factors in the etiology of the disease. Gastric cancer has the greatest incidence in Japan where survival rates are also the highest. Of interest, while the overall incidence of gastric cancer has decreased, there is an increase in the number of proximal tumors in the past 2 decades.

RISK FACTORS AND PATHOGENESIS

Environmental and genetic factors both appear to play a role in the pathogenesis of gastric cancer. Diets high in salts, preserved or smoked fish, or other meats (as in the Japanese diet) are associated with an increased risk of gastric cancer, while diets high in fresh fruits and antioxidants (vitamin C and ß-carotene) may have a protective role. Cigarette smoking has been found to be associated not only with ulcerative disease but with gastric cancer. Infectious agents, particularly *H. pylori* which has a high prevalence in Eastern Europe and Asia, also lead to an increased risk of gastric cancer over time. Gender influences the relative risk, with gastric cancer being more common in males, as does race, with Blacks more frequently afflicted with the disease in the United States. Other factors, including blood type A (which only marginally increases the relative risk), prior gastric resection, chronic gastritis as in pernicious anemia, or Menetrier's disease, also pose an increased risk. Various genes, including p53, of CDH1 which encodes E-cadherin, and the tumor suppressor RUNX3[27] whose expression levels are reduced in a large number of gastric cancers, may have an important involvement in the etiology of some gastric cancers.

Gastric cancer is divided into 2 major histologic types: intestinal and diffuse. The intestinal type tends to occur in older patients in the distal portion of the stomach and is characterized by a more differentiated cell morphology. This type displays considerable geographic variation and has shown a decrease in the United States in the past several decades. The diffuse type conversely tends to afflict younger patients, is characterized by a poorly differentiated cell pattern and a more aggressive nature, and shows less geographic and temporal variability. A rare form of gastric cancer in which the entire stomach is diseased, known as linitis plastica, displays particularly high virulence and compromises approximately 9% to 10% of patients with gastric carcinoma.

CLINICAL PRESENTATION, DIAGNOSIS, PREOPERATIVE EVALUATION, AND STAGING

Evaluation of patients with gastric cancer begins with a thorough history and physical. A large study conducted by the American College of Surgeons[29] in 1993 that looked at clinical presentation, diagnosis, and outcomes of 18,365 gastric cancer patients found that weight loss, abdominal pain, and nausea (61.6%, 51.6%, and 34.3%, respectively) were the most common presenting symptoms of patients with gastric cancer. Other symptoms such as anorexia (32.0%) and early satiety (17.5%) were reported less frequently. Rarely intestinal or colonic obstruction or severe GI bleed was the presenting symptom. Physical exam may reveal a palpable abdominal mass in a minority of patients, and evidence of metastatic disease in an even smaller fraction of patients by way of a palpable supraclavicular node (Virchow's node), periumbilical node (Sister Mary Joseph's node), or mass on rectal examination. Frequently, the physical exam may be normal or notable for cachexia.

Initial work-up of the patient with gastric cancer entails routine blood work, including serum electrolytes, CBC, liver function tests, and chest x-ray. As gastric carcinoma spreads both through the lymphatics and hematogenously, a thorough evaluation of not only local disease but of metastatic disease is necessary in the preoperative assessment. CT scan of the abdomen and pelvis is routinely obtained and is useful in the evaluation of intra-abdominal metastases. This diagnostic modality is limited though by its resolution, with lesions <5 mm in diameter often being missed. Accuracy in assessing tumor thickness or depth of penetration (tumor stage) by CT ranges from 42% (dynamic CT) to 76% (helical CT), with accurate nodal staging by this modality reported from 48% to 70%.[31,32] Determination of gastric wall penetration is often poorly assessable by CT scan.[32] For more proximal tumors or if suggested by physical exam or chest x-ray, a CT scan of the chest is often obtained.

In addition to CT scan, we routinely obtain esophagogastroduodenoscopy (EGD) and EUS in evaluating patients with gastric cancer. EGD can provide a tissue diagnosis and if the mass does not obstruct the lumen of the stomach, can provide the proximal and distal borders of the tumor. EUS provides important information regarding the depth of penetration of the tumor, achieving a resolution of 0.1 mm. Accurate T staging of gastric cancers has been reported as high as 78% to 86% with this modality,[31,33] although the figure for T2 tumors or those invading the muscular propria or subserosa may be less (63%).[33] Reports of accuracy of EUS in regional nodal staging range from 69% to 90%,[31,34] although lower figures have been reported (<60%), and limitations exist for detecting more distant nodes by this method. Clearly, experience and training of the user play a role in the accuracy of this modality. EUS in conjunction with FNA also offers the possibility of a tissue diagnosis.

Because of the incidence of metastatic disease undetected by CT or EUS that would otherwise be identified only upon laparotomy, the use of minimally-invasive surgery or laparoscopy has routinely become integrated into the staging of patients with gastric cancer and has been recommended by the National Comprehensive Cancer Network. A study performed at Memorial Sloan-Kettering Cancer Center[35] examined 111 gastric cancer patients with laparoscopy who were deemed to be free of metastatic disease by CT scan, and found 37% to have CT occult metastases. Twenty-four (22%) of the patients were spared a laparotomy on the basis of the laparoscopic findings. This led to shorter hospitalization stays (1.4 vs 6.5 days) for such patients who, on follow-up, did not re-present for further (palliative) surgery. These investigators argue that in the absence of bleeding, obstruction, or perforation, laparoscopy may help to avoid more extensive surgery in patients with an already grim prognosis.

PET scanning is used in some centers in the preoperative evaluation of patients with gastric cancer as a means of noninvasively increasing the sensitivity of detecting metastatic disease over conventional imaging modalities. In one study[36] that looked at peritoneal carcinomatosis from gastric and other cancers, PET scanning displayed a sensitivity of 57% alone and 78% when combined with CT scan. Because of the relatively high costs and inaccessibility of this modality, as well as its limitation in distinguishing regional nodal disease from the primary tumor, we do not routinely use PET scanning in our evaluation of patients with gastric cancer.

Peritoneal cytology obtained by laparotomy, laparoscopy, or percutaneous aspiration, particularly in cases of gastric cancers with serosal invasion, can provide useful information about dissemination of disease. Several studies show significantly worse survival rates[37,38] in patients with serosal invasion and positive cytology. Reverse-transcriptase polymerase chain reaction (RT-PCR) CEA mRNA can increase the sensitivity over cytology alone of detecting intraperitoneal disease and hence the accuracy of staging. Concern still exists as to the significance of free intraperitoneal cells and as to how they should precisely affect staging and further surgical management.

Multiple staging classifications have been offered for gastric cancer, with the most recent TNM staging scheme displayed in Appendix B. This classification incorporates depth of tumor penetration, the number of involved lymph nodes (a change from prior schemes which also took into account location of nodes) and the presence or absence of distant metastatic disease. Several studies corroborate the prognostic value of the new classification scheme,[39,40] although debate still exists as to the precise number of lymph nodes needed to be obtained for accurate staging ranging from 5 to 15.[39,41,42]

SURGICAL APPROACH TO GASTRIC CANCER

Surgery remains the mainstay for definitive curative treatment of localized gastric cancer. A growing amount of literature exists (particularly from Japan) supporting the use of minimally invasive endoscopic approaches for the resection of gastric cancers limited to the mucosa or submucosa (early gastric cancers). Endoscopic mucosal resection (EMR) for select T1 lesions with certain size and morphology characteristics has proved to be quite successful and is widely used in Japan.[43] Laparoscopic gastric resections for select early gastric cancers and submucosal lesions have also begun to be performed with some success.[44] While not undermining the growing importance of these minimally invasive techniques and their ability to reduce extensive surgical dissection, we will focus primarily on open laparotomy techniques currently recommended by the American Joint Committee on Cancer (AJCC) and those from our own experience. This chapter will moreover focus on surgical techniques for gastric cancer with curative intent, while not underemphasizing the large and important role that exists for palliative surgical procedures, particularly given the advanced stage of presentation of many patients with gastric cancer.

The 2 standard resective procedures generally performed for localized gastric cancer are subtotal and total gastrectomy with regional lymph node dissection. For proximal gastric cancers (which portend a worse prognosis) and mid-body lesions or lesions diffuse in nature or in which 6 cm of proximal margin cannot be obtained by partial gastrectomy, a total gastrectomy is performed. We generally reserve a subtotal gastrectomy for distal cancers. A French prospective study demonstrated no significant difference in postoperative mortality or 5-year survival between patients receiving a total versus subtotal gastrectomy for gastric antral tumors.[45] This study was corroborated more recently by an Italian randomized trial with 624 patients which demonstrated the 5-year survival probability for subtotal and total gastrectomy was 65.3% and 62.4%, respectively.[46]

A total gastrectomy is generally performed through either a midline or bilateral subcostal incision. After assessing for metastatic disease, attention is then turned toward mobilizing the stomach, which generally entails dissecting the omentum from the mesocolon, dividing the short gastric arteries, ligating the left gastric artery, and kocherizing the proximal duodenum. The duodenum is divided a couple of centimeters distal to the pylorus and the esophagus is transected several centimeters proximal to the GE junction. Negative surgical margins are confirmed by frozen sections. Regional lymphadenectomy is performed, and if there is evidence of encroachment into adjacent organs, these organs are resected. We do not routinely perform a splenectomy, as this has not been shown to improve survival outcome and increases morbidity.[47] Indications for a splenectomy include splenic involvement by the tumor or some locally advanced tumors on the greater curvature in the proximal third of the stomach. If splenectomy is indicated, the pancreas should be preserved (pancreatic resection is only indicated for tumor invasion of this organ).

A subtotal gastrectomy is performed in a similar manner to total gastrectomy, although approximately 20% to 25% of the proximal stomach is preserved (at least 6 cm proximal margins), with some short gastrics preserved to supply the remnant stomach. In both subtotal and total gastrectomy, the goal for curative intent is to achieve an R0 dissection (no residual macroscopic or microscopic disease).

There are several mechanisms of reconstruction following subtotal and total gastrectomy. Reconstruction following distal gastrectomy can be achieved by Billroth I or Billroth II procedures, which were found to have no significant difference in hospital mortality or 5-year survival outcome by randomized trial.[48] The standard reconstruction for a total gastrectomy is a Roux-en-Y esophagojejunostomy. Various more involved reconstructions with Hunt-Lawrence pouch replacement for the stomach have been developed with or without maintaining duodenal passage in efforts to reduce symptoms of early satiety, bloating, and weight loss, although no convincing data support them to have a significant benefit long-term. We generally recommend Roux-en-Y esophagojejunostomy reconstruction and frequently place a jejunostomy feeding tube for postoperative alimentary feeding.

One of the largest controversies in the surgical management of gastric cancer is the extent of lymph node dissection. Surgeons in Japan largely support a more radical lymphadenectomy, pointing to literature that shows a significant survival benefit for patients undergoing more extensive dissection involving not only perigastric nodes (N1), but nodes of the celiac axis and the major branches (N2) and hepatoduodenal ligament, celiac plexus, superior mesenteric artery (N3), and even in some instances of the periaortic area (N4). These encouraging results from Japanese literature have unfortunately failed to be consistently reproduced in Western studies. The reasons for this are unclear, although the possibility that differential staging practices and even differences in tumor biology may contribute to this phenomenon is raised. A recent large Dutch multicenter trial[49] with 996 patients found no significant survival difference at 5 years between patients undergoing removal of nodal tissue within 3 cm of the primary tumor (D1) and those also undergoing resection of splenic, hepatic, left gastric, and celiac nodes (D2) (45% vs 47%). The study, however, demonstrated a higher morbidity and postoperative mortality in the group undergoing the D2 dissection. In our practice, we generally perform gastrectomy with D1 dissection with an attempt to obtain at least 15 lymph nodes.

Five-year overall survival rates for patients with gastric cancer range from 10% to 20%, with survival rates for patients undergoing surgical resection with curative intent reported as high as 47%.[50] Higher survival figures have been reported in the Japanese literature where more aggressive screening programs may lead to earlier cancer detection. A recent large randomized Italian study[51] comparing morbidity and mortality from D1 and D2 dissections in experienced centers found overall postoperative morbidity to be about 13.6%, with overall postoperative mortality less than 1%. Complications after gastrectomy include anastomotic leak, which can be associated with significant morbidity and mortality. In a large series of 1114 patients who underwent total gastrectomy and esophagojejunostomy, the leak rate was 7.5%.[52] The majority of these were managed conservatively, although of the 30% that required re-exploration, the mortality was noted to be 64%.

NONSURGICAL TREATMENTS OF GASTRIC CANCER

Given the relatively poor prognosis of patients with gastric cancer undergoing surgical resection, adjuvant and neoadjuvant therapies have been investigated. Postoperative chemotherapy alone has not provided significant benefit in survival outcome. Two large meta-analyses[53,55] performed incorporate the data from several randomized trials. Hermans and colleagues reviewed 2096 patients from 11 clinical trials finding no statistical benefit from adjuvant chemotherapy. In a comment to the study,[54] a small benefit in survival was identified when further studies were included in the meta-analysis. A more recent meta-analysis including 13 trials in non-Asian countries[55] showed similarly at best a marginal improvement in survival benefit with adjuvant chemotherapy.

The value of adding radiation to chemotherapy in adjuvant therapy yielded conflicting and inconclusive results until a recent multi-institutional trial[56] demonstrated a significant survival benefit of this multi-modal approach. The study enrolled 556 patients and demonstrated an increase in median survival of 9 months (from 27 to 36 months) in patients undergoing surgical resection with adjuvant chemoradiation versus surgery alone. Patients in the chemoradiation arm received fluorouracil and leucovorin rescue for 5 days followed by 4500 cGy of external beam radiation over 5 weeks with modification of the chemotherapy regimen around the time of radiation, followed by two more 5-day cycles of fluorouracil and leucovorin 1 month upon completion of radiation treatment. Chemoradiation has largely become integrated into the postoperative regimen of patients with locally advanced gastric cancer.

Because of the prognostic importance of achieving an R0 resection, neoadjuvant chemotherapy has been explored as a means of improving outcome in patients with gastric cancer. Recent results from the ongoing MAGIC trial[57] comparing surgery alone to surgery plus preoperative chemotherapy with epirubicin, cisplatin, and 5-FU, demonstrated an increase in R0 resection rates, although survival outcome did not seem to be significantly affected. Other studies are currently underway investigating the potential benefit of neoadjuvant therapy.

Clearly, given the poor survival outcomes of patients with gastric cancer, there is still much to be learned about the biology of the disease, and a more thorough understanding of the molecular underpinnings of the disease will help to continue to guide more effective therapy.

REFERENCES

1. Jemal A, Murray T, et al. Cancer statistics, 2003. *CA Cancer J Clin.* 2003;53:5-26.

2. Daly JM, et al. Esophageal cancer: results of an American College of Surgeons Patient Care Evaluation Study. *J Am Coll Surg.* 2000;190(5):562-572; discussion 572-3.

3. Genkins GJ, et al. Genetic pathways involved in the progression of Barrett's metaplasia to adenocarcinoma. *Br J Surg.* 2002;89(7):824-837.

4. Hu N, et al. Evaluation of BRCA2 in the genetic susceptibility of familial esophageal cancer. *Oncogene.* 2004 Jan 22;23(3):852-858.

5. Hourihan RN. Transcriptional gene expression profiles of oesophageal adenocarcinoma and normal oesophageal tissues. *Anticancer Res.* 2003;23(1A):161-165.

6. Massari M, et al. Endoscopic ultrasonography for preoperative staging of esophageal carcinoma. *Surg Laparosc Endosc.* 1997;7(2):162-165.

7. Kienle P, et al. Prospective comparison of endoscopy, endosonography and computed tomography for staging of tumours of the oesophagus and gastric cardia. *Digestion.* 2002;66(4):230-236.

8. Chak A, et al. Prognosis of esophageal cancers preoperatively staged to be locally invasive (T4) by endoscopic ultrasound (EUS): a multicenter retrospective cohort study. *Gastrointest Endosc.* 1995;42(6):501-506.

9. Rasanen JV, et al. Prospective analysis of accuracy of positron emission tomography, computed tomography, and endoscopic ultrasonography in staging of adenocarcinoma of the esophagus and the esophagogastric junction. *Ann Surg Oncol.* 2003;10(8):954-960.

10. Nguyen NT, et al. Evaluation of minimally invasive surgical staging for esophageal cancer. *Am J Surg.* 2001;182(6):702-706.

11. Yeung HW, et al. FDG-PET in esophageal cancer. Incremental value over computed tomography. *Clin Positron Imaging.* 1999;2(5):255-260.

12. Hulscher JB, et al. Extended transthoracic resection compared with limited transhiatal resection for adenocarcinoma of the esophagus. *N Engl J Med.* 2002 Nov 21;347(21):1662-1669.

13. Lerut T, et al. Reflections on three field lymphadenectomy in carcinoma of the esophagus and gastroesophageal junction. *Hepatogastroenterology.* 1999;46(26):717-725.

14. Chu KM, et al. A prospective randomized comparison of transhiatal and transthoracic resection for lower-third esophageal carcinoma. *Am J Surg.* 1997;174(3):320-324.

15. Goldminc, et al. Oesophagectomy by a transhiatal approach or thoracotomy: a prospective randomized trial. *Br J Surg.* 1993;80(3):367-370.

16. Kelsen DP, et al. Chemotherapy followed by surgery compared with surgery alone for localized esophageal cancer. *N Engl J Med.* 1998;339(27):1979-1984.

17. Maraveyas A, et al. Surgical resection with and without chemotherapy in oesophageal cancer. *Lancet.* 2002;360(9340):1174-1175.

18. Walsh TN, et al. A comparison of multimodal therapy and surgery for esophageal adenocarcinoma. *N Engl J Med.* 1996;335(7):462-467.

19. Urschel JD, et al. A meta-analysis of randomized controlled trials that compared neoadjuvant chemoradiation and surgery to surgery alone for resectable esophageal cancer. *Am J Surg.* 2003;185(6):538-543.

20. Cooper JS, et al. Chemoradiotherapy of locally advanced esophageal cancer: long-term follow-up of a prospective randomized trial (RTOG 85-01). Radiation Therapy Oncology Group. *JAMA.* 1999;281(17):1623-1627.

21. Minsky BD, et al. INT 0123 (Radiation Therapy Oncology Group 94-05) phase III trial of combined-modality therapy for esophageal cancer: high-dose versus standard-dose radiation therapy. *J Clin Oncol.* 2002;20(5):1167-1174.

22. Baker RJ, Fischer JE. *Mastery of Surgery.* Philadelphia: Lippincott, Williams & Wilkins; 2001:813-827.

23. Feig BW, et al (eds.) *The MD Anderson Surgical Oncology Handbook.* 3rd ed. Philadelphia: Lippincott, Williams & Wilkins, 2002.

24. Enzinger PC, Mayer, RJ. Esophageal cancer. *N Engl J Med.* 2003;349(23):2241-2252.

25. Wu PC, Posner MC. The role of surgery in the management of oesophageal cancer. *Lancet Oncology.* 2003;(4):481-488.

26. Hulscher JB, van Sandwick JW, et al. Extended transthoracic resection compared with limited transhiatal resection for adenocarcinoma of the esophagus. *N Engl J Med.* 2002; 347:2241-2252.

27. Wong JEL, Ito Y, et al. Therapeutic strategies in gastric cancer. *J Clin Oncology.* 2003; 21(issue 90230):267s-269s.

28. Norton J, et al. *Essential Practice of Surgery: Basic Science and Clinical Evidence.* New York: Springer-Verlag; 2003.

29. Wanebo HJ, et al. Cancer of the stomach. A patient care study by the American College of Surgeons. *Ann Surg.* 1993;218:583-592.

30. Botet JF, et al. Preoperative staging of gastric cancer: comparison of endoscopic US and dynamic CT. *Radiology.* 1991;181(2):426-432.

31. Habermann CR, Weiss F, Riecken R, et al. Preoperative staging of gastric adenocarcinoma: comparison of helical CT and endoscopic US. *Radiology.* 2004;230(2):465-471.

32. Greenberg J, et al. Computed tomography or endoscopic ultrasonography in preoperative staging of gastric and esophageal tumors. *Surgery.* 1994;116(4):696-701; discussion 701-2.

33. Willis, S. et al. Endoscopic ultrasonography in the preoperative staging of gastric cancer: accuracy and impact on surgical therapy. *Surg Endosc.* 2000;14(10):951-954.

34. Xi WD, et al. Endoscopic ultrasonography in preoperative staging of gastric cancer: determination of tumor invasion depth, nodal involvement and surgical resectability. *World J Gastroenterol.* 2003;9(2):254-257.

35. Burke EC, Karpeh MS, Conlon KC, Brennan MF. Laparoscopy in the management of gastric adenocarcinoma. *Ann Surg.* 1997;225(3):262-267. Review.

36. Turlakow A, et al. Peritoneal carcinomatosis: role of (18)F-FDG PET. *J Nucl Med.* 2003;44(9):1407-1412.

37. Yoshikawa T, et al. Peritoneal cytology in patients with gastric cancer exposed to the serosa—a proposed new classification based on the local and distant cytology. *Hepatogastroenterology.* 2003;50(52):1183-1186.

38. Fujimoto T, et al. Evaluation of intraoperative intraperitoneal cytology for advanced gastric carcinoma. *Oncology.* 2002;62(3):201-208.

39. Klein EK, Hermans J, van Krieken JH, van de Velde CJ. Evaluation of the 5th edition of the TNM classification for gastric cancer: improved prognostic value. *Br J Cancer.* 2001;84(1):64-71.

40. Katai H, et al. Evaluation of the New International Union against Cancer TNM staging for gastric carcinoma. *Cancer.* 2000;88(8):1796-1800.

41. Minimum number of lymph nodes that should be examined for the International Union against Cancer/American Joint Committee on Cancer TNM classification of gastric carcinoma. *World J Surg.* 2003;27(3):330-333.

42. Bouvier AM. How many nodes must be examined to accurately stage gastric carcinomas? Results from a population based study. *Cancer.* 2002;94(11):2862-2866.

43. Ono H, et al. Endoscopic mucosal resection for treatment of early gastric cancer. *Gut.* 2001;48(2):225-229.

44. Shimizu S, et al. Laparoscopic gastric surgery in a Japanese institution: analysis of the initial 100 procedures. *J Am Coll Surg.* 2003;197(3):372-378.

45. Gouzi JL, et al. Total versus subtotal gastrectomy for adenocarcinoma of the gastric antrum. A French prospective controlled study. *Ann Surg.* 1989;209(2):162-166.

46. Bozzetti F, et al. Subtotal versus total gastrectomy for gastric cancer: five-year survival rates in a multicenter randomized Italian trial. Italian Gastrointestinal Tumor Study Group. *Ann Surg.* 1999;230(2):170-178.

47. Brady MS, et al. Effect of splenectomy on morbidity and survival following curative gastrectomy for carcinoma. *Arch Surg.* 1991;126(3):359-364.

48. Chareton B, et al. Prospective randomized trial comparing Billroth I and Billroth II procedures for carcinoma of the gastric antrum. *J Am Coll Surg.* 1996;183(3):190-194.

49. Bonenkamp JJ, et al. Extended lymph-node dissection for gastric cancer. Dutch Gastric Cancer Group. *N Engl J Med.* 1999;340(12):908-914.

50. Cady B, et al. Gastric adenocarcinoma. A disease in transition. *Arch Surg.* 1989; 124(3):303-308.

51. Degiuli M, et al. Morbidity and mortality after D1 and D2 gastrectomy for cancer: Interim analysis of the Italian Gastric Cancer Study Group (IGCSG) randomised surgical trial. *Eur J Surg Oncol.* 2004;30(3):303-308.

52. Lang H, et al. Management and results of proximal anastomotic leaks in a series of 1114 total gastrectomies for gastric carcinoma. *Eur J Surg Oncol.* 2000;26(2):168-171.

53. Hermans J, et al. Adjuvant therapy after curative resection for gastric cancer: meta-analysis of randomized trials. *J Clin Oncol.* 1993;11(8):1441-1447.

54. Hermans J, Bonenkamp JJ.. Meta-analysis of adjuvant chemotherapy in gastric cancer: a critical reappraisal [letter]. *J Clin Oncol.* 1994 Apr; 12:877-880.

55. Earle CC, Maroun JA. Adjuvant chemotherapy after curative resection for gastric cancer in non-Asian patients: revisiting a meta-analysis of randomised trials. *Eur J Cancer.* 1999;35(7):1059-1064.

56. MacDonald JS et al. Chemoradiotherapy after surgery compared with surgery alone for adenocarcinoma of the stomach or gastroesophageal junction. *N Engl J Med.* 2001; 345(10):725-730.

57. Allum W, Cunningham D, Weeden S for the UK NCRI Upper GI Clinical Studies Group. Preoperative chemotherapy in operable gastric and lower esophageal cancer: randomized controlled trial (the MAGIC trial) *Proc Am Soc Clin Oncol.* 2003;22:A998.

chapter **5**

Identification and Management of Familial Pancreatic Cancer

Stephen J. Rulyak, MD, MPH

INTRODUCTION

Epidemiologic studies have demonstrated that family history is an important risk factor for the development of pancreatic cancer. Families with multiple members diagnosed with pancreatic cancer are not infrequently encountered in clinical practice, and recent estimates suggest that up to 10% of pancreatic carcinomas may be inherited. In some families, the risk of pancreatic cancer may approach 50%. However, the identification of families predisposed to pancreatic cancer can be difficult, and the absence of a widely accepted screening test for pancreatic cancer presents a formidable challenge to the clinicians caring for members of these families. This chapter will review current knowledge about the etiology of familial pancreatic cancer, and provide insight into the clinical management of these high-risk patients with an emphasis on evolving approaches to screening and surveillance.

EPIDEMIOLOGY

The incidence of pancreatic cancer in the United States is 30,700 cases per year, and pancreatic cancer is the fourth leading cause of cancer death among both men and women, with a mortality rate nearly equal to its incidence rate. The cause of most pancreatic cancer cases remains unknown, and rapid and nearly uniform fatality of the disease presents a significant obstacle to epidemiologic investigation. However, studies have identified several risk factors for pancreatic cancer (Table 5-1). Tobacco smoking is the most consistently identified epidemiologic risk factor for pancreatic cancer, although the approximately 2-fold increase in risk associated with smoking is modest. Pancreatic cancer is also more common with advancing age, and male gender and Black race appear to be associated with a slight increase in risk. Dietary factors such as increased caloric intake, increased carbohydrate intake, and decreased dietary fiber have been associated with pancreatic cancer, although these epidemiologic relationships have been inconsistent. The association with other environmental factors such as occupation

Table 5-1

EPIDEMIOLOGIC RISK FACTORS FOR PANCREATIC CANCER

Factors Consistently Associated With the Risk of Pancreatic Cancer

Advancing age

Tobacco

Family history of pancreatic cancer

Cancer syndromes

- Familial breast cancer
- Hereditary breast/ovarian cancer
- Familial atypical multiple mole melanoma syndrome
- Peutz-Jeghers syndrome
- Familial adenomatous polyposis

Hereditary pancreatitis

Factors Possibly Associated With the Risk of Pancreatic Cancer

Diabetes mellitus

Black race

Male gender

Occupation

Diet

Chronic pancreatitis

Other genetic syndromes

- Hereditary nonpolyposis colorectal cancer
- Li-Fraumeni syndrome
- Ataxia-telangiectasia
- Fanconi's anemia

Factors Unlikely to Increase the Risk of Pancreatic Cancer

Moderate alcohol consumption

Coffee consumption

is even less certain. Diabetes mellitus does appear to be associated with pancreatic cancer. However, despite multiple epidemiologic studies, it remains difficult to conclude whether diabetes is cause or effect of the disease as glucose intolerance can result from pancreatic cancer by several mechanisms, including peripheral insulin resistance or impaired insulin release from islet cells. Early epidemiologic studies suggested an increase in the risk of pancreatic cancer associated with alcohol, but subsequent studies controlling for concurrent tobacco use have found no increase in the risk of pancreatic cancer. Nonetheless, heavy consumption may increase the risk of pancreatic cancer in some individuals if they develop chronic pancreatitis.

A family history of pancreatic cancer has been identified as a risk factor for pancreatic cancer in several epidemiologic studies. At least 5 cross-sectional studies report a significantly increased risk associated with family history, with risk estimates ranging from 1.5-fold to 15-fold depending on the population studied. One population-based case control study including 247 cases found that a family history of pancreatic cancer was associated with a 2.5-fold increase in the risk of pancreatic cancer, and that risk was further magnified by either smoking or by having a family member who was diagnosed with pancreatic cancer before age 60. Another study using the National Familial Pancreas Tumor Registry found an 18-fold increase in risk among persons with 2 or more first-degree relatives diagnosed with pancreatic cancer. Thus, while the magnitude of risk associated with family history varies from study to study, a family history appears to be one of the strongest and most consistently identified risk factors for pancreatic cancer.

GENETICS OF PANCREATIC CARCINOMA

Pancreatic adenocarcinomas are believed to arise from ductal epithelium, and there is increasing evidence that neoplastic transformation progresses through a precursor lesion known as pancreatic intraepithelial neoplasia (PanIN). It also appears that tumorigenesis occurs via a multistep process whereby oncogenes are activated and tumor suppressor genes are inactivated, similar to the adenoma-carcinoma that results in colorectal cancer. A number of molecular genetic alterations have been identified in pancreatic adenocarcinomas, and many of these same alterations are also present in PanIN although the sequence in which they occur has yet to be fully characterized. Some inherited pancreatic cancers are the result of germline mutations in the genes associated with sporadic pancreatic cancer.

GENETICS OF SPORADIC PANCREATIC CANCER

Activation of the K-*ras* oncogene appears to be one of the earliest molecular events in pancreatic tumorigenesis, and gene activation appears to lead to multiple cellular events, including proliferation, enhanced survival, and invasion. Mutations in K-*ras* are nearly ubiquitous in pancreatic adenocarcinomas (Table 5-2), and they are also common in PanIN. Mutations in *p16* also play an important role in pancreatic tumorigenesis. *p16* is a low molecular weight tumor suppressor protein encoded by the *CDKN2A* gene. The majority of pancreatic cancers harbor mutations in *CDKN2A*, although preliminary evidence suggests that these mutations may cause a later event in pancreatic tumorigenesis compared with K-*ras* mutations. Mutations in the *p53* tumor suppressor gene are also present in more than half of pancreatic adenocarcinomas and may represent a still later event in pancreatic tumorigenesis, although a limited number of studies of molecular alterations in PanIN have been conducted. Finally, SMAD4 (also known as DPC4 [deleted in pancreatic cancer locus 4]) encodes a transcription factor involved in transforming growth factor ß signaling pathway that may inhibit pancreatic epithelial proliferation. SMAD4 mutations are found in only a fraction of sporadic pancreatic adenocarcinomas and also appear to be a late event in tumorigenesis.

Chromosomal instability is another important finding in most pancreatic adenocarcinomas, and recent studies have identified telomere dysfunction as an important molecular event in pancreatic carcinogenesis. Telomeres are hexameric DNA repeat sequences (TTAGGG) at the end of chromosomes, which prevent fusions between chromosome ends. Telomere dysfunction usually arises in the setting of shortening of the telomere. This in turn results in chromosomal instability via fusion and formation of chromoso-

Table 5-2

GENETIC ALTERATIONS IN SPORADIC PANCREATIC ADENOCARCINOMA

Gene or Chromosomal Alteration	Function	Proportion of Pancreatic Adenocarcinomas With Mutation or Alteration
K-*ras*	oncogene	>95%
CDKN2A (p16)	tumor suppressor	63% to 100%
p53	tumor suppressor	50% to 75%
SMAD4 (DPC4)	tumor suppressor	30% to 50%
MLH1, MSH2	DNA mismatch repair	13%
Telomere shortening	chromosomal stability	>90%

mal bridges during anaphase of mitosis, with subsequent breakage of those bridges, and repeat fusion in an ongoing cycle. Telomere shortening and activation of the associated enzyme telomerase are relatively common findings in pancreatic cancer. Telomere shortening is also an early and very common finding in PanIN.

Still other molecular events may have the potential to result in pancreatic carcinoma. For example, one recent study identified high-frequency microsatellite instability (MSI) among a subset of patients with pancreatic cancers but without hereditary nonpolyposis colorectal cancer. Interestingly, patients with MSI-positive tumors had a significantly improved survival compared to patients with MSI-negative tumors.

GENETICS OF INHERITED PANCREATIC CANCER

Pancreatic cancer appears to be an integral lesion in a number of inherited cancer syndromes with well-defined genetic defects (Table 5-3). These syndromes include hereditary breast/ovarian cancer syndrome, familial atypical multiple mole melanoma syndrome (FAMMM), Peutz-Jeghers syndrome, FAP, and possibly the HNPCC. However, it is likely that the majority of inherited pancreatic cancers in the population occur in patients without one of these syndromes. These inherited cancers are referred to as *familial pancreatic cancers*. The gene or genes that result in most familial pancreatic cancers have yet to be discovered.

BRCA2 is a key regulator of gene transcription, and mutations in the gene appear to result in faulty DNA repair leading to susceptibility to breast, ovarian, and other cancers. Some families that inherit breast cancer in association with *BRCA2* mutations have also been reported to have an excess of pancreatic cancers. One recent study suggests that up to 19% of families with 2 or more first-degree members with pancreatic cancer may segregate germline mutations in *BRCA2*, although the prevalence of *BRCA2* mutations in a population-based sample of familial pancreatic cancer kindreds has yet to be determined. Interestingly, some of these families appear to inherit pancreatic cancers in the absence of breast or ovarian cancers. However, the penetrance of *BRCA2* mutations for

Table 5-3

GENETIC SYNDROMES ASSOCIATED WITH INCREASED RISK OF PANCREATIC CANCER

Syndrome	Gene(s)	Locus	Increase in Pancreatic Cancer Risk (RR or OR [95% CI])
Hereditary breast/ovarian cancer	BRCA2	13q12-13	7 (n/a)
FAMMM	CDKN2A	9p21	22 (9-45)
Peutz-Jeghers syndrome	Serine-threonine kinase (STK 11)	19p13.3	132 (44-261)
FAP	APC	5q21-22	4 (1.2-11)
HNPCC	DNA mismatch repair genes (MSH2, MLH1, MSH6)	2p21-22;3p21-23; 2p16	n/a
Hereditary pancreatitis	Cationic trypsinogen (PRSS1)	7q35	53 (23-105)
Cystic fibrosis	CFTR	7q31.2	32 (5-205)

pancreatic cancer is considerably lower than for breast or ovarian cancers, as only about 5% of *BRCA2* mutation carriers will develop pancreatic cancer. The explanation for reduced penetrance is not yet known, although there is some evidence to suggest that *BRCA2* mutations are a late event in pancreatic tumorigenesis and that other molecular alterations may be required to initiate pancreatic neoplasia. It is also possible that interactions with other genes or environmental factors may be required for *BRCA2* mutations to result in pancreatic cancer.

Members of FAMMM kindreds inherit a predisposition to develop multiple (>50) atypical cutaneous nevi and melanomas, and a subset of these families also appears to inherit pancreatic cancer. The most common mutations in FAMMM kindreds are found in the CDKN2A gene on chromosome 9p21. Mutations in CDKN2A are also frequently identified in sporadic pancreatic adenocarcinomas. CDKN2A encodes *p16*, which acts as a tumor suppressor protein by inhibition of the cyclin D1-cyclin-dependent kinase complex (CDK4). If not inhibited, the CDK4 complex in turn phosphorylates the retinoblastoma protein, allowing a cell to progress unchecked through the G1 phase of the cell cycle, resulting in unregulated cell growth. Lynch and colleagues first reported a melanoma kindred predisposed to PC in 1968, and a number of additional families have since been identified. Several studies of FAMMM kindreds have found a 10- to 40-fold increase in the risk of nonmelanoma cancers, and the cumulative risk of pancreatic cancer has been estimated to be 17% by age 75. Growing epidemiologic evidence supports the observation that pancreatic cancer is inherited as an autosomal dominant trait in at least some families that inherit CDKN2A mutations.

Peutz-Jeghers syndrome is an autosomal dominant disease that results in hamartomatous gastrointestinal polyps and mucocutaneous pigmentation. The disease is caused by germline mutations in the serine threonine kinase 11 gene (STK11), and patients are predisposed to a variety of cancers, including pancreatic cancer. There appears to be more than a 100-fold increase in the relative risk of pancreatic cancer in these families (RR=132; 95% CI 44-261) and the lifetime risk of pancreatic cancer in these patients may exceed 36%.

FAP and HNPCC are cancer syndromes most closely associated with increased risk of colorectal adenomas and cancers, but affected patients are also predisposed to a number of extracolonic cancers, including pancreatic cancer. FAP results from a mutation in the tumor suppressor gene APC, which normally controls cell proliferation by inhibition of beta-catenin. In addition to colorectal cancers, affected patients can develop small intestinal cancers, desmoid tumors, and papillary thyroid carcinoma. The risk of pancreatic cancer in FAP patients is increased approximately 4-fold, although the absolute risk of pancreatic cancer seems to be lower than the risk of other extracolonic cancers. HNPCC is the most common form of hereditary colorectal cancer and is caused by defects in DNA mismatch repair genes. Mutations in 2 mismatch repair genes (*MSH2* and *MLH1*) may account for up to 90% of cases, although defects in other mismatch repair genes result in a similar phenotype. Patients with HNPCC are also predisposed to a number of extracolonic cancers of the endometrium, ovary, small intestine, stomach, and genitourinary tract. One study suggests that HNPCC families may also be predisposed to pancreatic cancers, but population-based data to support this association are lacking.

In addition to cancer syndromes, other hereditary diseases can predispose affected individuals to pancreatic cancer. Hereditary pancreatitis is an autosomal dominant disorder associated with mutations in the cationic trypsinogen gene, PRSS1. Patients with hereditary pancreatitis are among those at greatest risk of pancreatic cancer, as they have been found to have a 50-fold increase in the risk of pancreatic cancer with a lifetime cumulative incidence of pancreatic cancer in excess of 40%. Epidemiologic studies suggest that patients with cystic fibrosis are also at increased risk to develop digestive cancers, including cancer of the pancreas, although the absolute risk of pancreatic cancer in these patients appears to be low. One recent study has identified mutations in the genes associated with Fanconi's anemia in apparently sporadic pancreatic cancers, although the importance of these mutations in either sporadic or familial pancreatic cancers remains to be defined. Finally, there are preliminary data to suggest mutations in the ATM gene that results in ataxia-telangiectasia may play a role in pancreatic cancer.

FAMILIAL PANCREATIC CANCER

The majority of cases of inherited pancreatic cancer do not result from a known clinical syndrome. These *familial pancreatic cancers* are a clinically heterogeneous group of cancers characterized by variability in the age of cancer onset, gender distribution, and the presence of pancreatic endocrine or exocrine dysfunction. It is possible that the familial pancreatic cancers may be genetically heterogeneous disorders caused by mutations in multiple oncogenes and/or modifier genes. However, 2 recent studies using genetic segregation analysis suggest the existence of a single major pancreatic cancer gene with autosomal dominant transmission. This familial pancreatic cancer gene has yet to be identified, but a study of one large familial pancreatic cancer kindred that inherits pancreatic cancer as an autosomal dominant trait has mapped a pancreatic cancer susceptibility locus to chromosome 4q32-34. This unique locus does not encompass any of the genes that result in cancer syndromes associated with pancreatic cancer, and efforts to localize a pancreatic cancer gene in this region are ongoing.

ENVIRONMENTAL RISK FACTORS AND FAMILIAL PANCREATIC CANCER

Relatively few environmental risk factors have been identified for sporadic pancreatic cancer and still fewer have been identified for familial pancreatic cancer. Cigarette smoking is the most consistently identified of these factors. In a population-based case-control study, Schenk found significant interaction between smoking and family history, particularly in families with a relative diagnosed with pancreatic cancer before the age of 60 (relative risk [RR], 8.2; 95% confidence interval [CI], 2.2 to 31.1). In a study of nearly 500 patients with hereditary pancreatitis, Lowenfels and colleagues reported a 2-fold increase in the risk of pancreatic cancer in patients who had never smoked (odds ratio [OR], 2.1; 95% CI, 0.7 to 6.1). A study of members of familial pancreatic cancer kindreds without a known cancer syndrome found a nearly 4-fold increase in risk (OR, 3.7; 95% CI, 1.8 to 7.6) associated with smoking, and the onset of cancer was one decade earlier in smokers compared to nonsmokers (Figure 5-1). In this study, there was no significant association between diabetes and pancreatic cancer. Interestingly, this study found that up to one-third of familial pancreatic cancer kindreds demonstrate genetic anticipation, which is the occurrence of a genetic condition with an earlier age of onset in successive generations. If confirmed in subsequent studies, genetic anticipation would have major implications for the screening of familial pancreatic cancer kindreds as the mean decrease in the age of onset between generations was approximately

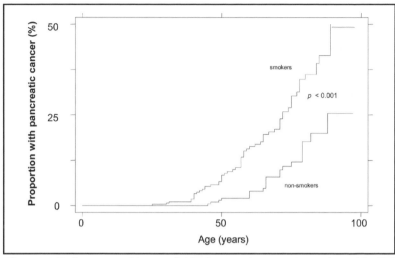

Figure 5-1. Earlier onset and increased risk of pancreatic cancer in members of familial pancreatic cancer kindreds who smoke. (Reprinted from *Gastroenterology*, Vol. 124(5), 1292-9, Rulyak SJ, et al, Risk factors for the development of pancreatic cancer in familial pancreatic cancer kindreds, Copyright 2003, with permission from the American Gastroenterological Association.)

20 years. The roles of other potential risk factors such as race, gender, diet, or occupation have yet to be examined in the familial setting. Nonetheless, all patients with a family history of pancreatic cancer should be advised not to smoke.

IDENTIFICATION OF PATIENTS AT RISK FOR FAMILIAL PANCREATIC CANCER

The identification of patients at increased risk for familial pancreatic cancer can be challenging because familial aggregation of pancreatic cancer may be influenced by a number of factors, including chance, family size, shared environmental exposures, and incomplete gene penetrance. For example, a shared environmental factor could hypothetically result in multiple first-degree relatives with pancreatic cancer. Conversely, if a parent with a pancreatic cancer gene with complete penetrance has 4 children, there is a 6.25% chance that none of the children will be affected. If this hypothetical gene is also incompletely penetrant, the chance that no offspring will be affected is even greater. Furthermore, it can be difficult or impossible to obtain accurate family history data for such a rapidly and uniformly fatal disease, and the clinician is often unable to elicit an accurate family history for more than one or two generations of a family.

For these reasons, there is currently no clear consensus on the definition of familial pancreatic cancer. However, families known to segregate mutations associated with cancer syndromes and those patients with hereditary pancreatitis should be considered at increased risk. It also appears that the absolute number of affected first-degree relatives is correlated with increased cancer risk, and most experts would agree the families that

Table 5-4

CRITERIA FOR THE IDENTIFICATION OF PATIENTS AT RISK FOR INHERITED PANCREATIC CANCER

Increased Risk for Inherited Pancreatic Cancer

1. Patients with 2 or more first- degree relatives with pancreatic cancer
2. Patients known to harbor mutations that result in cancer syndromes associated with pancreatic cancer
   - Familial breast cancer (*BRCA2*)
   - Familial atypical multiple mole melanoma syndrome (CDKN2A)
   - Peutz-Jeghers syndrome (STK 11)
   - Familial adenomatous polyposis (APC)
   - Patients with hereditary pancreatitis*

Possibly Increased Risk for Inherited Pancreatic Cancer

1. Individuals with one first-degree relative and one or more second-degree relative(s) diagnosed with pancreatic cancer
2. Individuals with one first-degree relative diagnosed with pancreatic cancer at an early age (under the age of 50)
3. Individuals with 2 or more second-degree relatives with pancreatic cancer, one of whom developed it at an early age
4. Patients meeting clinical criteria for one of the above cancer syndromes without a clearly defined mutation
5. Members of HNPCC families

*Endoscopic screening is of uncertain utility as the findings of chronic pancreatitis are similar to the findings of dysplasia.

include 2 or more first degree relatives with pancreatic cancer should be considered to have familial pancreatic cancer until proven otherwise. Families that include multiple second-degree relatives with pancreatic cancer and/or those with an unusually young age of onset (<50 years of age) may also be at increased risk, although these criteria are more controversial. These latter criteria may be most useful in evaluating small families and/or those with limited family history data.

It is important for the clinician to recognize that the risk to an individual patient varies by both the number *and* relationship of affected relatives. For example, a patient whose mother and brother have been diagnosed with pancreatic cancer is likely to be at much higher risk of developing pancreatic cancer than if his or her uncle or first cousin were affected. Table 5-4 gives criteria that may prompt a clinician to consider the diagnosis of familial pancreatic cancer, although it is important to emphasize that estimation of risk for an individual patient is likely to be imprecise and that listed criteria have not been validated prospectively.

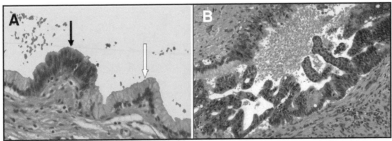

Figure 5-2. Histology of PanIN. (A) PanIN-1 (open arrow) is characterized by elongation of epithelial cells with abundant supranuclear mucin and PanIN-2 (solid arrow) is defined by nuclear abnormalities including enlargement and crowding, hyperchromatism, and stratification. (B) In PanIN-3, there are lush papillary projections, loss of nuclear polarity, and nuclear atypia with mitoses. (Photomicrographs courtesy of Dr. Teresa Brentnall.) *For a full-color version, see page CA-IV of the Color Atlas.*

SCREENING FOR PANCREATIC CARCINOMA IN FAMILIAL PANCREATIC CANCER

Pancreatic cancer is most often asymptomatic until it has progressed to an incurable stage. The nearly uniform lethality of pancreatic cancer is in part due to the lack of an acceptable screening test for pancreatic cancer. At present, there are no adequate radiographic, endoscopic, or laboratory tests for use in population-based pancreatic cancer screening. However, the risk of familial pancreatic cancer approaches 50% in some kindreds, and methods for early detection of pancreatic cancer and precancer in such families are clearly needed. The goal of such strategies is to identify family members with pancreatic dysplasia or very early pancreatic cancers before they progress to invasive disease.

DYSPLASIA AS A PRECURSOR TO PANCREATIC CANCER

The discovery of a dysplastic precursor lesion has been critical to the development of screening and surveillance tests for other gastrointestinal cancers including those arising in the colon, esophagus, and stomach. Pancreatic adenocarcinomas also appear to arise from dysplasia, which is more correctly referred to as PanIN. There are different grades of PanIN, which appear to represent a continuum of neoplastic progression (Figure 5-2). PanIN-1 is also referred to as intraepithelial ductal hyperplasia and is characterized by elongation of epithelial cells with abundant supranuclear mucin (PanIN-1A), sometimes with papillary architecture (PanIN-1B). PanIN-2, or LGD, is defined by nuclear abnormalities including enlargement and crowding, hyperchromatism, and stratification. PanIN-3, also referred to as HGD or carcinoma in-situ, is characterized by papillary projections, loss of nuclear polarity, nuclear atypia, and mitoses. The prevalence of PanIN in the general population is currently unknown, but a recent study of a referral population of familial pancreatic cancer kindreds suggests that the prevalence of PanIN-2 and PanIN-3 may be as high as 34% if stringent criteria are used to select family members for screening.

There are several important limitations in the literature regarding PanIN lesions and their progression to cancer. First, the absolute risk of pancreatic cancer in patients with pancreatic dysplasia has yet to be determined, as does the prevalence of PanIN in the general population. Second, the time course for progression from PanIN to cancer is as yet unknown. In one series of 3 patients who underwent pancreatic surgery for non-malignant indications and were found to have dysplasia at the resection margins, all patients progressed to cancer within 10 years. Clearly, larger studies of the natural history of PanIN are needed to confirm this finding. Finally, it is important to note that the accurate pathologic diagnosis of PanIN can be difficult. In one study, interobserver agreement among expert gastrointestinal pathologists was found to be only fair for PanIN 1 and PanIN 3 (kappa=0.43 and kappa=0.42, respectively) and poor for PanIN 2 lesions (kappa=0.14). Accurate diagnosis of PanIN is critical because PanIN is a multifocal or diffuse process and total pancreatectomy is necessary to ensure removal of all dysplastic tissue. It is likely that the accuracy of PanIN diagnoses will improve as pathologists accrue additional experience with this lesion.

While the natural history of pancreatic dysplasia is difficult to study and incompletely characterized, PanIN represents a curable precursor lesion and thus it is possible that effective screening tests can be developed. Potential screening methods may involve the use of imaging modalities such as endoscopy or radiography. Ultimately, a biomarker in serum or pancreatic juice may be most attractive option for screening. PanINs share many of the molecular genetic alterations found in adenocarcinomas. Because these molecular alterations appear to be acquired in a step-wise fashion, it may eventually be possible to detect the highest risk precursor lesions shortly before cancer develops.

ENDOSCOPIC APPROACHES FOR SCREENING

Endoscopic techniques have been used to detect PanIN or early pancreatic cancer, and endoscopic screening protocols for high-risk members of familial pancreatic cancer kindreds are ongoing at several institutions in the United States and abroad. At present, EUS appears to be the most promising screening test for identifying pancreatic dysplasia and early pancreatic cancer because it is relatively non-invasive and has the ability to discriminate subtle abnormalities in the pancreatic parenchyma. The pancreatic abnormalities on EUS that are associated with dysplasia are the same findings that are present on EUS in patients with chronic pancreatitis. These changes include the presence of hyperechoic strands, hyperechoic foci, lobules (sometimes referred to as hypoechoic nodules), echogenic pancreatic duct walls, and irregularity of the pancreatic duct (Figure 5-3). Several of these findings have been reported to be more common in relatives of patients with pancreatic cancer compared to controls undergoing EUS for another indication (Table 5-5). More importantly, Brentnall and colleagues have shown that these findings can be used to identify members of familial pancreatic kindreds with histopathologically-confirmed PanIN on pancreatic biopsy specimens.

The findings seen on EUS should not be mistaken to represent endosonographic imaging of PanIN lesions, as EUS does not permit resolution of cellular details. Instead, these findings should be thought of as endoscopic markers associated with dysplasia. These changes may represent inflammation, fibrosis, or fatty replacement of the pancreas associated with PanIN, although the precise anatomic correlates of these findings have yet to be determined. One important limitation of EUS in screening is that identical findings can be found in patients with chronic pancreatitis, patients who consume alcohol, and occasionally in otherwise healthy adults undergoing EUS for other indications.

Figure 5-3. EUS findings associated with pancreatic dysplasia in familial pancreatic cancer kindreds. Radial imaging of the pancreas reveals hyperechoic strands (small arrows) and hypoechoic lobules (larger arrows) in a patient subsequently diagnosed with PanIN 3. (Image courtesy of Dr. Michael Kimmey.)

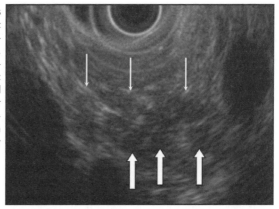

Table 5-5

Findings of EUS Examinations of Members of Families With 3 or More Members With Pancreatic Cancer (n=30) Compared to Controls Undergoing EUS for Other Indications (n=103)

Finding	FPC relatives (%)	Controls (%)	p-value
Nodules*	46	1	0.0001
Prominent septae	33	10	0.003
Dilated side branch	33	14	0.03
Echogenic foci	70	52	0.09
Echogenic strands	67	48	0.09
Mass	10	2	0.08
Irregular main duct	17	7	0.14
Echogenic duct wall	7	4	0.62

*These findings, also known as "lobules," are multifocal hypoechoic areas throughout the pancreatic parenchyma measuring between 2 mm and 8 mm. The term *lobule* is used to distinguish these findings from those of a discrete mass lesion within the pancreas

Adapted from Jagannath S, et al. Endoscopic ultrasound abnormalities in at-risk relatives from familial pancreatic cancer kindreds: a prospective, controlled pilot cohort study. *Gastrointest Endosc.* 2002;56(Suppl):S120.

ERCP may also have utility in detecting pancreatic dysplasia, although few would advocate this as a first-line screening test given the potential for complications, including pancreatitis. As with EUS findings, the ERCP findings associated with dysplasia can also be seen in patients with chronic pancreatitis. However, in selected members of familial pancreatic cancer kindreds without clinical evidence for pancreatitis, several ERCP findings have been associated with dysplasia. These include irregularity of main

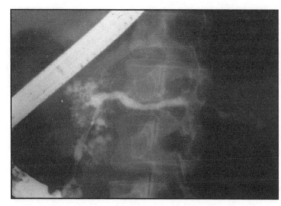

Figure 5-4. ERCP findings associated with pancreatic dysplasia in familial pancreatic cancer kindreds. Markedly abnormal pancreatogram reveals an irregular, dilated main pancreatic duct with multiple side branch sacculations within the pancreatic head. (Image courtesy of Dr. Michael Kimmey.)

pancreatic duct or side branches, ectasia of pancreatic duct side branches, sacculations of pancreatic ducts, and early acinarization of pancreatic head during pancreatic duct injection with inability to completely fill the pancreatic tail (Figure 5-4). ERCP should be used primarily as a confirmatory test when abnormalities on EUS are identified, although one potential advantage of ERCP is ability to obtain pure pancreatic juice or pancreatic duct brushings, which may provide material for screening if an accurate molecular screening assay can be developed. It is important to emphasize that the use of endoscopic screening tests in familial pancreatic cancer is a field under development, and all screening should be conducted in the context of an approved clinical protocol.

RADIOGRAPHIC APPROACHES FOR SCREENING

If the goal of a screening program is to detect PanIN, it is unlikely that currently available radiographic imaging modalities such as helical CT or magnetic resonance cholangiopancreatography (MRCP) have the ability to resolve either the histopathologic abnormalities seen in PanIN or the fibroinflammatory changes detected with EUS. However, improvements in technology may eventually allow detection of pancreatic cancers at a very early stage where the potential of cure is reasonable. However, until the clinical utility of radiographic tests is demonstrated, their use outside of research protocol is inadvisable unless patients report symptoms that warrant cross-sectional imaging.

MOLECULAR APPROACHES TO SCREENING

The detection of molecular alterations in either blood or pancreatic juice may have the potential for the early detection of pancreatic cancer or PanIN. Mutations in k-*ras* have been the most widely studied of these alterations. While k-*ras* can be detected in pancreatic juice, pancreatic brushings, or fine needle aspirates of the pancreas, none of these assays have adequate specificity for the diagnosis of adenocarcinoma or dysplasia because k-*ras* mutation are also present in benign conditions, including chronic pancreatitis. *p53* mutations can also be detected in pancreatic juice. However, *p53* mutations appear to be a late event in pancreatic carcinogenesis and these mutations are absent in up to 50% of adenocarcinomas, thereby limiting sensitivity for the detection of pancreatic cancers or dysplasia. Mutations in *CDKN2A (p16)* and *SMAD4 (DPC4)* can be identified from pancreatic juice, but one recent study suggests that testing for these mutations adds little additional diagnostic information to the detection of K-*ras*. It is possible that combinations of screening markers may improve the accuracy of molecular testing for pancreatic cancers. There has been one study to suggest that combining assays for K-*ras* and *p53* may improve diagnostic accuracy for pancreatic adenocarcinoma. However, no published studies have utilized combinations of molecular tests for the diagnosis of PanIN lesions.

Telomere dysfunction is another promising molecular marker for screening of familial pancreatic cancer kindreds because it is an early and nearly ubiquitous alteration in PanIN. Telomere length shortening has been reported to be present in 96% in PanIN specimens. Assays of telomere length currently require histologically normal tissue as a control, and such tissue cannot be readily obtained by sampling pancreatic juice or by fine needle aspiration because PanIN is a diffuse and frequently multifocal process. However, telomerase activity is a surrogate for telomere shortening, and preliminary reports suggest that telomerase activity can be determined from either pancreatic juice or fine needle aspirates. It is important to recognize that telomere dysfunction is presently not only seen in low grade dysplasia (PanIN-2) and high grade dysplasia (PanIN-3), but also in pancreatic duct hyperplasia (PanIN-1). Therefore, any potential assay for telomere dysfunction is likely to have high sensitivity but low specificity for the diagnosis of dysplasia, although sensitivity is arguably the most important feature of a screening assay. If a suitable assay for telomere dysfunction can be developed, it may be most useful to select a subset of patients who warrant more intensive screening with EUS or other modalities.

In patients with a family history suggestive of one of the defined cancer syndromes that result in pancreatic cancer, testing for germline mutations may represent an important tool for identifying family members at risk for pancreatic cancer. The yield of routine testing of familial pancreatic cancer kindreds for most of these mutations is likely to be low. One exception may be testing for *BRCA2*, as recent studies suggest that up to 19% of familial pancreatic cancer kindreds may harbor a *BRCA2* mutation in the absence of a family history of breast or ovarian cancer. However, future studies to confirm the prevalence of *BRCA2* mutations among familial pancreatic cancer kindreds are needed before such testing can be widely recommended.

As the pathways that lead to pancreatic adenocarcinoma are better understood, molecular approaches may assume an increasing role in screening and surveillance of high-risk family members. With the advent of proteomic technology, it is likely that newer markers with improved sensitivity and specificity will become available. While molecular techniques hold great promise, there are presently few studies to suggest that testing for single molecular genetic alterations or combinations thereof have utility in clinical detection of PanIN or early pancreatic cancer. As with other screening modalities, their use should be restricted to investigational protocols.

APPROACH TO PATIENTS WITH A FAMILY HISTORY OF PANCREATIC CANCER

The management of members of familial pancreatic cancer kindreds presents a formidable challenge to the clinician because clinical experience with screening among high-risk pancreatic cancer patients is limited and currently evolving. However, several centers across the United States have initiated protocols to study the role of screening and surveillance for high-risk family members, and early results from these studies are promising. One protocol using endoscopic screening has been developed at the University of Washington Medical Center in Seattle. To date, 73 patients from 50 different familial pancreatic cancer kindreds have been enrolled and follow-up extends to 9 years. From this cohort, 9 patients have been diagnosed with PanIN 3 and 7 have been diagnosed with PanIN 2. Thirteen of these patients have elected to undergo total pancreatectomy, with no operative deaths. Most importantly, no patient enrolled in the protocol has developed pancreatic cancer while under surveillance.

While these results are encouraging, it must be emphasized that experience with endoscopic screening is limited, and endoscopic tests such as EUS are operator dependent. Therefore, screening with EUS should only be entertained in patients at greatest risk for pancreatic dysplasia, and patients should be well-informed, active participants in the decision to proceed with screening. The findings of EUS should be corroborated by other studies, including ERCP and ultimately laparoscopic biopsy of the pancreatic tail, prior to proceeding with total pancreatectomy. Finally, it cannot be overemphasized that the natural history of pancreatic dysplasia is uncertain and the performance characteristics of endoscopic tests such as EUS and ERCP have yet to be determined. However, a recent decision analysis that assumed a 90% sensitivity of EUS for dysplasia suggested that a strategy employing EUS to screen members of familial pancreatic cancer kindreds is cost-effective, although the benefit appears to be limited to patients with a pre-test probability of pancreatic dysplasia of 16% or greater.

In all patients with a family history of pancreatic cancer, evaluation should begin with a careful history and physical examination in order to determine if alarm symptoms such as abdominal or back pain, diarrhea, weight loss, or recent onset diabetes are present. A history of smoking, alcohol consumption, or occupational exposures should also be elicited. All patients with a family history of pancreatic cancer should be counseled not to smoke. A careful family history should be obtained in order to construct a detailed family pedigree, which can then be used to select patients who may be candidates for screening. Patients with 2 or more first-degree family members diagnosed with pancreatic cancer are considered at increased risk of pancreatic cancer, as are patients who are known to harbor a germline mutation associated with pancreatic cancer. Patients with less compelling family histories may also be at increased risk of pancreatic cancer, although the utility of screening in such patients is far less certain. Table 5-4 lists proposed criteria for pancreatic cancer risk stratification, with the understanding that such criteria have yet to be prospectively validated. Patients with hereditary or acquired chronic pancreatitis represent a particular challenge, because the EUS and ERCP findings in patients with these conditions are indistinguishable from the findings of dysplasia. Therefore, endoscopic screening patients with chronic pancreatitis cannot be widely recommended, although experience with this population of patients is limited.

Once a patient is deemed to be at increased risk for pancreatic cancer, extensive counseling regarding the uncertainties about the natural history of PanIN and lack of clearly validated methods for screening and surveillance for pancreatic neoplasia should then be undertaken. Counseling must include a frank discussion about the outcome of screening if abnormalities are uncovered, specifically total pancreatectomy. In patients with family histories suggestive of a known cancer syndrome, genetic counseling and mutational analysis should be considered. Patients who remain interested after a thorough discussion of risks and benefits are then offered screening.

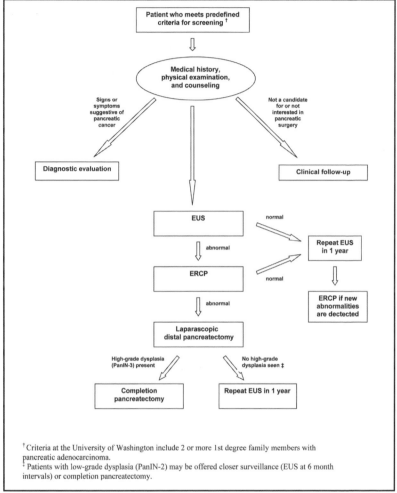

Figure 5-5. Approach to screening for pancreatic cancer in familial pancreatic cancer kindreds.

The algorithm used at the University of Washington for screening patients who meet criteria for familial pancreatic cancer is shown in Figure 5-5. Interested patients are offered EUS as the initial screening test, beginning either at the age of 50 years or 10 years prior to the earliest age at which pancreatic cancer was diagnosed in an affected family member. If EUS is abnormal and there is no recent history of alcohol use, the patient is then offered ERCP to confirm the pancreatic abnormalities noted on EUS. However, if the patient actively consumes alcohol, he or she is advised to abstain from alcohol for 6 months and the EUS is repeated to confirm that abnormalities persist. If both EUS and ERCP display characteristic abnormalities, the patient is referred for laparascopic distal pancreatectomy to confirm the presence of dysplasia. Patients with high-grade dysplasia (PanIN-3) are advised to undergo completion total pancreatectomy, which is required to ensure removal of all dysplastic tissue. Postoperatively, these patients require lifelong pancreatic enzyme replacement and close follow-up by a diabetologist for diabetes mellitus. Experience with the management of patients with LGD (PanIN-2) limited, and patients are offered the choice of pancreatectomy or continued close surveillance. To date, several patients with PanIN-2 have elected to undergo pancreatectomy, while others have chosen to continue surveillance with EUS and/or ERCP.

Patients with normal findings on EUS are advised to undergo repeat examination on a yearly basis, as at least one case of progression from a normal EUS to cancer in less than 12 months has occurred. It remains to be determined whether the surveillance interval may be lengthened after several normal examinations. Patients with an abnormal EUS examination but normal findings at ERCP are recommended to undergo repeat EUS in 1 year with close comparison of findings. Patients with progression of endosonographic changes undergo repeat ERCP, with laparoscopic biopsy reserved for patients with abnormalities on ERCP. However, if the abnormal EUS findings are stable in such patients, the examination is repeated on a yearly basis.

CONCLUSION

Approximately 10% of pancreatic cancers are inherited. A number of genetic syndromes can predispose mutation carriers to pancreatic cancer, including FAP, FAMMM, Peutz-Jeghers syndrome, hereditary breast/ovarian cancer syndrome, hereditary pancreatitis, and possibly HNPCC. However, the gene or genes involved in the majority of inherited pancreatic cancers have yet to be determined, although the molecular pathways of pancreatic tumorigenesis are beginning to be better understood. Smoking appears to be an important modifier of familial pancreatic cancer risk, but the role of other environmental factors in such families has yet to be determined. Screening and surveillance protocols using endoscopic techniques such as EUS and ERCP have been developed, but their use should be restricted to approved research protocols. Molecular genetic testing may have the greatest potential for screening and surveillance, although tests with improved sensitivity and specificity will need to be developed. Most importantly, what is learned from familial pancreatic cancer kindreds will have important implications for screening and prevention of pancreatic cancer in the general population.

BIBLIOGRAPHY

Banke MG, Mulvihill JJ, Aston CE. Inheritance of pancreatic cancer in pancreatic cancer-prone families. *Med Clin North Am.* 2000;84(3):677-690.

Brat DJ LK, Yeo CJ, Warfield PB, Hruban RH. Progression of pancreatic intraductal neoplasias to infiltrating adenocarcinoma of the pancreas. *Am J Surg Pathol.* 1998;22:163-169.

Brentnall TA, Bronner MP, Byrd DR, Haggitt RC, Kimmey MB. Early diagnosis and treatment of pancreatic dysplasia in patients with a family history of pancreatic cancer. *Ann Intern Med.* 1999;131(4):247-255.

Eberle MA, Pfutzer R, Pogue-Geile KL, et al. A new susceptibility locus for autosomal dominant pancreatic cancer maps to chromosome 4q32-34. *Am J Hum Genet.* 2002;70(4):1044-1048.

Giardiello FM, Welsh SB, Hamilton SR, et al. Increased risk of cancer in the Peutz-Jeghers syndrome. *N Engl J Med.* 1987;316:1511-1514.

Giardiello FM, Offerhaus GJ, Lee DH, et al. Increased risk of thyroid and pancreatic carcinoma in familial adenomatous polyposis. *Gut.* 1993;34(10):1394-1396.

Goldstein AM, Fraser MC, Struewing JP, et al. Increased risk of pancreatic cancer in melanoma-prone kindreds with p16INK4 mutations. *N Engl J Med.* 1995;333(15): 970-974.

Goldstein AM, Struewing JP, Chidambaram A, Fraser MC, Tucker MA. Genotype-phenotype relationships in U.S. melanoma-prone families with CDKN2A and CDK4 mutations. *J Natl Cancer Inst.* 2000;92(12):1006-1010.

Hahn SA, Greenhalf B, Ellis I, et al. BRCA2 germline mutations in familial pancreatic carcinoma. *J Natl Cancer Inst.* 2003;95(3):214-221.

Hruban RH, Adsay NV, Albores-Saavedra J, et al. Pancreatic intraepithelial neoplasia: a new nomenclature and classification system for pancreatic duct lesions. *Am J Surg Pathol.* 2001;25(5):579-586.

Kimmey MB, Bronner MP, Byrd DR, Brentnall TA. Screening and surveillance for hereditary pancreatic cancer. *Gastrointest Endosc.* 2002;56(4 Suppl):S82-86.

Klein AP, Beaty TH, Bailey-Wilson JE, Brune KA, Hruban RH, Petersen GM. Evidence for a major gene influencing risk of pancreatic cancer. *Genet Epidemiol.* 2002;23(2):133-149.

Lowenfels AB, Maisonneuve P, DiMagno EP, et al. Hereditary pancreatitis and the risk of pancreatic cancer. International Hereditary Pancreatitis Study Group. *J Natl Cancer Inst.* 1997;89:442-446.

Lowenfels AB, Maisonneuve P, Whitcomb DC, Lerch MM, DiMagno EP. Cigarette smoking as a risk factor for pancreatic cancer in patients with hereditary pancreatitis. *JAMA.* 2001;286(2):169-170.

Lowenfels AB, Maisonneuve P. Epidemiologic and etiologic factors of pancreatic cancer. *Hematol Oncol Clin North Am.* 2002;16(1):1-16.

Lynch HT, Smyrk T, Kern SE, et al. Familial pancreatic cancer: a review. *Semin Oncol.* 1996; 23:251-255.

Lynch HT, Voorhees G, Lanspa S, McGreevy PS, Lynch JF. Pancreatic carcinoma and hereditary nonpolyposis colorectal cancer: A family study. *Br J Cancer.* 1985;52:27-28.

Lynch HT, Brand RE, Hogg D, et al. Phenotypic variation in eight extended CDKN2A germline mutation familial atypical multiple mole melanoma-pancreatic carcinoma-prone families: the familial atypical mole melanoma-pancreatic carcinoma syndrome. *Cancer.* 2002;94(1):84-96.

Murphy KM, Brune KA, Griffin C, et al. Evaluation of candidate genes MAP2K4, MADH4, ACVR1B, and BRCA2 in familial pancreatic cancer: deleterious BRCA2 mutations in 17%. *Cancer Res.* 2002;62(13):3789-3793.

Neglia JP, FitzSimmons SC, Maisonneuve P, et al. The risk of cancer among patients with cystic fibrosis. Cystic Fibrosis and Cancer Study Group. *N Engl J Med.* 1995;332:494-499.

Ozcelik H, Schmocker B, DiNicola N, et al. Germline BRCA2 617delT mutations in Ashkenazi Jewish pancreatic cancer patients. *Nat Genet.* 1997;16:17-18.

Rulyak SJ, Brentnall TA. Inherited pancreatic cancer: surveillance and treatment strategies for affected families. *Pancreatology.* 2001;1:477-485.

Rulyak SJ, Lowenfels AB, Maisonneuve P, Brentnall TA. Risk factors for the development of pancreatic cancer in familial pancreatic cancer kindreds. *Gastroenterology.* 2003;124(5): 1292-1299.

Rulyak SJ, Kimmey MB, Veenstra DL, Brentnall TA. Cost-effectiveness of pancreatic cancer screening in familial pancreatic cancer kindreds. *Gastrointest Endosc.* 2003;57(1):23-29.

Rulyak SJ, Brentnall TA, Lynch HT, Austin MA. Characterization of the neoplastic phenotype in the familial atypical multiple-mole melanoma-pancreatic carcinoma syndrome. *Cancer.* 2003;98(4):798-804.

Schenk M, Schwartz AG, O'Neal E, et al. Familial risk of pancreatic cancer. *J Natl Cancer Inst.* 2001;93(8):640-644.

Schutte M, Hruban RH, Geradts J, et al. Abrogation of the Rb/p16 tumor-suppressive pathway in virtually all pancreatic carcinomas. *Cancer Res.* 1997;57:3126-3130.

Tersmette AC, Petersen GM, Offerhaus GJ, et al. Increased risk of incident pancreatic cancer among first-degree relatives of patients with familial pancreatic cancer. *Clin Cancer Res.* 2001;7:738-744.

van der Heijden MS, Yeo CJ, Hruban RH, Kern SE. Fanconi anemia gene mutations in young-onset pancreatic cancer. *Cancer Res.* 2003;63(10):2585-2588.

van Heek NT, Meeker AK, Kern SE, et al. Telomere shortening is nearly universal in pancreatic intraepithelial neoplasia. *Am J Pathol.* 2002;161(5):1541-1547.

chapter **6**

Surgical Approach to Ampullary and Pancreatic Neoplasia

Kristoffel R. Dumon, MD; Robert J. Canter, MD;
and Noel N. Williams, MD

INTRODUCTION

Carcinoma of the exocrine pancreas is a significant health problem in the United States and other Western nations. It is one of the most lethal malignancies with an overall 5-year survival rate of approximately 3% and an incident rate nearly equivalent to its mortality rate. Although a minority of patients are resectable at the time of diagnosis, surgical resection offers the only potentially curative treatment, and surgical treatment clearly provides the best long-term results. For patients in whom curative resection is not possible, surgical intervention remains important as a means of palliation, particularly in patients with locally advanced disease.

This chapter reviews the various roles of surgical intervention in the curative and palliative treatment of patients with pancreatic cancer, focusing on patients with carcinoma of the exocrine pancreas. Preoperative evaluation, with an emphasis on the controversial and evolving approaches to preoperative staging and determination of resectability, is discussed.

PANCREATIC NEOPLASIA

Pancreatic neoplasia can be subdivided into 3 clinical entities: 1) pancreatic duct cell adenocarcinoma—frequently referred to as adenocarcinoma of the pancreas; 2) non-pancreatic periampullary cancer, which includes distal bile duct tumors, tumors originating in the ampulla of Vater, and periampullary duodenal tumors; and 3) rare pancreatic neoplasms, which include acinus cell carcinoma (a tumor that occurs more frequently in the tail of the pancreas), primary pancreatic lymphoma, cystic neoplasms of the pancreas including intraductal papillary mucinous tumors (IPMT), solid and papillary pancreatic neoplasms, and pancreatic neuroendocrine tumors. The clinical presentation of these various entities is frequently similar. Since the decision for resection is often made without a tissue diagnosis, the surgical approach to these different neoplasms is generally the same, although the prognosis and role for adjuvant therapy varies depending on the histology.

Table 6-1

PANCREATIC CANCER STAGE AND OVERALL PROGNOSIS AT THE TIME OF DIAGNOSIS

Stage	Percent of Patients	5-Year Survival	Median Survival
Localized nonmetastatic	9.8%	17%	12 to 20 months
Regional	28%	7%	8 to 9 months
Distant	62.2%	2%	4 to 6 months
All stages	100%	4%	6 to 8 months

Patients who undergo surgical resection for localized nonmetastatic adenocarcinoma of the pancreatic head have a long-term survival rate of approximately 20% and a median survival of 12 to 20 months (Table 6-1). Disease recurrence following a potentially curative pancreaticoduodenectomy remains common. In patients who undergo surgery alone, local recurrence occurs in up to 86% of patients, peritoneal recurrence in 25%, and liver metastases in 50%. When surgery and chemoradiation are used to maximize local regional tumor control, liver metastases become the dominant form of tumor recurrence and occur in 25% to 53% of patients.

Among patients with periampullary adenocarcinoma treated by pancreaticoduodenectomy, those with duodenal adenocarcinoma are most likely to be long-term survivors. Five-year survival is less likely for patients with ampullary, distal bile duct, and pancreatic primaries, in declining order. Resection margin status, resected lymph node status, and degree of tumor differentiation also significantly influence long-term outcome. Particularly for patients with pancreatic adenocarcinoma, 5-year survival is not equated with cure, because many patients die of recurrent disease >5 years after resection (Table 6-2).

Pancreatic periampullary cancer is felt to have an improved prognosis compared to adenocarcinoma of the exocrine pancreas. This may be secondary to both earlier diagnosis and more favorable tumor biology. Neoplasms of the ampullary region cause biliary obstruction when the primary tumor is relatively small. Patients who undergo pancreaticoduodenectomy for localized periampullary adenocarcinoma of nonpancreatic origin have an improved survival duration compared with similarly treated patients who have adenocarcinoma of pancreatic origin.

INTRADUCTAL PAPILLARY MUCINOUS TUMOR

Cystic neoplasms of the exocrine pancreas comprise a small fraction of pancreatic tumors. Within this group, awareness of intraductal papillary mucinous tumor (IPMT), a disease heretofore commonly confused with chronic pancreatitis, has increased since the WHO classified these tumors as a separate group in 1996. This disease is characterized by dilation of the main pancreatic duct or branch ducts associated with mucin overproduction. There may be peripheral lesions consisting of ectatic branch ducts connected to the main duct or cysts that do not connect with the main duct. Either of these can

Table 6-2

SURGICAL RESULTS FOR PATIENTS UNDERGOING PANCREATICODUODENECTOMY FOR PANCREATIC CARCINOMA

Author	Yeo	Sohn	Conlon	Richter	Billingsley
Year	1999	2000	2001	2003	2003
No. of patients	650	564	409	194	462
Morbitity (%)	–	31	54	30	45.9
Mortality (%)	1.4	2.3	3	3	9.3
5-year survival	–	17	–	25	–
Median survival (months)	20	17	17.2	–	–

mimic so-called mucinous cystic neoplasm (MCN). Because the incidence of invasive cancer at surgery is 25 to 50%, it is important to distinguish this entity from chronic pancreatitis. This is usually done on the basis of typical changes evident on CT and ERCP. The ERCP examination may reveal mucus exuding from the papilla or characteristic intraductal filling defects. The lesion, even if it does not contain invasive cancer, is premalignant, and benign lesions contain several genetic mutations associated with pancreatic cancer. Because of their favorable prognosis, an extensive diagnostic workup for IPMTs should be performed in patients presenting with cystic lesions of the pancreas. Surgical resection is the therapy of choice for IPMTs. The type of resection depends upon the extent of the ductal involvement. Total pancreatectomy is currently the recommended treatment for an IPMT that comprises the entire main duct.

PREOPERATIVE EVALUATION

Accurate preoperative assessment of resectability is the most critical aspect of the diagnostic and treatment sequence for patients with pancreatic cancer. Imaging includes nonoperative techniques, such as abdominal ultrasonography, CT scan, MRI, angiography, and a variety of invasive techniques, such as laparoscopy and laparoscopic or intraoperative ultrasonography.

The studies for the diagnosis and staging of pancreatic cancer differ considerably from center to center. The challenge to this process is that a high percentage of patients who currently undergo surgery with curative intent have unresectable disease. The goal of preoperative imaging is to spare patients a nontherapeutic laparotomy in those with unresectable pancreatic cancer. However, this must be taken in the context of possible palliative surgery.

HISTORY AND PHYSICAL EXAMINATION

Virtually all patients with periampullary neoplasms and approximately 50% of patients with pancreatic cancer have jaundice due to extrahepatic biliary obstruction at the time of diagnosis. The classical presentation is painless jaundice in association with a palpable gallbladder (Courvoisier's sign). Tumors arising in the ampulla of Vater or within the intrapancreatic portion of the common bile duct typically cause biliary obstruction early in the course of disease and therefore may be associated with a better prognosis. Small tumors of the pancreatic head located near the intrapancreatic portion of the bile duct may also obstruct the bile duct and cause the patient to seek medical attention when the tumor is still localized and potentially resectable. In contrast, adenocarcinomas arising in the pancreas that do not cause obstruction of the intrapancreatic portion of the bile duct are often not diagnosed until locally advanced or metastatic. In the absence of extrahepatic biliary obstruction, few pancreatic cancer patients present with potentially resectable disease.

If jaundice is not present, patient complaints are often nonspecific, as are clinical signs on physical examination. The pain typical of locally advanced pancreatic cancer is a dull, fairly constant pain of visceral origin localized to the region of the middle and upper back. Some patients have vague, intermittent epigastric pain. Fatigue, weight loss, and anorexia are common even in the absence of mechanical gastric outlet obstruction. Pancreatic exocrine insufficiency due to obstruction of the pancreatic duct may result in malabsorption and steatorrhea. Although malabsorption and mild changes in stool frequency are common, diarrhea is uncommon. Onset of diabetes mellitus may herald the appearance of pancreatic cancer, particularly if the diabetes occurs during or beyond the sixth decade. Diabetes mellitus is present in 60% to 81% of patients with pancreatic cancer, and the majority of patients receive the diagnosis within 2 years of recognition of pancreatic cancer.

There is a postulated increased association of thromboembolic disorder and pancreatic carcinoma (Trousseau's syndrome) as well as an association with cutaneous manifestations such as pancreatic panniculitis (Weber-Christian disease).

Since 7% to 8% of patients with pancreatic cancer have a family history of pancreatic cancer (first-degree relative), family history is a key element in the detection of risk groups.

The importance of the clinical examination cannot be overstated. This has 2 objectives: to assess fitness for operation and to detect evidence of metastatic disease. Clinical factors such as the patient's performance status and cardiopulmonary function can indicate that the perioperative risk is prohibitive. The presence of left supraclavicular adenopathy, umbilical nodes, peritoneal carcinomatosis, or ascites can provide evidence of diffuse malignant disease. Clinically apparent disseminated disease is an obvious contraindication to attempted pancreatic resection.

LABORATORY TESTS/TUMOR MARKERS

Several tumor markers have been evaluated for pancreatic cancer. These include serum mucins (such as CA 19.9), pancreatic amyloid (IAPP), and genetic markers (K-*ras*, p53, p15/MTS2). Because of the limited sensitivity and specificity, tumor markers are currently not widely used in clinical practice but some studies suggest that tumor markers may have a useful role in monitoring clinical response after surgical resection or chemotherapy.

The most widely used marker is the serum concentration of cancer-associated antigen 19-9 (CA 19-9), which was found to have the greatest sensitivity (70%) and specificity (87%) for diagnosis of pancreatic cancer with a cutoff value of 70 U/mL. With a lower cutoff of 37 U/mL, sensitivity was somewhat higher (86%) and specificity was identical (87%). However, biliary tract obstruction with cholangitis caused by a lesion other than cancer causes high levels of CA 19-9.

Genetic markers may be used to detect pancreatic cancer, but the clinical value of these markers remains unproven. The most common gene abnormality (90%) described in pancreatic cancer is a K-*ras* mutation. Mutations of the p53 tumor cell suppressor gene are found in 50% to 70% of pancreatic cancers, and approximately 50% have reduced expression of the DCC gene. A number of other gene deletions are less frequent in pancreatic cancer, including alterations of tumor suppressor genes FHIT, 16/MTS1 and p15/MTS2.

K-*ras* mutation is the most widely studied genetic marker. K-*ras* in pancreatic secretions may be an early marker for pancreatic cancer, but whether K-*ras* mutations found in duodenal or pancreatic juice or stools of patients with chronic pancreatitis herald pancreatic cancer is not clear.

ULTRASOUND

Abdominal ultrasonography (US) is the initial screening technique because of its low cost and easy availability. US will confirm the presence of gallstones, assess the liver for metastatic deposits, detect abdominal ascites, and identify the level of biliary obstruction. In certain patients, US can enable one to manage the patient without any further investigation. Patients with malignant ascites and liver deposits require confirmatory biopsy and no further investigation.

In addition, patients presenting with biliary obstruction are usually evaluated with abdominal US to confirm the mechanical nature of the obstruction and to determine whether the site of obstruction is the intrahepatic or extrahepatic portion of the biliary tree. Obstruction of the intrapancreatic portion of the bile duct is then evaluated with a combination of CT, ERCP, and EUS/MRCP.

However, there remain many limitations to abdominal US in the evaluation of patients with pancreatic cancer. Bowel gas obscures the image in up to 15% of patients. US is notoriously operator-dependent and not accurate in assessing central abdominal and retroperitoneal structures.

CROSS-SECTIONAL IMAGING/COMPUTED TOMOGRAPHY SCAN

CT scan has undergone a rapid evolution over the last 2 decades, with each new development enhancing the imaging capability of the technique. Conventional CT has been superceded by dynamic thin section CT, spiral CT, and multidetector CT (MDCT). These new techniques have dramatically improved the ability of CT to diagnose and stage pancreatic cancer (Table 6-3). High-quality CT can identify the majority of pancreatic tumors and accurately define the relationship of the tumor to the celiac axis and superior mesenteric vessels.

The use of standardized, objective radiologic criteria for preoperative tumor staging is critical for treatment planning. The following CT criteria definine a potentially resectable pancreatic cancer:

- The absence of extrapancreatic disease
- No evidence of arterial encasement/no direct tumor extension to the celiac axis or superior mesenteric artery
- A patent superior mesenteric-portal venous (SMPV) confluence, assuming the technical ability to resect isolated involvement of the superior mesenteric vein (SMV) or SMPV confluence

Table 6-3

PREOPERATIVE IMAGING OF PANCREATIC CANCER

Study	Sensitivity (%)	Specificity (%)	Accuracy (%)
US	67 to 74	40 to 87	69
CT	72	80	–
Spiral CT	85 to 92	87 to 95	70 to 76
UMRI	95	93	80
MRCP	84	97	–
ERCP	70	95	–
EUS	75 to 87	77	–
EUS-FNA	84 to 92	96 to 100	85
PET Scan	85 to 93	84 to 88	85 to 91

US=ultrasound; CT=computer tomography; UMRI=ultrafast magnetic resonance imaging; EUS=endoscopic ultrasound; EUS-FNA=endoscopic ultrasound-guided fine needle aspiration; PET Scan=positron emission tomography

A patient is deemed to have locally advanced, unresectable disease when there is clear evidence on CT scans of the following:

- Hepatic and distant metastasis
- Locally advanced disease (eg, peripancreatic extension of tumor to locally contiguous structures, vascular encasement or invasion of the SMA or celiac axis)
- Occlusion of the SMPV confluence

Despite the wide application of conventional CT scan in the assessment of resectability, it remains inaccurate in assessing local vascular invasion. Therefore, most efforts have been directed to improving its ability to assess this factor.

The value of conventional CT in predicting unresectability has been reviewed in some studies. In a study by McCarthy et al comparing CT assessment of resectability with surgical findings, the sensitivity and specificity for CT prediction of resectability were 72% and 80%, respectively. Positive predictive value and negative predictive value were 77% and 76%, respectively (see Table 6-3). Of concern are false-positive and false-negative scans. Most studies confirm that CT cannot be relied on entirely because some criteria of unresectability—such as venous encasement, dorsal extension, and lymphadenopathy—are too inaccurate with this imaging modality.

The advent of dual-phase thin-cut spiral CT scan has offered the potential of improved accuracy. Spiral CT can generate highly detailed images that enable a greater appreciation of the relationship between the tumor and surrounding vascular structures. Spiral CT performed with contrast enhancement and a thin-section technique can accurately assess the relationship of the low-density tumor to the celiac axis, SMA, and superior mesenteric–portal vein (SMPV) confluence. Several authors have shown spiral CT to be more accurate for diagnosing pancreatic cancer and for predicting resectability.

In the latest advance in spiral CT technology, volume rendering of spiral CT data can be combined with a 3-dimensional display and is referred to as multi detector CT (MDCT). It allows the user to modify parameters to optimize visualization of structures. The viewing plane can be altered to allow inclusion of key elements of anatomy that might have been missed. This provides CT angiography, which rivals the images obtained by conventional angiography. Visualization of the bile and pancreatic ducts is also optimized. Some authors have demonstrated the incredibly accurate images that MDCT can provide. They believe that MDCT accurately assesses the patency of the superior mesenteric artery, celiac axis, and portal venous system. Although software for this technology is not currently widely available, it is likely to be in the near future. Its accuracy and reliability remain to be proven.

MAGNETIC RESONANCE IMAGING

Magnetic resonance imaging in the evaluation of pancreatic neoplasia was initially limited by image artifacts from respiration, aortic pulsation, bowel peristalsis, and a lack of suitable contrast material for the gut lumen. The introduction of ultrafast MRI (UMRI) has increased the usefulness of the technique (see Table 6-3). UMRI is more accurate than both US and CT in predicting resectability, with sensitivity, specificity, and overall accuracy of 95.7%, 93.5%, and 80.4%, respectively. Some authors maintain that UMRI may be superior to other imaging modalities, avoiding endoscopy, vascular cannulation, allergic reactions, and ionizing radiation. The use of MRI to visualize the biliary system without the administration of intravenous contrast is known as MRCP. MRCP had a sensitivity and specificity of 84% and 97%, respectively, for the diagnosis of pancreatic carcinoma. Although some authors believe that MRCP is not as accurate as spiral CT for assessment of respectability, the ability of MRI to combine pancreatography and angiography in one sitting without exposure to ionizing radiation makes it attractive as a potential replacement to spiral CT scan as the imaging modality of choice for pancreatic cancer.

ENDOSCOPIC RETROGRADE CHOLANGIOPANCREATOGRAPHY

If a low-density mass is not seen on CT scans, patients with extrahepatic biliary obstruction undergo diagnostic and therapeutic ERCP. A malignant obstruction of the intrapancreatic portion of the common bile duct is characterized by the double-duct sign, which represents proximal obstruction of the common bile and pancreatic ducts. A malignant obstruction can often be accurately differentiated from choledocholithiasis and the long, smooth tapering bile duct stricture seen with chronic pancreatitis. Conversely, a normal pancreatogram does not entirely exclude malignancy. Potentially "silent areas" on ERCP are the uncinate process, the accessory duct, and the tail. Small tumors just below the papilla will dilate the entire duct and are often missed on ERCP. It can also be difficult to differentiate between chronic pancreatitis and pancreatic cancer on ERCP.

ERCP also permits the sampling of pancreatic fluid for cytologic examination. This can help establish a definitive preoperative diagnosis. However, a benign or nondiagnostic result by ERCP-guided aspiration should not be interpreted as an indication to not operate.

POSITRON EMISSION TOMOGRAPHY

Positron emission tomography (PET) provides an alternative in tumors less than 2 cm in diameter. In lesions of this size, it is often difficult to distinguish focal pancreatitis from tumor. Preliminary studies indicate that PET has a positive predictive value for tumor of 92% compared with 91% for CT. PET may also be able to differentiate between otherwise unclear pancreatic masses and may be superior to CT scan in distinguishing benign from malignant cystic neoplasms of the pancreas. Nevertheless, the true diagnostic value for this image modality remains unclear and results from larger studies are needed.

ENDOSCOPIC ULTRASONOGRAPHY

EUS allows an ultrasound probe to be placed in close proximity to the pancreas. This eliminates interference from overlying bowel gas and allows higher frequencies to be used, resulting in markedly improved resolution of images of the pancreas and surrounding structures. EUS is not as widely available as spiral CT and requires extensive experience and knowledge of pancreatic ultrasonographic anatomy. Although EUS gives superior results compared with conventional CT scan, it appears to be equivalent to spiral CT scan in detecting tumors >3 cm and in assessing venous invasion and lymph node involvement. However, its assessment of arterial invasion is limited. Although it allows the pancreas to be assessed for small tumors (<3 cm) that may be missed on CT scan, EUS is an invasive procedure that requires sedation and is highly operator dependent. Moreover, it is the most reliable method to obtain accurate tissue for histologic diagnosis.

ENDOSCOPIC ULTRASOUND-GUIDED FINE NEEDLE ASPIRATION AND PREOPERATIVE TISSUE DIAGNOSIS

In most patients, accurate staging and biliary decompression are achieved with CT and ERCP, but these modalities cannot reliably distinguish nodal metastases from inflammatory lymphadenopathy or differentiate focal pancreatitis from tumor. To obtain a cytologic diagnosis of malignancy, EUS-guided fine-needle aspiration (FNA) is currently the procedure of choice. If neoadjuvant chemotherapy or radiotherapy is proposed, a firm tissue diagnosis is imperative. Since a negative FNA result does not absolutely exclude a malignancy and since some studies have raised the possibility of peritoneal seeding of malignant cells along the needle tract during biopsy, many centers with an experienced surgical team forego a preoperative biopsy in potentially resectable tumors.

In a patient who presents with extrahepatic biliary obstruction, a malignant-appearing stricture of the intrapancreatic portion of the common bile duct, and no history of recurrent pancreatitis or alcohol abuse, the absence of a mass on CT or EUS should not rule out the possibility of a carcinoma of the pancreas or bile duct. Similarly, negative results of EUS-guided FNA should not be considered definitive proof that a malignancy does not exist. The results of EUS, with or without FNA, should be considered in the context of the clinical picture and as a complement to CT and ERCP findings.

DIAGNOSTIC LAPAROSCOPY

For the past decade, laparoscopy has been used in patients who have radiologic evidence of localized pancreatic cancer to detect extrapancreatic tumor not visualized on CT scan. This allows laparotomy to be limited to patients who truly have localized disease. In a recent study of 398 patients with pancreatic or periampullary cancer evaluated preoperatively with high-quality CT, ERCP, and angiography, 194 of the 398 patients had tumors that were deemed to have a high probability of being resectable. Of the 194 patients, 172 (89%) underwent successful pancreaticoduodenectomy, and only 9 (5%) of the 194 patients thought to have resectable tumors were found to have occult metastatic disease at laparotomy. This indicates that only a small group of patients would benefit from laparoscopy.

The extent to which laparoscopy should be used remains controversial. Laparoscopy is reasonable to consider prior to laparotomy (during the same anesthesia induction) in patients with biopsy-proven or suspected potentially resectable pancreatic cancer in whom a decision has been made to proceed with pancreaticoduodenectomy. However, we do not recommend the routine use of laparoscopy as a staging procedure under a separate anesthesia induction.

DIAGNOSTIC APPROACH TO ASSESS SURGICAL MANAGEMENT

There seems to be an overall trend that spiral CT is the most useful initial investigative tool in the assessment and staging of pancreatic cancer (Figure 6-1). Although spiral CT can reliably predict nonresectability, there are limitations.

If no mass is seen on spiral CT or in a patient who presents with extrahepatic biliary obstruction, ERCP with biliary decompression is the second diagnostic step. With a malignant-appearing stricture of the intrapancreatic portion of the common bile duct and no history of recurrent pancreatitis or alcohol abuse, the absence of a mass on CT or EUS should not rule out the possibility of a carcinoma of the pancreas or bile duct. Concern remains about the potential for false-positive diagnosis of unresectability and the inappropriate denial of potentially curative surgery. Therefore, many experienced pancreatic surgeons feel comfortable proceeding to resection without histology. This also allows the use of an operative imaging modality such as laparoscopic ultrasonography in questionable cases. Local expertise and resources will determine the optimal policy.

TECHNIQUES OF PRIMARY RESECTION

The fundamental principle in surgery for pancreatic cancer is an en bloc resection of the primary tumor with adequate margins. However, given its highly vascular network as well as its close proximity to the major mesenteric and hepatic vessels, pancreatic resection is a technically challenging surgical procedure. In fact, Dr. Whipple's original series of pancreaticoduodenectomy published in the 1930s was complicated by a mortality rate approaching 50%. Even during the 1980s, perioperative mortality following the Whipple procedure remained near 20%, which, in light of the poor long-term survival for patients with pancreatic cancer, prompted some prominent clinicians to adopt the nihilistic view that the risk of pancreatic resection outweighed the potential benefits. With the improvements in perioperative anesthetic management and postoperative intensive care, contemporary series and large epidemiologic data report acceptable mortality rates in the 1% to 4% range (see Table 6-2). Nevertheless, pancreatic resection

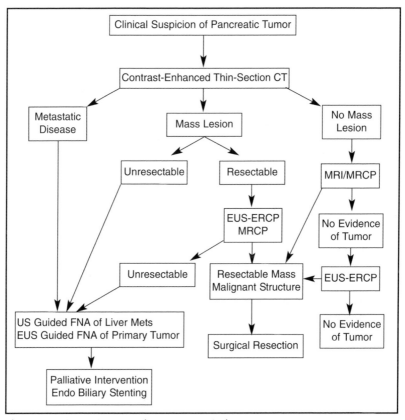

Figure 6-1. Diagnostic approach to assess surgical management.

remains a formidable procedure, and as extensive outcomes data have demonstrated, one that should only be performed by well-trained surgeons at high-volume centers.

Anatomically, the pancreas is divided into 4 sections: the head, neck, body, and tail. The head lies within the C loop of the duodenum and extends to the border of the superior mesenteric vein (Figure 6-2). The head also includes the uncinate process, which passes caudad and to the left and is the only part of the gland that lies posterior to the mesenteric vessels. The neck typically refers to the portion of the gland that lies directly over the superior mesenteric artery and vein. The body and tail of the pancreas lie to the left of the superior mesenteric artery and extend to the splenic hilum. Despite these anatomic boundaries, in practice, the key clinical distinction is whether a tumor is located to the right or left of the mesenteric vessels, since tumors to the right are typically treated by pancreaticoduodenectomy and tumors to the left by distal pancreatectomy.

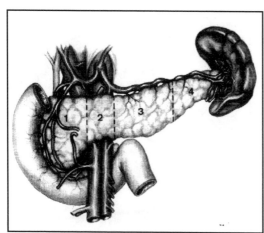

Figure 6-2. Surgical anatomy of the pancreas. The pancreas is divided into 4 sections: 1) head, 2) neck, 3) body, and 4) tail. Clinically, the principal determination is whether a tumor lies to the right or the left of the mesenteric vessels since tumors to the right are treated by pancreaticoduodenectomy and tumors to the left are treated by distal pancreatectomy. (Reprinted with permission from Etala E. *Atlas of Gastrointestinal Surgery.* Baltimore: Williams and Wilkins; 1997:469.)

WHIPPLE VS PYLORUS-PRESERVING PANCREATICODUODENECTOMY

Pancreaticoduodenectomy for carcinoma of the head of the pancreas was first described by Whipple in 1935. It includes resection of the head of the pancreas and entire duodenum, along with the distal stomach, the proximal jejunum, the gallbladder, and the distal common bile duct. Classically, a bilateral truncal vagotomy is also performed, although in recent practice, this has been less commonly employed. A modified procedure, pylorus-preserving pancreaticoduodenectomy (PPPD), was introduced in the 1970s. PPPD differs from the classic Whipple procedure by avoiding gastric resection to conserve the pylorus and the first few centimeters of the duodenum. Advocates of this procedure maintain that an intact stomach is more physiologic, allowing improved GI tract function and nutritional status, and avoids the potential complications of a gastrojejunal anastomosis, including alkaline reflux, dumping syndrome, and jejunal ulceration. There is, however, little rigorous data to conclusively favor one procedure over the other because the prospective series that have compared these 2 operations are limited by methodology, most significantly by small-sample size which leaves them underpowered to demonstrate any conclusive differences. Other methodologic shortcomings of these studies include nonrandomized designs, limited follow-up, and single-institution experiences which limit their generalizability.

However, a consistent finding among the majority of studies comparing classic Whipple to PPPD is that delayed gastric emptying is more common following PPPD. This is manifested by nausea, vomiting, and abdominal distension leading to an inability to tolerate oral alimentation up to 14 days following surgery. This complication occurs 2 to 5 times more frequently in patients undergoing PPPD and leads to a slightly prolonged length of stay, typically 4 to 5 days, for those patients. Other morbidities are generally equivalent between the 2 operations, and intraoperative variables, such as blood loss and duration of surgery, are also comparable. Since these series involve limited numbers of patients, it is possible that other small but potentially clinically significant differences between the classic Whipple and PPPD exist but have not been demonstrated.

Figure 6-3. Drawing depicting the extent of resection in a classic Whipple procedure including the head and neck of the pancreas along with the entire duodenum, the distal stomach, the proximal jejunum, the gallbladder, and the distal common bile duct. (Reprinted with permission from Etala E. *Atlas of Gastrointestinal Surgery*. Baltimore: Williams and Wilkins; 1997: 607.)

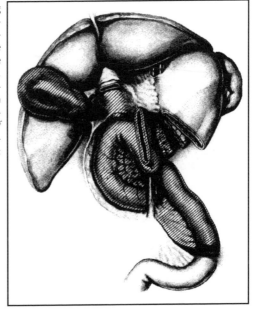

There exists even fewer data regarding the long-term nutritional outcome for patients following classic versus pylorus-preserving pancreaticoduodenectomy. There are no randomized trials, and the few published series are limited by significant numbers of patients lost to follow-up. Moreover, the nutritional data that are available are confounded by the inclusion of patients with disease progression who have significant weight loss and malnutrition secondary to their advanced disease rather than the type of resection that was performed. Consequently, insufficient evidence exists to definitively favor one surgical technique over another. The classic Whipple procedure (Figure 6-3) likely leads to a more rapid return of bowel function with a consequent shorter postoperative hospital stay, but there is probably little long-term difference between the 2 operations. Ultimately, the choice of procedure becomes one of the surgeon's experience, and as with other aspects of surgical outcomes, surgeon and hospital volume are the overriding factors to obtain the best results.

Pancreaticoduodenectomy (Figure 6-4) can be performed through either a subcostal or midline incision. Some surgeons routinely begin the operation with laparoscopy to rule out occult intraperitoneal spread of cancer and thereby spare patients unnecessary laparotomy. The number of patients who may be spared laparotomy by this approach varies among series from 4% to 25%, largely because of differences in preoperative staging algorithms and because of institutional differences in approaches to palliative procedures. However, even in institutions where resectability rates are high because of extensive preoperative cross-sectional imaging or where an aggressive approach to surgical palliation is adopted, laparoscopy prior to formal laparotomy is quick to perform and will identify the occasional patient with carcinomatosis or unsuspected liver metastases who is unresectable and therefore not an appropriate candidate for surgical palliation. These patients will benefit from avoiding unnecessary laparotomy.

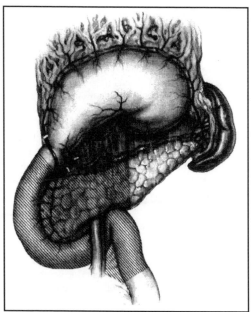

Figure 6-4. Drawing depicting the extent of resection in a pylorus-preserving pancreatico-duodenectomy. The duodenum is transected 2 to 3 cm distal to the pylorus. Proponents of this procedure maintain that an intact stomach and pylorus lead to improved nutritional parameters in this patient population. (Reprinted with permission from Etala E. *Atlas of Gastrointestinal Surgery*. Baltimore: Williams and Wilkins; 1997:687.)

Extensive laparoscopic exploration of the retroperitoneum seems unjustified since patients who do not have disseminated disease will need laparotomy for either resection for cure or for a palliative procedure. In addition, although several case series have described successful laparoscopic pancreaticoduodenectomy, these reports involve small numbers of highly selected patients. Given that there are few patients who come to operation with tumors clearly in an early stage, it seems unlikely that laparoscopic pancreaticoduodenectomy will gain a major role in the surgical treatment of tumors in the head of the pancreas.

VASCULAR INVOLVEMENT

For those patients who do undergo abdominal exploration, pancreaticoduodenectomy is begun by mobilizing the second and third portions of the duodenum from its retroperitoneal attachments in the so-called Kocher maneuver. This permits the head of the pancreas to be elevated from the retroperitoneum, thereby exposing the vena cava, the aorta, and the origin of the superior mesenteric artery. This maneuver allows the mesenteric vessels, in particular the superior mesenteric artery, to be assessed for tumor encasement and enables the surgeon to make a decision regarding resectability for cure. Arterial encasement or invasion is generally accepted as an absolute contraindication to resection. In contrast, many authors do not consider venous involvement by local tumor extension to be a contraindication to pancreatic resection. Although the published series involve relatively few patients, resection of the portal and/or superior mesenteric vein has been shown to be technically possible and safe in experienced hands. In addition, patient survival in these studies has been comparable to patients undergoing standard pancreaticoduodenectomy without venous reconstruction, suggesting that venous invasion is not an independent risk factor for a worse prognosis and should not be considered a contraindication to resection.

Following inspection of the mesenteric vessels, the gastrohepatic omentum and the porta hepatis are then examined to determine if lymph node metastases outside the field of resection are present. It is also very important to identify or confirm (since many patients will have preoperative magnetic resonance or CT angiography) aberrant arterial anatomy since these variations are not uncommon, and ligation of incorrectly identified hepatic arteries can lead to devastating postoperative complications. The peritoneum overlying the superior and inferior portion of the gland is then incised so that the surgeon may place his or her fingers around the dorsal aspect of the gland and establish a potential plane for transection. If the tumor is deemed resectable, the pancreas is typically transected at this point. The exact line of transection varies from surgeon to surgeon, but typically lies to the left of the superior mesenteric artery so that an adequate margin of non-neoplastic pancreatic tissue can be obtained.

METHODS OF PANCREATICO-JEJUNAL RECONSTRUCTION

Once the resection is complete, reconstruction of the GI tract is performed. Numerous techniques have been advocated, particularly for the pancreatico-enteric anastomosis, reflecting the technical difficulty of re-establishing pancreatico-enteric continuity and concern for pancreatic leak. Both pancreaticojejunal and pancreaticogastric anastomoses have been described, and these anastomoses can be divided into two methods, one that relies on intussuscepting or "dunking" the pancreatic stump into the intestinal lumen, and one that relies on direct pancreatic duct to intestinal mucosa anastomosis. Intussusception is generally favored when a normal pancreas is present, since a normal pancreas is soft and fragile and will not hold sutures well. In contrast, a duct-to-mucosa anastomosis is preferred when biliary obstruction has led to a dilated, easily visualized pancreatic duct with a thickened gland that retains sutures.

INDICATIONS FOR TOTAL PANCREATECTOMY

Although some authors have claimed that total pancreatectomy provides better long-term survival rates for carcinoma of the head of the pancreas, data to support this contention are lacking. Moreover, although perioperative morbidity and mortality for total pancreatectomy have declined in recent years, there is evidence that long-term complications following total pancreatectomy are significant. The most significant disadvantage of total pancreatectomy is that it frequently leads to a brittle diabetic state with unpredictable glycemic control. In addition, exocrine secretion of the pancreas is lacking, and patients require careful oral replacement of pancreatic enzymes to ensure adequate digestion and absorption of food. Consequently, given the equivalent oncologic outcomes between pancreaticoduodenectomy and total pancreatectomy combined with the increased morbidity following total pancreatectomy, total pancreatectomy should be reserved for those patients in whom intraoperative frozen section fails to obtain an adequate distal pancreatic margin and who have a performance status good enough to tolerate the significant morbidity of complete pancreatic exocrine and endocrine insufficiency.

INDICATION FOR DISTAL PANCREATECTOMY

Patients with carcinomas located in the body and tail of the pancreas often present with advanced disease because these tumors fail to produce symptoms until late in their clinical course. Tumors in this location, if amenable to surgical resection, are best treated by distal pancreatectomy. This is a more straightforward procedure than pancreatico-duodenectomy since it is not necessary to reconstruct any part of the GI tract. The gastrocolic ligaments are divided to provide exposure to the lesser sac. The retroperitoneum is incised over both the superior and inferior borders of the pancreas, with care taken to identify and ligate the inferior mesenteric vein inferiorly and the splenic artery and vein superiorly. The tumor is then identified by palpation, and if all gross disease is confined to the field of resection, the pancreas is transected, typically with the use of automatic stapling devices. The cut edge of the gland is then frequently oversewn to control bleeding and minimize the risk of fistula formation. The spleen can also be preserved in this procedure by dissecting the splenic hilum away from the tail of the pancreas, with care taken to avoid injury to the short gastric vessels on which blood supply to the spleen will be based. Although theoretically appealing given the spleen's role in preventing infection by encapsulated organisms, there has been little proven benefit to splenic preservation.

PALLIATIVE INTERVENTION

Although surgical resection offers the only potential chance for cure in patients with pancreatic cancer, the majority of patients are not candidates for resection because of the presence of locally advanced or metastatic disease at the time of presentation. For those patients with unresectable disease, the question becomes how to best palliate the symptoms of biliary obstruction, gastric outlet obstruction, and persistent abdominal pain. Different approaches to these entities depend on the overall clinical picture of the patient as well as institutional variation toward palliation.

Patients who are diagnosed with metastatic disease on preoperative imaging or at the time of diagnostic laparoscopy are not considered candidates for curative resection. Although chemotherapy has limited efficacy in this setting, it is often the only therapeutic modality available to patients. Since recovery from a laparotomy delays initiation of this treatment, many surgeons are reluctant to perform surgical palliative procedures in the setting of metastatic disease. Palliation of biliary obstruction can be successfully accomplished in these patients by the placement of expandable metal stents. These stents, which can be placed either endoscopically or percutaneously by interventional radiology, are effective. Randomized trials have shown similar overall survival between patients undergoing biliary stenting and those undergoing surgical biliary-enteric bypass. Stented patients have a higher incidence of later morbidity such as stent occlusion with recurrent jaundice and cholangitis, while biliary-enteric bypass patients have a higher procedure-related morbidity and mortality. For example, in one recent series, palliative bypass carried a 3% mortality and 22% morbidity rate.

Many surgeons adopt a somewhat more aggressive approach to the palliation of jaundice for patients who undergo abdominal exploration for possible resection and are found to be unresectable based on locally advanced disease, such as vascular invasion. These patients have already been subjected to the greater short-term morbidity of a laparotomy, so the completion of a more durable biliary-enteric bypass, usually in the form of a choledochojejunostomy, seems indicated. This is illustrated by a recent randomized trial comparing endoscopic stent insertion with surgical biliary bypass where recurrent jaundice developed in only 2% of the bypass patients compared to 36% of the stented patients.

Another advantage of surgical bypass is the ability to perform a concomitant gastrojejunostomy to treat or prevent gastric outlet obstruction. Patients who have symptoms of gastric outlet obstruction at the time of exploration should be treated with therapeutic gastrojejunostomy. Prophylactic gastrojejunostomy is more questionable since fewer than 20% of patients with pancreatic cancer will develop duodenal obstruction, and for most of these patients, this occurs late in the course of their disease. Endoscopically-placed intraluminal stents have emerged as a potential minimally-invasive method to treat patients with gastric outlet obstruction. Although experience with these devices is limited, they hold promise as a potentially effective palliative procedure for the minority of patients who develop late gastric outlet obstruction secondary to unresectable pancreatic cancer.

Intractable pain can be a significant problem for many patients with pancreatic cancer. Although narcotic analgesics are effective for many patients, some patients will have unremitting abdominal and back pain with significant effects on quality of life. An increasingly employed approach is celiac-plexus block, which involves ablation of the intra-abdominal pain fibers usually by the injection of 98% alcohol. This can be performed surgically, percutaneously, or more recently by endoscopic ultrasound. Results of celiac-plexus block appear to show a benefit to this approach. A randomized trial of surgical splanchnectomy in conjunction with "double bypass" for patients with unresectable pancreatic cancer demonstrated greater pain relief in the celiac-block group. This translated into improved nutritional parameters for the celiac-block group with a trend towards longer survival.

POSTOPERATIVE CARE

Although pancreatic fistula remains a relatively frequent occurrence following pancreatic resection, with fistula rates of 5% to 10% in most series, it is no longer the dreaded complication it once was. With the use of closed-suction drains placed at the time of surgery, or alternatively with percutaneous drains placed postoperatively into suspicious peripancreatic collections, pancreatic fistulae are easily controlled, and almost always resolve spontaneously. In fact, many surgeons no longer consider the presence of a postoperative pancreatic fistula an absolute indication for bowel rest and total parenteral nutrition, and patients are allowed to take a diet as tolerated as long as fistulous drainage does not increase.

SUMMARY

Pancreatic cancer is the fourth leading cause of cancer-related mortality in the United States. Since surgical resection remains the only potentially curative option, an aggressive approach to surgical exploration is indicated even though only a minority of patients are resectable. Preoperative staging should include high resolution cross-sectional imaging as well as endoscopic ultrasound for tissue sampling and assessment of locoregional spread. Preoperative laparoscopy is used in the treatment of patients with pancreatic cancer since the occasional patient will be diagnosed with unsuspected disseminated disease and spared the morbidity of a formal laparotomy. For patients who undergo abdominal exploration, careful assessment of the mesenteric vessels should be performed since extensive vascular invasion is a contraindication to resection. In the absence of disseminated disease or vascular invasion, en bloc pancreatic resection along with removal of the regional lymph nodes should be undertaken with the type of resection depending on the location of the primary tumor. For patients with unresectable disease, palliative procedures can provide significant relief, although newer minimally invasive techniques may replace surgical palliative procedures.

BIBLIOGRAPHY

Adamek HE, Albert J, Breer H, et al. Pancreatic cancer detection with magnetic resonance cholangiopancreatography and endoscopic retrograde cholangiopancreatography: a prospective controlled study. *Lancet.* 2000;356:190-193.

Adler DG, Baron TH. Endoscopic palliation of malignant gastric outlet obstruction using self-expanding metal stents: experience in 36 patients. *Am J Gastroenterol.* 2002;97:72-78.

Alazraki N. Imaging of pancreatic cancer using fluorine-18 fluorodeoxyglucose positron emission tomography. *J Gastrointest Surg.* 2002;6:136-138.

Billingsley KG, Hur K, Henderson WG, et al. Outcome after pancreaticoduodenectomy for periampullary cancer: an analysis from the Veterans Affairs National Surgical Quality Improvement Program. *J Gastrointest Surg.* 2003;7:484-491.

Birkmeyer JD, Finlayson SR, Tosteson AN, et al. Effect of hospital volume on in-hospital mortality with pancreaticoduodenectomy. *Surgery.* 1999;125:250-256.

Birkmeyer JD, Siewers AE, Finlayson EV, et al. Hospital volume and surgical mortality in the United States. *N Engl J Med.* 2002;346:1128-1137.

Bold RJ, Charnsangavej C, Cleary KR, et al. Major vascular resection as part of pancreaticoduodenectomy for cancer: radiologic, intraoperative, and pathologic analysis. *J Gastrointest Surg.* 1999;3:233-243.

Chou FF, Sheen-Chen SM, Chen YS, Chen MC, Chen CL. Postoperative morbidity and mortality of pancreaticoduodenectomy for periampullary cancer. *Eur J Surg.* 1996;162: 477-481.

Clarke DL, Thomson SR, Madiba TE, Sanyika C. Preoperative imaging of pancreatic cancer: a management-oriented approach. *J Am Coll Surg.* 2003;196:119-129.

Conlon KC, Labow D, Leung D, et al. Prospective randomized clinical trial of the value of intraperitoneal drainage after pancreatic resection. *Ann Surg.* 2001;234:487-493.

Doberneck RC, Berndt GA. Delayed gastric emptying after palliative gastrojejunostomy for carcinoma of the pancreas. *Arch Surg.* 1987;122:827-829.

Eisenberg E, Carr DB, Chalmers TC. Neurolytic celiac plexus block for treatment of cancer pain: a meta-analysis. *Anesth Analg.* 1995;80:290-295.

Espat NJ, Brennan MF, Conlon KC. Patients with laparoscopically staged unresectable pancreatic adenocarcinoma do not require subsequent surgical biliary or gastric bypass. *J Am Coll Surg.* 1999;188:649-655.

Fernandez-del Castillo C, Rattner DW, Warshaw AL. Standards for pancreatic resection in the 1990s. *Arch Surg.* 1995;130:295-299;discussion 299-300.

Freeny PC. Pancreatic carcinoma: what is the best imaging test? *Pancreatology.* 2001;1:604-609.

Friess H, Kleeff J, Silva JC, et al. The role of diagnostic laparoscopy in pancreatic and periampullary malignancies. *J Am Coll Surg.* 1998;186:675-682.

Grile G Jr. The advantages of bypass operations over radical pancreatoduodenectomy in the treatment of pancreatic carcinoma. *Surg Gynecol Obstet.* 1970;130:1049-1053.

Gullo L, Pezzilli R, Morselli-Labate AM. Diabetes and the risk of pancreatic cancer. Italian Pancreatic Cancer Study Group. *N Engl J Med.* 1994;331:81-84.

Gunaratnam NT, Sarma AV, Norton ID, Wiersema MJ. A prospective study of EUS-guided celiac plexus neurolysis for pancreatic cancer pain. *Gastrointest Endosc.* 2001;54:316-324.

Harada N, Wiersema MJ, Wiersema LM. Endosonography-guided celiac plexus neurolysis. *Gastrointest Endosc Clin N Am.* 1997;7:237-245.

Heinemann V, Schermuly MM, Stieber P, et al. CA19-9: a predictor of response in pancreatic cancer treated with gemcitabine and cisplatin. *Anticancer Res.* 1999;19:2433-2435.

Hennig R, Tempia-Caliera AA, Hartel M, Buchler MW, Friess H. Staging laparoscopy and its indications in pancreatic cancer patients. *Dig Surg.* 2002;19:484-488.

Hilgers W, Rosty C, Hahn SA. Molecular pathogenesis of pancreatic cancer. *Hematol Oncol Clin North Am.* 2002;16:17-35,v.

Jemal A, Tiwari RC, Murray T, et al. Cancer statistics, 2004. *CA Cancer J Clin.* 2004;54:8-29.

Kahl S, Glasbrenner B, Zimmermann S, Malfertheiner P. Endoscopic ultrasound in pancreatic diseases. *Dig Dis.* 2002;20:120-126.

Kalra MK, Maher MM, Mueller PR, Saini S. State-of-the-art imaging of pancreatic neoplasms. *Br J Radiol.* 2003;76:857-865.

Kim HS, Lee DK, Kim HG, et al. J. Features of malignant biliary obstruction affecting the patency of metallic stents: a multicenter study. *Gastrointest Endosc.* 2002;55:359-365.

Leach SD, Lee JE, Charnsangave JC, et al. Survival following pancreaticoduodenectomy with resection of the superior mesenteric-portal vein confluence for adenocarcinoma of the pancreatic head. *Br J Surg.* 1998;85:611-617.

Lieberman MD, Kilburn H, Lindsey M, Brennan MF. Relation of perioperative deaths to hospital volume among patients undergoing pancreatic resection for malignancy. *Ann Surg.* 1995;222:638-645.

Lillemoe KD, Cameron JL, Hardacre JM, et al. Is prophylactic gastrojejunostomy indicated for unresectable periampullary cancer? A prospective randomized trial. *Ann Surg.* 1999;230:322-328;discussion 328-330.

Lillemoe KD, Cameron JL, Kaufman HS, et al. Chemical splanchnicectomy in patients with unresectable pancreatic cancer. A prospective randomized trial. *Ann Surg.* 1993;217:447-455;discussion 456-447.

Lillemoe KD, Kaushal S, Cameron JL, et al. Distal pancreatectomy: indications and outcomes in 235 patients. *Ann Surg.* 1999;229:693-698;discussion 698-700.

Lim JE, Chien MW, Earle CC. Prognostic factors following curative resection for pancreatic adenocarcinoma: a population-based, linked database analysis of 396 patients. *Ann Surg.* 2003;237:74-85.

Lin PW, Lin YJ. Prospective randomized comparison between pylorus-preserving and standard pancreaticoduodenectomy. *Br J Surg.* 1999;86:603-607.

Loftus EV Jr, Olivares-Pakzad BA, Batts KP, et al. Intraductal papillary-mucinous tumors of the pancreas: clinicopathologic features, outcome, and nomenclature. Members of the Pancreas Clinic, and Pancreatic Surgeons of Mayo Clinic. *Gastroenterology.* 1996;110:1909-1918.

Lynch HT, Brand RE, Lynch JF, Fusaro RM, Kern SE. Hereditary factors in pancreatic cancer. *J Hepatobiliary Pancreat Surg.* 2002;9:12-31.

McCarthy MJ, Evans J, Sagar G, Neoptolemos JP. Prediction of resectability of pancreatic malignancy by computed tomography. *Br J Surg.* 1998;85:320-325.

Midwinter MJ, Beveridge CJ, Wilsdon JB, et al. Correlation between spiral computed tomography, endoscopic ultrasonography and findings at operation in pancreatic and ampullary tumours. *Br J Surg.* 1999;86:189-193.

Polati E, Finco G, Gottin L, et al. Prospective randomized double-blind trial of neurolytic coeliac plexus block in patients with pancreatic cancer. *Br J Surg.* 1998;85:199-201.

Richter A, Niedergethmann M, Sturm JW, et al. Long-term results of partial pancreaticoduodenectomy for ductal adenocarcinoma of the pancreatic head: 25-year experience. *World J Surg.* 2003;27:324-329.

Rivera JA, Fernandez-del Castillo C, Pins M, et al. Pancreatic mucinous ductal ectasia and intraductal papillary neoplasms. A single malignant clinicopathologic entity. *Ann Surg.* 1997;225:637-644;discussion 644-636.

Rocha Lima CM, Centeno B. Update on pancreatic cancer. *Curr Opin Oncol.* 2002;14:424-430.

Rumstadt B, Schwab M, Schuster K, Hagmuller E, Trede M. The role of laparoscopy in the preoperative staging of pancreatic carcinoma. *J Gastrointest Surg.* 1997;1:245-250.

Sarmiento JM, Sarr MG. Staging strategies for pancreatic adenocarcinoma: what the surgeon really wants to know. *Curr Gastroenterol Rep.* 2003;5:117-124.

Schmitz-Winnenthal FH, Z'Graggen K, Volk C, Schmied BM, Buchler MW. Intraductal papillary mucinous tumors of the pancreas. *Curr Gastroenterol Rep.* 2003;5:133-140.

Seiler CA, Wagner M, Sadowski C, Kulli C, Buchler MW. Randomized prospective trial of pylorus-preserving vs. classic duodenopancreatectomy (Whipple procedure): initial clinical results. *J Gastrointest Surg.* 2000;4:443-452.

Sohn TA, Lillemoe KD. Surgical palliation of pancreatic cancer. *Adv Surg.* 2000;34:249-271.

Sohn TA, Yeo CJ, Cameron JL, et al. Resected adenocarcinoma of the pancreas-616 patients: results, outcomes, and prognostic indicators. *J Gastrointest Surg.* 2000;4:567-579.

Stojadinovic A, Brooks A, Hoos A, et al. An evidence-based approach to the surgical management of resectable pancreatic adenocarcinoma. *J Am Coll Surg.* 2003;196:954-964.

Strasberg SM, Drebin JA, Mokadam NA, et al. Prospective trial of a blood supply-based technique of pancreaticojejunostomy: effect on anastomotic failure in the Whipple procedure. *J Am Coll Surg.* 2002;194:746-758; discussion 759-760.

Trede M, Rumstadt B, Wendl K, et al. Ultrafast magnetic resonance imaging improves the staging of pancreatic tumors. *Ann Surg.* 1997;226:393-405; discussion 405-397.

van Berge Henegouwen MI, Moojen TM, van Gulik TM, et al. Postoperative weight gain after standard Whipple's procedure versus pylorus-preserving pancreatoduodenectomy: the influence of tumour status. *Br J Surg.* 1998;85:922-926.

Van Hoe L, Baert AL. Pancreatic carcinoma: applications for helical computed tomography. *Endoscopy.* 1997;29:539-560.

Weaver DW, Wiencek RG, Bouwman DL, Walt AJ. Gastrojejunostomy: is it helpful for patients with pancreatic cancer? *Surgery.* 1987;102:608-613.

Williams DB, Sahai AV, Aabakken L, et al. Endoscopic ultrasound guided fine needle aspiration biopsy: a large single centre experience. *Gut.* 1999;44:720-726.

Yeo CJ. The Whipple procedure in the 1990s. *Adv Surg.* 1999;32:271-303.

Yeo CJ, Sohn TA, Cameron JL, Hruban RH, Lillemoe KD, Pitt HA. Periampullary adenocarcinoma: analysis of 5-year survivors. *Ann Surg.* 1998;227:821-831.

Yeo TP, Hruban RH, Leach SD, et al. Pancreatic cancer. *Curr Probl Cancer.* 2002;26:176-275.

Zerbi A, Balzano G, Patuzzo R, et al. Comparison between pylorus-preserving and Whipple pancreatoduodenectomy. *Br J Surg.* 1995;82:975-979.

chapter 7

Chemotherapy and Radiation in the Treatment of Pancreatic Cancer

Bapsi Chak, MD and Jordan Berlin, MD

INTRODUCTION

This chapter will review neoplasms from the sites referred to by the term *pancreaticobiliary malignancy*. This term refers to several primary sites often considered together. Pancreas cancer is the most common of the pancreaticobiliary malignancies representing an estimated 31,860 new cases and 31,270 deaths in the United States in 2004, making it the fourth leading cause of cancer death in the United States.[1] Finally, there are many rare histologic subtypes that occur in the pancreas, but this chapter will only focus on the most common cell type, adenocarcinoma.

PANCREATIC CANCER

Pancreatic cancer is a devastating illness with <5% of all patients surviving 5 years. Clinical decision making for therapy of pancreatic cancer patients is determined by classifying these tumors into one of 3 categories: metastatic disease, locally advanced and unresectable, and resectable disease. To introduce the chemotherapy drugs, this chapter will work backward from metastatic disease to resectable disease.

CHEMOTHERAPY FOR METASTATIC DISEASE

For metastatic disease, the current goal of chemotherapy is control of disease and/or its symptoms. In many cancers, the expectations from chemotherapy are much greater. For example, response rates for first-line colorectal cancer therapy range from 40% to 50%. However, with pancreatic cancer, response rates of only 5% to 10% may indicate activity.

The original chemotherapy drug for metastatic disease was 5-FU, a fluorinated pyrimidine. The mechanisms of action for 5-FU include incorporation into RNA and disruption of DNA synthesis by inhibiting thymidylate synthase (TS). Data suggests that administering 5-FU as a quick bolus (intravenous injection over a few minutes) favors RNA incorporation and using prolonged infusions, which can last up to several

Table 7-1

SCHEDULES USED FOR 5-FU ADMINISTRATION

Drug	Dose (mg/m²)	Duration of Infusion	Schedule of Cycle	Duration of Cycle
Leucovorin[1]	20	Bolus	Daily x 5	4 to 5 weeks
5-FU	425	Bolus		
Leucovorin[1]	500	2 hours	Once weekly x 6	8 weeks
5-FU	500	Bolus		
Leucovorin[1]	200	2 hours	Day 1	2 weeks
5-FU	400	Bolus		
5-FU	2000 to 2400	46 hours		
5-FU	2600	24 hours	Once weekly x 4	4 weeks
Leucovorin[1]	500	2 hours	Once weekly x 4	4 weeks
5-FU	2200 to 2600	24 hours		
Capecitabine*	1250	Oral	Twice daily x 2 weeks	3 weeks

[1]Leucovorin is always given prior to 5-FU.
*Capectabine is an oral prodrug of 5-FU.

weeks, favors TS inhibition. It is clear that altering the administration schedule alters the toxicity profile. For example, infusional schedules have higher rates of hand and foot rash (palmar plantar erythrodysesthesia), while bolus injections have higher rates of diarrhea or hematologic toxicity. The metabolite of 5-FU (5-fluorodeoxyuridine monophosphate or FdUMP) that binds to TS requires a reduced folate as a cofactor. Therefore, folinic acid or leucovorin is often coadministered with 5-FU. Studies demonstrated that 5-FU-based therapy significantly improved the average survival for pancreatic cancer patients compared to palliative care alone.[2,3] In addition, 5-FU maintained quality of life better than supportive care alone.[2] When using 5-FU, there are a number of doses and schedules for administration, including an oral prodrug, capecitabine, that is converted in vivo to 5-FU. Table 7-1 provides several schedules for 5-FU with or without leucovorin.

Gemcitabine (2',2'-diflorodeoxycytidine), another pyrimidine analogue, demonstrated efficacy early in clinical trials. Although response rates on the phase II trials were low (<10%), investigators noted that pancreatic cancer patients receiving gemcitabine appeared to have improvements in disease-related symptoms out of proportion to objective response rates.[4-6] Common and serious side effects of gemcitabine are listed in Table 7-2. When the phase III trial comparing gemcitabine to 5-FU was designed, the investigators used a new parameter called "clinical benefit response" as the primary endpoint.[7] The clinical benefit response attempted to objectively measure the effects of gemcitabine on symptoms common to pancreatic cancer patients: pain (pain score and analgesic con-

Table 7-2	
SIDE EFFECTS OF GEMCITABINE	
Frequency	*Side Effect*
Common (>0% of patients)	Nausea/vomiting (mildly emetogenic)
	Leukopenia
	Thrombocytopenia
	Anemia
	Erythematous rash
	Mild elevations in transaminases
	Fatigue
	Flu-like symptoms (fever, myalgia, headache, back pain, chills, asthenia, anorexia)
	Sweats
	Edema
Uncommon (1% to 10%)	Diarrhea
	Constipation
	Mucositis
	Short-term dyspnea
	Pruritis
Rare (≤1%)	Pulmonary infiltrates or fatal dyspnea
	Desquamation, ulceration
	Alopecia
	Uncontrollable nausea/vomiting

sumption), fatigue (Karnofsky performance status), and weight loss. To have clinical benefit response, a patient had to have and maintain improvement in one parameter without a decline in any other symptoms. Clinical benefit response evaluates specific symptoms and is not a measure of global quality of life. The secondary parameters studied included response rate, median survival and 1-year survival. Results are shown in Table 7-3. Gemcitabine was superior to 5-FU in terms of clinical benefit response, time to tumor progression, overall survival, and 1-year survival. Neither regimen produced many objective responses. With these results, gemcitabine became the standard treatment for pancreatic cancer and the control arm for future studies. However, like 5-FU, there may be rationale for administering gemcitabine by different schedules. Gemcitabine is a prodrug that needs to be phosphorylated for activation. The rate-limiting enzyme, deoxycytidine kinase, is saturable in laboratory studies at a rate of 10 mg/m^2/min. The standard regimen infuses gemcitabine 1000 mg/m^2 over 30 minutes, which far exceeds the saturation rate. A single randomized phase II study compared a 30-minute infusion of high-dose gemcitabine to a "fixed-dose rate" of gemcitabine in which the infusion rate was kept at 10 mg/m^2/min.[8] With a total of 92 patients enrolled, there was a suggestion that fixed-dose rate gemcitabine had better median (8 months vs 5 months, respectively) and 1-year survival rates than the 30-minute arm. In addition, higher levels of gemcitabine triphosphate were measured in peripheral blood mononu-

---

Table 7-3

RESULTS OF GEMCITABINE VS 5-FU RANDOMIZED PHASE III TRIAL

Parameter	5-FU (n=63)	Gemcitabine (n=63)
Clinical benefit response	4.8%	23.8% (p=0.0022)
Time to tumor progression	4 weeks	9 weeks (p=0.0002)
Response rate	0%	5.4%
Median survival	4.4 months	5.6 months (p=0.0025)
1-year survival	2%	18%

Table 7-4

PHASE III TRIALS OF GEMCITABINE VS NEW DRUG X

Reference	Study Arms	# of Patients	Time to Tumor Progress.	Median Survival	1-Year Survival
Richards (2004)	Gemcitabine	170	4.4 mos	6.6 mos	22.1%
	Exactecan	169	2.8 mos	5.0 mos	17.9%
Moore (2003)	Gemcitabine	139	3.5 mos*	6.6 mos	25%
	BAY 12-9666	138	1.7 mos (p<0.001)	3.7 mos (p<0.001)	10%
Bramall (2001)	Gemcitabine	103		5.6 mos	20%
	Marimastat 5 mg	104		3.7 mos	14%
	Marimastat 10 mg	105		3.5 mos	14%
	Marimastat 25 mg	102		4.2 mos	19%

*Progression-free survival data

---

clear cells of patients treated with fixed-dose rate gemcitabine than those treated with a higher total dose of gemcitabine given as a 30-minute infusion.

Current and recent randomized trials largely follow one of 2 designs: gemcitabine vs drug X or gemcitabine + drug X vs gemcitabine alone. Results for these trials are shown in Tables 7-4 and 7-5 and discussed in the following text. Table 7-6 provides a list of gemcitabine-based regimens.

Adding gemcitabine to 5-FU has produced variable results. Several factors play a role, including patient selection, small sample size, inclusion of locally advanced disease patients with metastatic disease patients, and possibly the use of different schedules of 5-FU in combination with gemcitabine. Median survival times on some of the phase II trials have varied from as low as 4 months to >10 months, although response rates have remained <10% throughout.[9-11] Thus far, one randomized trial has been reported comparing gemcitabine to gemcitabine + bolus 5-FU (see Table 7-5).[12] There was a statisti-

Table 7-5

FURTHER PHASE III TRIALS OF GEMCITABINE VS NEW DRUG X

Reference	Study Arms	# of Patients	Time to Tumor Progress.	Median Survival	1-Year Survival
Berlin (2002)	Gemcitabine	162	2.2 mos	5.4 mos	N/A
	Gemcitabine + 5-FU	160	3.4 mos (p<0.022)	6.7 mos (p<0.09)	N/A
Richards (2004)	Gemcitabine	282	3.6 mos	6.3 mos	20.1%
	Gemcitabine + Pemetrexed	283	5.2 mos (p<0.42)	6.2 mos (p<0.85)	21.4% (p<0.72)
Louvet (2004)	Gemcitabine	156	3.7 mos*	7.1 mos	27.8%
	Gemcitabine + Oxaliplatin	157	5.5 mos (p<0.04)	9.0 mos (p<0.13)	34.7%
Heineman (2003)	Gemcitabine	97	2.5 mos	6.0 mos	N/A
	Gemcitabine + Cisplatin	95	4.6 mos (p<0.016)	7.6 mos (p<0.12)	
Rocha Lima (2004)	Gemcitabine	169	3.0 mos	6.6 mos	20%
	Gemcitabine + Irinotecan	173	3.5 mos (p<0.35)	6.3 mos (p<0.79)	20%
O'Reilly (2004)	Gemcitabine	174	3.8 mos	6.2 mos	21%
	Gemcitabine + Exatecan	175	3.7 mos (p<0.22)	6.7 mos (p<0.52)	23%
Bramall (2002)	Gemcitabine	119	–	5.5 mos	18%
	Gemcitabine + Marimastat	120	–	5.5 mos (p<NS)	17% (p<NS)
VanCutsem (2004)	Gemcitabine	341	3.6 mos*	6.0 mos	24%
	Gemcitabine + Tipifarnib	347	3.7 mos	6.4 mos (p<0.75)	27%

*Progression-free survival data; NS=not significant

cally significant improvement in progression-free survival (PFS), one of two methods of measuring the time from start of study until tumor grows, the other being time to tumor progression (TTP). (The difference between TTP and PFS is how they assess patients who die without progressive disease.) The median survival for patients receiving gemcitabine alone was 5.4 months compared to 6.7 months for the combination of gemcitabine + 5-FU, but this did not reach statistical significance so this regimen is not considered part of pancreatic cancer standard therapy (see Table 7-5). Other combinations of gemcitabine with 5-FU are still under investigation. Gemcitabine and 5-FU are part of a broader class of chemotherapy drugs called antimetabolites. Another antimetabolite, pemetrexed, did not add to the efficacy of gemcitabine (see Table 7-5).[13]

Table 7-6

A SAMPLE OF GEMCITABINE-BASED REGIMENS

Agent	Dose (mg/m²)	Frequency	Cycle Duration
Gemcitabine[1]	1000 over 30 mins	Weekly x 3 weeks	4 weeks
Gemcitabine	1500 over 150 mins	Weekly x 3 weeks	4 weeks
Gemcitabine	1000 over 30 mins	Weekly x 3 weeks	4 weeks
Leucovorin	25 bolus	Weekly x 3 weeks	
5-FU	600 bolus	Weekly x 3 weeks	
Gemcitabine	1000 over 30 mins	Every 2 weeks	4 weeks
Cisplatin	50	Every 2 weeks	
Gemcitabine	1000 over 100 mins	Day 1	2 weeks
Oxaliplatin	100 over 2 hours	Day 2	
Cetuximab[2]	250 over 1 hour, then wait 60 mins	Weekly	4 weeks
Gemcitabine[1]	1000 over 30 mins	Weekly x 3 weeks	
Gemcitabine	1000 over 30 mins	Weekly x 3 weeks	4 weeks
Bevacizumab[3]	10 mg/kg over 1 hour	Every 2 weeks	

The first regimen only is considered standard care in pancreatic cancer. Others have been or are being studied in phase III trials. The first drug administered is always listed on top.

[1]The first cycle is usually given as 7 weekly infusions followed by 1 week of rest (total duration is 8 weeks).
[2]The first dose is 400 mg/m² over 2 hours and subsequent doses are given over 60 mins.
[3]The first dose is given over 2 hours and infusion time is shortened to 1 hour over time.

Exatecan, rubitecan, and irinotecan are camptothecin analogues. Like camptothecin, these agents inhibit the enzyme topoisomerase I as it nicks and unwinds DNA prior to replication. As demonstrated in Tables 7-2 and 7-3, neither irinotecan nor exatecan added benefit to gemcitabine, and exatecan alone was inferior to gemcitabine. Phase III rubitecan trials are pending.[14-16]

Cisplatin and oxaliplatin, 2 platinum derivatives, appear to be synergistic with several chemotherapy agents including gemcitabine. Similar to gemcitabine + 5-FU, the combination of gemcitabine and platinum increased TTP (4.6 months) compared to gemcitabine alone (2.5 months).[17] Despite initial reports of high response rates, gemcitabine + cisplatin only produced a 10% response rate. Although these 2 parameters were encouraging, the survival difference did not reach statistical significance (see Table 7-5). The combination of gemcitabine + oxaliplatin was tested in a phase III trial comparing gemcitabine + oxaliplatin versus gemcitabine alone.[18] This combination of gemcitabine + oxaliplatin uses a fixed-dose rate infusion of gemcitabine on day 1 followed by oxaliplatin on day 2, both given every other week. The results demonstrated significant improvements for gemcitabine + oxaliplatin vs gemcitabine alone in response rate (26.8% vs 17.3%, p<0.04), progression free survival (5.8 months vs 3.7 months, p=0.04) and clinical benefit response rate (38.2% vs 26.9%, p=0.03). However, survival did not reach statistical significance (9 vs 7.1 months, p=0.12). Of note, the overall survival of 7.1 months on the control arm is higher than expected for gemcitabine alone and may be due to the 30% of enrolled patients having locally advanced disease. Combined with this question, this randomized trial had enough parameters that differed between arms to warrant further study in a larger trial. The larger trial will complete accrual in February 2005.

BEYOND CHEMOTHERAPY

Because standard cytotoxic chemotherapy has had limited effects in pancreatic cancer, other approaches need to be sought. Rather than blocking DNA synthesis at various levels, the so-called "targeted" therapies inhibit proteins in signaling pathways that promote tumorigenic phenotypes. For example, the epidermal growth factor receptor (EGFR or HER1) is a member of the HER family of transmembrane tyrosine kinases. It has 4 domains. The external receptor portion binds a ligand that results in homodimerization or heterodimerization with another member of the HER family. Dimerization activates the internal tyrosine kinase portion, which initiates 2 kinase pathways that produce cellular growth, proliferation, and metastasis. Antibodies to EGFR block activation of the external receptor portion and small molecules inhibit the activity of the internal tyrosine kinase domain. Cetuximab is a chimerized (70% human, 30% mouse) antibody to the EGFR that was tested in combination with gemcitabine in a phase II trial.[19] Of 41 patients enrolled, 5 (12.2%) responded and 63.4% had stable disease. Median survival was 7.1 months with 31.7% of patients alive at 1 year. These promising data have led to a large phase III trial in the Southwest Oncology Group (SWOG). Of the small molecule inhibitors, erlotinib has been tested in pancreatic cancer in a phase III trial conducted by the National Cancer Institute of Canada (NCIC), randomly assigning patients to gemcitabine alone or in combination with erlotinib. Patients were randomized to gemcitabine + placebo vs gemcitabine + erlotinib given orally as either 100 mg or 150 mg/day.[20] Only 48 of the 569 patients enrolled were randomized to placebo vs 150 mg/day. The data have not been published or presented in a scientific forum as of the beginning of 2005, but have been released on the Genentech Web site (www.biooncology.com). When compared to gemcitabine alone, gemcitabine + erlotinib improved median survival from 5.9 to 6.4 months. One-year survival was 25.6% for gemcitabine + erlotinib compared to 19.6% for gemcitabine + placebo. When converted to a hazard ratio of 0.81, this data was statistically significant (p=0.025). There were no differences in response rates in the 2 arms and little is noted of extra side effects on the erlotinib arm, although diarrhea and rash are known side effects. This trial needs to undergo peer review to evaluate whether or not the apparent small benefits outweigh the risks of adding erlotinib to pancreatic cancer therapy.

Another cell signaling pathway that stimulates cellular growth is the *ras* pathway. K-*ras*, one of the subtypes of *Ras*, has an activating mutation in >90% of pancreatic cancers that leaves the *Ras* pathway permanently "on." The *Ras* proteins require posttranslational modification, including farnesylation, to get to the transmembrane position required for its activity. Farnesyl transferase inhibitors were tested as inhibitors of the *Ras* pathway in an attempt to improve upon gemcitabine, but tipifarnib (R115777) did not add to the efficacy of single agent gemcitabine (see Table 7-5).[21] The lack of efficacy of farnesyl transferase inhibitors do not prove that K-*ras* is not a good target, but may be due to the fact that K-*ras* can undergo other forms of post-translational modification than farnesylation.

The extracellular matrix in which cancer develops is now known to interact with the cancer. In order to metastasize, cancer cells have to break free of their primary location, migrate, invade, and alter the environment to allow growth. At the center of this development is an enhanced understanding of tumor angiogenesis, the process by which tumors break down the extracellular matrix and stimulate new blood vessel growth to allow for larger sized masses to develop.

Matrix metalloproteinases (MMPs) are proteins that degrade components of the extracellular matrix. The activity of some of these MMPs allows for invasion and angiogenesis to occur. Two matrix metalloproteinase inhibitors (MMPIs) were tested in pancreatic cancer patients. Both marimastat and BAY 12-9566 were less effective than gemcitabine (see Table 7-4).[22,23] When added to gemcitabine, marimastat did not improve upon single-agent gemcitabine results (see Table 7-5).[24] Since these trials, scientific understanding of MMPs has continued to develop. Whether this will lead to more effective therapy is not yet known.

More recently, promise has been shown by an inhibitor of vascular endothelial growth factor (VEGF). VEGF is produced by a variety of epithelial tumors, including pancreatic cancers. VEGF stimulates vascular growth and permeability as well as sustains survival of tumor vasculature. Bevacizumab is a humanized monoclonal antibody (95% human, 5% mouse) that binds VEGF, preventing it from activating its receptor. A multi-institutional phase II trial of bevacizumab + gemcitabine showed promising median survival of 8.7 months, 1-year survival of 29%, and an excellent response rate of 19%.[25] This data led to the development of the current Cancer and Leukemia group B (CALGB) trial randomly assigning patients to gemcitabine vs gemcitabine + bevacizumab.

Immune Therapy

The goal of immune therapy is to utilize the immune system to selectively kill cancer cells without harming normal cells. Two methods have recently shown promise in developing immune therapy. G17DT is a fusion protein consisting of gastrin 17 and diphtheria toxin. Through administration of G17DT, neutralizing antibodies to glycine-extended gastrin 17 may be formed. pancreatic cancers can be stimulated by amidated gastrin to increase expression of EGFR ligands, matrix metalloproteinases, and anti-apoptotic factors. A phase II randomized trial of G17DT versus placebo in patients unable to or unwilling to undergo chemotherapy was reported.[26] Median survival for G17DT was 5 months compared to 2.7 months for placebo (p=0.03). These data warrant further investigation.

An alternative immune therapy approach is to vaccinate the patient against proteins that are preferentially expressed by tumor cells. Two examples of such proteins are MUC-1 and CEA. A recently reported phase I trial vaccinated patients to CEA using a vaccinia CEA vaccine for one dose then a fowlpox CEA vaccine, both of which were co-administered with 3 T-cell costimulatory molecules.[27] Enhanced CEA-specific T cell responses were seen in the majority of patients and intriguing stable diseases were seen in a variety of cancers. This agent is currently being studied in a randomized trial vs 5-FU or irinotecan as treatment for pancreatic cancer patients who have progressed on gemcitabine.

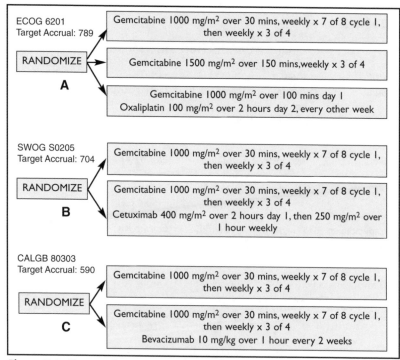

Figure 7-1. Cooperative group randomized trials open in the United States as of January 1, 2005.

CONCLUSION

Systemic therapy of pancreatic cancer has had limited impact on the natural history of disease. While oxaliplatin or altering the schedule of gemcitabine may still improve upon the results of single agent gemcitabine, future benefits from chemotherapy are likely to be limited. Therefore, newer "targeted" therapies and immune therapies provide hope for more significant improvements in disease control. Currently active United States cooperative group trials are depicted in Figure 7-1.

LOCALLY ADVANCED DISEASE

The patients in this category generally have no evidence of metastatic disease, but have involvement of major vascular trunks such as the superior mesenteric artery or vein, the celiac trunk, or the portal vein. The determination of operability of an individual cancer should be made by a multidisciplinary team and is not part of the scope of this chapter.

Because this is a localized setting, radiation therapy has been studied as the primary treatment modality in this setting. It has been studied alone and in combination with chemotherapy. Table 7-7 contains a list of schedules of chemotherapy + radiation used in trials for locally advanced disease.

Table 7-7

CHEMORADIATION REGIMENS

Agent	Dose	Schedule	Duration	# of Courses
5-FU	350 mg/m² bolus	Days 1 to 3	During XRT	2 courses separated by a 2 week break
XRT	1.8 Gy/day	Daily x 5 each week	2 weeks	
5-FU	200 mg/m²/day	Continuous infusion	During XRT	1 course
XRT	1.8 Gy/day	Daily x 5 each week	5.5 weeks (50.4 Gy)	
Capecitabine	825 mg/m²	Orally BID	During XRT	1 course
XRT	1.8 Gy/day	Daily x 5 each week	5.5 weeks (50.4 Gy)	
Gemcitabine	600 mg/m²/week	Weekly	During XRT	1 course
XRT[1]	1.8 Gy/day	Daily x 5 each week	5.5 weeks (50.4 Gy)	
Gemcitabine	1000 mg/m²/week	Weekly x 3	During XRT	1 course
XRT*	2.4 Gy/day	Daily x 5 each week	3 weeks (36 Gy)	

Radiosensitizing chemotherapy listed only. Postradiation regimens have consisted of 5-FU or gemcitabine regimens listed in Tables 7-1 and 7-5.

[1]Field size was reduced at 39.6 Gy; *Field size was much smaller than standard

In an attempt to improve upon overall disease control, chemotherapy was administered both during radiation therapy (chemoradiation) to sensitize cells to radiation for improved local control and after radiation to improve systemic control of pancreatic cancer. The Gastrointestinal Tumor Study Group (GITSG) performed a randomized trial comparing 60 Gy of radiation to either 40 Gy or 60 Gy of radiation in combination with 5-FU chemotherapy.[28] The radiation was given in 2-week blocks administering 2 Gy fractions 5 days per week for 2 weeks (total=20 Gy over 2 weeks) followed by 2-week breaks (Figure 7-2A). Therefore, the 40 Gy arm had 1 break during radiation and the 60 Gy arms had 2 breaks. Both chemotherapy + radiation arms performed significantly better than the radiation alone arm. Survival times for the high dose and low dose chemoradiation arms were 9.3 months and 9.7 months, respectively, while it was only 5.3 months for radiation alone.[29] This established chemoradiation as a standard against which to compare other treatments. In addition, using this administration schedule, this study established that higher doses of radiation were not better than 40 Gy. The GITSG

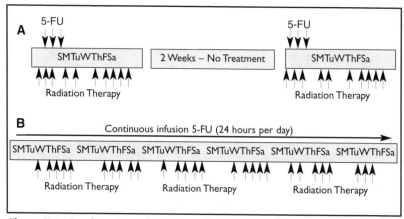

Figure 7-2. Graphic view of 5-FU + radiation schedules used in trials in pancreatic cancer.

also studied chemoradiation against chemotherapy alone. The chemoradiation included 5-FU during radiation and postradiation 5-FU in combination with 2 older agents now rarely used, mitomycin C and streptozocin (SMF). The study accrued 43 patients and found an improvement in survival of 9.7 months for chemoradiation vs 7.4 months for chemotherapy alone (p<0.02). While this study suggested chemoradiation was superior to chemotherapy alone, a second trial performed by ECOG randomly assigned 50 patients to 5-FU or to 5-FU + radiation.[30] The same median survivals were 8.2 and 8.3 months, respectively. Thus, with only these 2 trials of chemoradiation vs. chemotherapy, there is no certainty as to the standard care of locally advanced pancreatic cancer patients. Technology and understanding have both advanced. It is now possible to administer 5-FU with a continuous infusion outpatient pump, which theoretically optimizes the radiosensitization properties of 5-FU since it only has a 10-minute half-life. In addition, the 2 week breaks allowed in the GITSG trials theoretically negate the efficacy of the radiation by allowing tumor re-growth during the break. Current standards of radiation have led to a dose of 50.4 Gy in 1.8 Gy fractions as the dose for radiation to the pancreas. A phase I trial conducted by the Eastern Cooperative Oncology Group (ECOG) established a safe dose for continuous infusion 5-FU and radiation therapy to the current standard dosage of 50.4 Gy in patients with pancreatic cancer (Figure 7-2B).[31]

The current focus of clinical trials for locally advanced pancreatic cancer focus on testing new agents in combination with radiation therapy. Gemcitabine has undergone extensive testing since it supplanted 5-FU as the standard of care for metastatic disease. Using the weekly schedule of gemcitabine in combination with 50.4 Gy radiation in 1.8 Gy fractions, doses of 600 mg/m^2 have been administered compared to 1000 mg/m^2 when given without radiation.[32] This is despite the fact that the radiation field in this regimen is reduced from 3 cm around gross tumor volume (GTV) to 2 cm around GTV when the radiation dose is 39.6 Gy. However, some preclinical studies have suggested that gemcitabine radiosensitization is only effective for approximately 72 hours. Based on this data, studies of twice weekly gemcitabine in combination with full dose radiation were conducted. The CALGB phase II trial with 39 evaluable patients resulted in only an 8.2 month median survival at the expense of serious (grade 3 or 4) hematologic toxicity in 21% of patients and grade 3 gastrointestinal toxicity in 10% of patients. This survival was not felt to be long enough to further pursue the regimen. An interesting phase I approach was to administer the gemcitabine at full dose then escalate the radiation dose. In this case, weekly gemcitabine of 1000 mg/m^2 was used during a 3-week course of radiation therapy.[34] The dose per fraction of radiation for the phase II trial was 36 Gy over 15 fractions (2.4 Gy per fraction). This trial also employed smaller radiation fields than used on other studies, meaning that these data are not applicable to a standard field size. When 41 locally advanced, unresectable patients and preoperative resectable patients were treated, two patients responded to therapy and 25 had stable disease while 20% had grade 3 gastrointestinal toxicities. The investigators have now successfully added cisplatin to this gemcitabine + radiation regimen.[35] Finally, in at least one trial, adding gemcitabine to standard infusional 5-FU + radiation was not well tolerated.[36]

CONCLUSION

Locally advanced disease patients are currently treated with chemotherapy alone (included with patients on metastatic trials) or with chemotherapy + radiation. The current ECOG randomized trial will help to define the role of chemoradiation vs chemotherapy alone by testing gemcitabine with or without radiation therapy. Other groups are trying to improve upon chemoradiation by adding newer agents such as cetuximab, erlotinib, and bevacizumab.

RESECTABLE DISEASE

Patients with resectable disease represent a small subset (<10% of all patients) of pancreatic cancer patients. However, even if the cancer can be completely removed with negative margins (no microscopic or macroscopic residual disease at the cut edges), the majority still have recurrences, with only 20% of patients alive at 5 years.

Adjuvant therapy is the term used for treatment administered to patients who have completed a definitive primary therapy such as surgery. The purpose of adjuvant therapy is to eliminate microscopic residual disease and reduce risk of cancer recurrence. Patients with pancreatic cancer who have undergone complete resection with negative margins (R0) or with only microscopic residual disease (R1) have been studied to learn the benefits of either chemotherapy alone or in combination with radiation therapy for adjuvant treatment. Data on adjuvant therapy remain limited.

The GITSG compared surgery alone to a treatment arm consisting of surgery followed first by combined chemotherapy with radiation (chemoradiation) and subsequently by 24 months of weekly bolus 5-FU chemotherapy.[37] The chemoradiation consisted of bolus 5-FU on days 1 to 3 of each of two 2-week courses of 20 Gy of radiation, totaling 40 Gy. Forty-three patients were randomized over 8 years. Survival in the control arm was 11 months compared to 20 months in the adjuvant treatment arm (p=0.035). However, this trial was small and took a long time to accrue. To confirm the findings of the randomized trial, the GITSG subsequently enrolled 30 patients on a phase II adjuvant trial using the same regimen of chemoradiation followed by 2 years of weekly bolus 5-FU.[38] At 18 months, the median survival was similar to the treatment arm of the phase III trial. These results suggest that chemoradiation followed by chemotherapy can be considered a possible standard option for adjuvant therapy.

However, as discussed earlier, there is theoretical benefit for more continuous administration of both 5-FU and radiation, particularly in combination. In a large randomized trial of rectal cancer adjuvant therapy, continuous infusion 5-FU combined with radiation therapy significantly improved disease-free and overall survival compared to bolus administration of 5-FU. Although rectal cancer is a different disease, theoretically the principles hold for radiation sensitization between disease sites.

The EORTC conducted a randomized trial comparing continuous infusion 5-FU and 50.4 Gy radiation (Figure 7-2B) after surgery versus surgery alone.[39] No chemotherapy was given after completing chemoradiation. This trial enrolled 207 patients, of whom 114 were pancreatic cancer patients. The remaining patients had periampullary tumors. For the overall group, there was no difference in median survival between the surgery alone arm and the chemoradiation arm (19 months vs 24.5 months, respectively, p<NS). At 5 years, 28% of patients receiving chemoradiation were still alive compared to 22% of patients who did not have adjuvant therapy, which was also not statistically significant. However, when a subset analysis was performed, the pancreatic cancer patients had a trend toward improved survival favoring the chemoradiation arm (17.1 months vs 12.6 months, p=0.099), suggesting a need for further studies to be performed.

The most recently reported randomized trial, titled ESPAC-1, was designed to evaluate the roles of both chemotherapy and chemoradiation.[40,41] A 2-x-2 design was employed in which patients were randomized to either chemotherapy or no chemotherapy and chemoradiation or no chemoradiation (referring to chemotherapy during radiation only). If patients were randomized to chemoradiation or chemotherapy, then the chemoradiation was administered first. Chemotherapy consisted of bolus 5-FU for 6 months. Chemoradiation consisted of bolus 5-FU in combination with radiation administered in the same split-course therapy as in the GITSG trial (see Figure 7-2A). ESPAC-1 was designed to evaluate only the patients randomized in a 2-x-2 fashion, but some institutions were allowed to enroll patients in only one of the two randomizations.[40] These patients were never designed to be part of the primary evaluation. In the preliminary report of ESPAC-1, the patients randomized in a 2-x-2 fashion were combined with the subsets that were only randomized once. The data suggested that benefit came from chemotherapy compared to no chemotherapy but no benefit was derived from the use of chemoradiation. The final report was recently released with 47 months median follow-up for survivors.[41] Because the primary analysis was designed to evaluate only the 289 patients in the 2-x-2 randomization group, the subset randomized only once was not included in the final report. The patients randomized to chemotherapy had a statistically significantly longer median survival than patients not randomized to chemotherapy (20.1 months vs 15.5 months, respectively, p=0.0009). In contrast, those patients randomly assigned to chemoradiation had a nonsignificant shorter survival than those randomized to no chemoradiation (15.9 months vs 17.9 months, respectively, p<NS). Although this study suggested a possible detriment from chemoradiation, ESPAC-1 used a split-course radiation therapy with bolus 5-FU. The trial does not address the role of infusional 5-FU administered concurrently with a more continuous course of radiation.

Current clinical trials are attempting to integrate other agents into the adjuvant therapy of pancreatic cancer. Gemcitabine, 2',2'-difluorodeoxycytidine, is a cytidine analogue that is activated to a phosphorylated form and incorporated into DNA, resulting in chain termination (triphosphate form) and also inhibits the enzyme ribonucleotide reductase (diphosphate form). It is the current standard therapy for metastatic disease.

In Europe, ESPAC-3 is currently testing the regimen of 5-FU from ESPAC-1 vs 6 months of gemcitabine as adjuvant therapy. No radiation is included. A third arm of surgery alone was dropped based on the final results of ESPAC-1. In the United States, the intergroup (a collaboration of many of the cancer cooperative groups) completed a trial testing gemcitabine versus 5-FU with both administered before and after chemoradiation consisting of continuous infusion of 5-FU with 50.4 Gy of radiation. The data from this trial should be available in 2005. In a single institution study of this chemoimmunotherapy with radiation, ß-interferon, cisplatin, and infusional 5-FU were combined with radiation followed by postradiation 5-FU.[42] Actuarial survival for the 43 patients was estimated to be 95%, 64%, and 55% at 1, 2, and 5 years, respectively. The regimen, however, was very toxic, with 42% of patients hospitalized, but no deaths reported. Therefore, the ACOSOG is studying a slight modification of this chemoimmunotherapy + radiation regimen to better establish safety and efficacy.

CONCLUSION

Four randomized trials have been conducted in adjuvant therapy of pancreatic cancer thus far. ESPAC-1 has established a benefit to adjuvant chemotherapy with 5-FU and established that split course chemoradiation is ineffective. However, questions still remain as to the role of chemoradiation using more modern regimens, the role of neoadjuvant therapy, and the impact of newer systemic agents.

REFERENCES

1. Jemal A, Tiwari RC, Murray T, et al. Cancer statistics 2004. *CA Cancer J Clin.* 2004;54: 8-29.
2. Glimelius B, Hoffman K, Sjoden PO, et al. Chemotherapy improves survival and quality of life in advanced pancreatic and biliary cancer. *Ann Oncol.* 1996;7:593-600.
3. Palmer KR, Kerr M, Knowles G, et al. Chemotherapy prolongs survival in inoperable pancreatic carcinoma. *Br J Surg.* 1994;81:882-5.
4. Carmichael J, Fink U, Russell RC, et al. Phase II study of gemcitabine in patients with advanced pancreatic cancer. *Br J Cancer.* 1996;73:101-5.
5. Casper ES, Green MR, Kelsen DP, et al. Phase II trial of gemcitabine (2,2'-difluorodeoxycytidine) in patients with adenocarcinoma of the pancreas. *Investigational New Drugs.* 1994;12:29-34.
6. Rothenberg ML, Moore MJ, Cripps MC, et al. A phase II trial of gemcitabine in patients with 5-FU-refractory pancreas cancer. *Annals of Oncology.* 1996;7:347-53.
7. Burris HA 3rd, Moore MJ, Andersen J, et al. Improvements in survival and clinical benefit with gemcitabine as first-line therapy for patients with advanced pancreas cancer: a randomized trial. *J Clin Oncol.* 1997;15:2403-13.
8. Tempero M, Plunkett W, Ruiz van Haperen V, et al. Randomized phase II comparison of dose-intense gemcitabine: thirty-minute infusion and fixed dose rate infusion in patients with pancreatic adenocarcinoma. *J Clin Oncol.* 2003;21:3402-3408.
9. Berlin JD, Adak S, Vaughn DJ, et al. A phase II study of gemcitabine and 5-fluorouracil in metastatic pancreatic cancer: an Eastern Cooperative Oncology Group study (E3296). *Oncology.* 2000;58:215-218.
10. Oettle H, Pelzer U, Hochmuth K, et al. Phase I trial of gemcitabine (Gemzar), 24 h infusion 5-fluorouracil and folinic acid in patients with inoperable pancreatic cancer. *Anticancer Drugs.* 1999;10:699-704.

11. Hidalgo M, Castellano D, Paz-Ares L, et al. Phase I-II study of gemcitabine and fluorouracil as a continuous infusion in patients with pancreatic cancer. *J Clin Oncol.* 1999;17:585-592.

12. Berlin JD, Catalano P, Thomas JP, et al. Phase III study of gemcitabine in combination with fluorouracil versus gemcitabine alone in patients with advanced pancreatic carcinoma: Eastern Cooperative Oncology Group Trial E2297. *J Clin Oncol.* 2002; 20:3270-3275.

13. Richards DA, Kindler HL, Oettle H, et al. A randomized phase III study comparing gemcitabine + pemetrexed versus gemcitabine in patients with locally advanced and metastatic pancreas cancer. *J Clin Oncol.* 2004;22(14S):4005

14. Rocha Lima CM, Green MR, Rotche R, et al. Irinotecan plus gemcitabine results in no survival advantage compared with gemcitabine monotherapy in patients with locally advanced or metastatic pancreatic cancer despite increased tumor response rate. *J Clin Oncol.* 2004;22:3776-3783.

15. Cheverton P, Friess H, Andras C, et al. Phase III results of exatecan (DX-8951f) versus gemcitabine (Gem) in chemotherapy-naïve patients with advanced pancreatic cancer (APC). *J Clin Oncol.* 2004;22(14S):(abstr 4005).

16. O Reilly EM, Abou-Alfa GK, Letourneau R, et al. A randomized phase III trial of DX-8951f (exatecan mesylate; DX) and gemcitabine (GEM) vs gemcitabine alone in advanced pancreatic cancer (APC). *J Clin Oncol.* 2004;22(14S):(abstr 4006).

17. Heinemann V, Quietzsch D, Gieseler F, et al. A phase III trial comparing gemcitabine plus cisplatin vs. gemcitabine alone in advanced pancreatic carcinoma. *Proc Amer Soc Clin Oncol.* 2003;22:250 (updated from online presentation).

18. Louvet C, Labianca R, Hammel P, et al. GemOx (gemcitabine + oxaliplatin) versus Gem (gemcitabine) in non resectable pancreatic adenocarcinoma: final results of the GERCOR /GISCAD Intergroup Phase III. *J Clin Oncol.* 2004;22(14S):(abstr 4008).

19. Xiong HQ, Rosenberg A, LoBuglio A, et al. Cetuximab, a monoclonal antibody targeting the epidermal growth factor receptor, in combination with Gemcitabine for advanced pancreatic cancer: a multicenter phase II trial. *J Clin Oncol.* 2004;22:2610-2616

20. Genentech Press Release. Sept 20, 2004

21. Van Cutsem E, van de Velde H, Karasek P, et al. Phase III trial of gemcitabine plus tipifarnib compared with gemcitabine plus placebo in advanced pancreatic cancer. *J Clin Oncol.* 2004; 22:1430-1438.

22. Moore MJ, Hamm J, Dancey J, et al. Comparison of gemcitabine versus the matrix metalloproteinase inhibitor BAY 12-9566 in patients with advanced or metastatic adenocarcinoma of the pancreas: a phase III trial of the National Cancer Institute of Canada Clinical Trials Group. *J Clin Oncol.* 2003;21:3296-3302.

23. Bramhall SR, Rosemurgy A, Brown PD, Bowry C, Buckels JAC. Marimastat as first-line therapy for patients with unresectable pancreatic cancer: a randomized trial. *J Clin Oncol.* 2001;19:3447-3455.

24. Bramhall SR, Schulz J, Nemunaitis J, et al. A double-blind placebo-controlled, randomised study comparing gemcitabine and marimastat with gemcitabine and placebo as first line therapy in patients with advanced pancreatic cancer. *Br J Cancer.* 2002; 87:161-167.

25. Kindler HL, Friberg G, Stadler WM, et al. Bevacizumab (B) plus gemcitabine (G) in patient (pts) with advanced pancreatic cancer (PC): updated results of a multi-center phase II trial. *J Clin Oncol.* 2004;22(14S):4009.

26. Gilliam D, Topuzov EG, Garin AM, et al. Randomised, double blind, placebo-controlled, multi-centre, group-sequential trial of G17DT for patients with advanced pancreatic cancer unsuitable or unwilling to take chemotherapy. *J Clin Oncol.* 2004;22 (14S):2511.

27. John L. Marshall JL, Gulley JL, et al. Phase I study of sequential vaccinations with Fowlpox-CEA(6D)-TRICOM aone and sequentially with Vaccinia-CEA(6D)-TRI-COM, with and without granulocyte-macrophage colony-stimulating factor, in patients with carcinoembryonic antigen-expressing carcinomas. *J Clin Oncol.* 2005;23(early online release).

28. Moertel CG, Frytak S, Hahn RG, et al. Therapy of locally unresectable pancreatic carcinoma: A randomized comparison of high dose (6000 rads) radiation alone, moderate dose radiation (4000 Rads + 5-fluorouracil), and high dose radiation + 5-fluorouracil. *Cancer.* 1981;48:1705-1710.

29. Gastrointestinal Tumor Study Group. Treatment of locally unresecatble carcinoma of the pancreas: Comparison of combined-modality therapy (chemotherapy plus radiotherapy) to chemotherapy alone. *J Natl Cancer Inst.* 1988;80:751-754.

30. Klaasen DJ, MacIntyre JM, Catton GE, et al. Treatment of locally unresectable cancer of the stomach and pancreas: a randomized comparison of 5-fluorouracil alone with radiation plus concurrent and maintenance 5-fluorouracil. An Eastern Cooperative Oncology Group study. *J Clin Oncol.* 1985;3:373-378.

31. Whittington R, Neuberg D, Tester WJ, et al. Protracted intravenous fluorouracil infusion with radiation therapy in the management of localized pancreaticobiliary carcinoma: A phase I Eastern Cooperative Oncology Group trial. *J Clin Oncol.* 1995;13:227-232.

32. McGinn CJ, et al. A phase I study of gemcitabine (GEM) in combination with radiation therapy (RT) in patients with localized, unresectable pancreatic cancer. *Proc Amer Soc Clin Oncol.* 1998;17:A1091.

33. Blackstock AW, Tepper JE, Niedwiecki D, et al. Cancer and leukemia group B (CALGB) 89805: phase II chemoradiation trial using gemcitabine in patients with locoregional adenocarcinoma of the pancreas. *Int J Gastrointest Cancer.* 2003;34(2-3):107-116.

34. McGinn CJ, Zalupski MM, Shureiqi I, et al. Phase I trial of radiation dose escalation with concurrent weekly full-dose gemcitabine in patients with advanced pancreatic cancer. *J Clin Oncol.* 2001;19:4202-4208.

35. Muler JH, McGinn CJ, Normolle D, et al. Phase I trial using a time-to-event continual reassessment strategy for dose escalation of cisplatin combined with Gemcitabine and radiation therapy in pancreatic cancer. *J Clin Oncol.* 2004;22(2):238-243.

36. Talamonti MS, Catalano PJ, Vaughn DJ, et al. Eastern Cooperative Oncology Group phase I trial of protracted venous infusion fluorouracil plus weekly gemcitabine with concurrent radiation therapy in patients with locally advanced pancreas cancer: a regimen with unexpected early toxicity. *J Clin Oncol.* 2000;18:3384-3389.

37. Kalser MH, Ellenberg SS. Pancreatic cancer. Adjuvant combined radiation and chemotherapy following curative resection. *Arch Surg.* 1985;120:899-903 [erratum appears in *Arch Surg.* 1986;121(9):1045].

38. Gastrointestinal Tumor Study Group. Further evidence of effective adjuvant combined radiation and chemotherapy following curative resection of pancreatic cancer. *Cancer.* 1987;59:2006-10.

39. Klinkenbijl JH, Jeekel J, Sahmoud T, et al. Adjuvant radiotherapy and 5-fluorouracil after curative resection of cancer of the pancreas and periampullary region: phase III trial of the EORTC gastrointestinal tract cancer cooperative group. *Ann Surg.* 1999;230:776-782.

40. Neoptolemos JP, Dunn JA, Stocken DD. Adjuvant chemoradiotherapy and chemotherapy in resectable pancreatic cancer: a randomised controlled trial. *Lancet.* 2001;358: 1576-1585.

41. Neoptolemos JP, Stocken DD, Friess H, et al. A randomized trial of chemoradiotherapy and chemotherapy after resection of pancreatic cancer. *N Engl J Med.* 2004;350: 1200-10 [erratum appears in *N Engl J Med.* 2004;351(7):726].

42. Picozzi VJ, Kozarek RA, Traverso LW. Interferon-based adjuvant chemoradiation therapy after pancreaticoduodenectomy for pancreatic adenocarcinoma. *Am J Surg.* 2003; 185:476-80

Endoscopic Retrograde Cholangiopancreatography in the Management of Pancreaticobiliary Neoplasia

Ilias Scotiniotis, MD

INTRODUCTION

Pancreaticobiliary malignances can be divided into tumors of the ampulla of Vater, tumors of the bile ducts, tumors of the pancreas, and metastatic disease affecting the biliary system. Endoscopy had little role in the management of these conditions until 1968, when the first description of endoscopic cannulation of the ampulla of Vater was published, thus signaling the birth of ERCP. This was followed in 1979 by the first description of biliary stent placement, which greatly increased the therapeutic utility of pancreaticobiliary endoscopy. In the years that followed, ERCP became the "gold standard" for imaging and draining the pancreaticobiliary tree. At present, a large portion of the 30,000 cases of pancreatic cancer and 7000 cases of biliary cancer diagnosed each year in the United States undergo ERCP at some point in the course of their illness. The recent development of less invasive diagnostic modalities, such as dual-phase helical CT, MRCP, and EUS, results in a fine-tuning of the application of ERCP, such that a majority of these procedures are now performed with therapeutic rather than diagnostic intent. This chapter will discuss the role of ERCP in the evaluation and management of pancreaticobiliary malignancies.

TECHNIQUE OF ERCP

ERCP is a technically demanding procedure. In experienced hands, it is a safe and well-tolerated procedure that can usually be performed on an out-patient basis. The procedure is performed with the patient in a modified prone position to enhance visualization of the pancreaticobiliary tree, and imaging is obtained with a fluoroscopic unit. Conscious sedation is administered, typically with intravenous midazolam and meperidine or fentanyl. Propofol administration by an anesthesiologist is used increasingly for patients who are difficult to sedate. Duodenoscopes used for ERCP are specially designed with side-viewing orientation to offer an "en face" view of the major papilla. The outer diameter of a duodenoscope is 10.5 to 12.5 mm, as compared with a diameter of 9 mm for a diagnostic upper endoscope. It should be noted that the side-viewing orientation of the endoscopes used for ERCP allows for only a cursory examination of the esophagus, stomach, and duodenal bulb. Examination of the upper gastrointestinal tract with a side-viewing duodenoscope is therefore not a substitute for evaluation with a forward-viewing upper endoscope, except for those with experience.

In a patient with a prior gastrectomy and Billroth II anastomosis, reaching the ampulla of Vater can be a challenge, since the duodenoscope must ascend the length of the afferent limb in a retrograde direction. Pyloric or duodenal stenosis or a Roux-en-Y gastrojejunostomy may make it impossible to reach the papilla. Once the major papilla has been reached in the second portion of the duodenum, a cannulation catheter is passed through the working channel of the endoscope. By maneuvering the tip of the endoscope and angling the tip of the catheter with an "elevator" lever, selective cannulation of the bile duct or pancreatic duct is performed. Radiopaque dye is then injected under fluoroscopic inspection. Selective cannulation of the desired duct requires considerable endoscopic skill and experience. Successful cannulation should be achieved in more than 90% of cases. A variety of catheter designs and guidewires are available to assist in cannulation.

THE NORMAL CHOLANGIOGRAM

Once bile duct cannulation has been accomplished, care must be taken to define all aspects of the biliary tree, including intrahepatic and extrahepatic ducts, as well as the cystic duct and gallbladder if possible (Figure 8-1). The origin and course of the cystic duct are highly variable. The left hepatic duct is slightly longer than the right. With the patient in the usual prone position during ERCP, the left hepatic duct is in a dependent position and therefore fills preferentially when contrast material is injected into the common bile duct. The muscular wall of the distal common bile duct at the sphincter of Oddi can appear as a shelf-like "notch" in the cholangiogram, and this may be mistaken for a stricture. One differentiates this finding from a true distal stricture by watching the notch disappear as contrast medium empties from the duct, as opposed to the fixed appearance of a true stricture.

ENDOSCOPIC STENTING

The technique of endoscopic stent placement across an obstructive biliary lesion is relatively straightforward once the stricture has been traversed with a guidewire. In the majority of cases, it is not necessary to cut through the muscular fibers of the sphincter of Oddi (ie, sphincterotomy) prior to placing a biliary stent. On the other hand, sphincterotomy may be helpful if multiple stents are to be placed (which is sometimes done for lesions at the hepatic duct bifurcation) or if subsequent stent exchanges are anticipated. Similarly, dilation of the stricture is usually not performed, but may be necessary prior to stent placement for complex, tight strictures.

The stents most commonly used in patients with malignant obstruction are made of polyethylene and have flaps at both ends to prevent migration. They have a slightly curved shape to conform to the course of the bile duct. "Pigtail" stents are rarely used because they have been shown to have lower flow rates. The typical stent has an outside diameter of 10 French (3.3 mm), allowing it to fit through the channel of the endo-

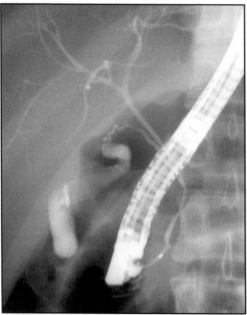

Figure 8-1A. Normal cholangiogram in a young patient. A catheter has been placed in the distal common bile duct for contrast injection. The cystic duct is seen leading to the gallbladder. The bifurcation of the common hepatic duct into left and right hepatic ducts is demonstrated.

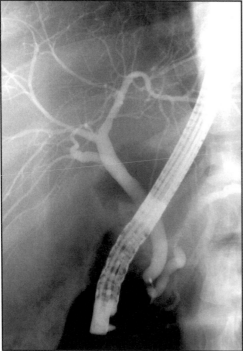

Figure 8-1B. Normal cholangiogram in elderly patient. Advanced age is associated with a 'fuller' appearance of the biliary system. The diameter of the bile duct can be compared to the 12 mm outer diameter of the duodenoscope. As seen, the left hepatic duct is often longer than the right. There is opacification of the distal pancreatic duct, seen coursing to the right of the distal common bile duct. The cystic duct and gallbladder have not filled with contrast.

scope. Unfortunately, once a plastic stent is placed, gradual occlusion is an inexorable process. This is initiated by the build-up of a bacterial biofilm on the inner surface of the stent, which eventually leads to stent occlusion within 4 to 6 months. Modifications in stent design trying to counter that process have not resulted in longer patency rates, including stents constructed out of smoother material (such as Teflon [DuPont, Wilmington, Del]), stents with inner surfaces that are coated with a hydrophilic polymer, or stents that are impregnated with antibiotics.[1]

A major breakthrough in stent technology has been the development of self-expanding metallic stents (SEMS), which have the advantage of longer patency due to greater diameter. They are delivered in a compressed state, allowing them to fit through the channel of the duodenoscope. Once they are placed across the stricture, they are allowed to expand, reaching an outer diameter of 30 French (10 mm). For metal stents, occlusion can occur as a result of tumor ingrowth through the mesh of the stent (which is currently being addressed by the testing of metal stents fitted with an inner covering of plastic) or the deposition of debris through the reflux of ingested food from the duodenum. The relative indications for their use are discussed later in the chapter.

It should be noted that stenting of the pancreatic duct has been shown to lead to rapid development of fibrotic changes along the duct wall. For that reason, as well as its technically demanding nature, pancreatic stent placement is not routinely performed. Most stents placed into the pancreatic duct should not be left in place for more than a few weeks.

COMPLICATIONS OF ERCP

Complications related to ERCP can be divided into those that are inherent to any prolonged endoscopic procedure and those that are specific to ERCP and sphinctorotomy. The former include aspiration pneumonia, adverse cardiovascular or neurologic events related to sedation, drug reactions, and perforation. The most common ERCP-specific complication is pancreatitis, occurring in 5% of patients and accounting for more that half of the total complications (Table 8-1). Typical pancreatitis-like pain is present in those cases. The mere elevation of serum levels of pancreatic enzymes is not diagnostic of post-ERCP pancreatitis, since 75% of uncomplicated ERCPs are followed by a transient "bump" in amylase or lipase levels. Sphincterotomy may be complicated by serious bleeding in 2% of cases, and this can be managed endoscopically in the great majority of cases. Cholangitis, occurring in about 1% of ERCP procedures, usually results from inadequate ductal drainage following contrast injection.

Complications specific to stent placement include stent migration and stent occlusion. The clinical picture of the 2 is indistinguishable, since they both result in recurrence of obstruction and possibly cholangitis. Stent migration may be spontaneous or caused by inappropriate placement. If a stent migrates proximally (into the bile duct), it has to be retrieved endoscopically, since a nondraining stent will form the nidus for infection. If a stent migrates distally, its distal end may compress and erode into the duodenal wall opposite the ampulla of Vater, causing hemorrhage or perforation. If it passes completely out of the bile duct into the duodenal lumen, it need not be retrieved and can be left to pass spontaneously.

Table 8-1

COMPLICATIONS OF ENDOSCOPIC SPHINCTEROTOMY

Type of Complication	Percent With Complication	Percent With Severe Complication
Pancreatitis	5.4	0.4
Hemorrhage	2.0	0.5
Perforation	0.3	0.2
Cholangitis	1.0	0.1
Cholecystitis	1.0	0.1
Miscellaneous*	1.1	0.3
Any complication	9.8	1.6

*Includes cardiopulmonary complications, ductal perforations by guidewire, stent malfunction, antibiotic-induced diarrhea, indeterminate fluid collection, and infection of pancreatic pseudocyst.

ERCP AS A DIAGNOSTIC TOOL IN PANCREATICOBILIARY MALIGNANCY

In patients who present with painless jaundice due to malignancy, 85% of tumors are pancreatic carcinomas, 6% are cholangiocarcinomas, and 4.5% each are duodenal and ampullary carcinomas. Making the distinction between these is important, since duodenal and ampullary lesions have a significantly better prognosis. Until fairly recently, ERCP represented the most effective method of imaging the pancreaticobiliary system. The emergence of helical CT in the past decade has resulted in a reassessment of that role. A helical CT performed with a 'pancreatic protocol' provides fine cuts through the pancreas during both the arterial and venous phases, and is a sensitive means of detecting tumors of the pancreatic head, the most common type of pancreaticobiliary malignancy. A helical CT should therefore be obtained early in the evaluation of a patient with suspected pancreaticobiliary malignancy, preferably with a dual-phase, fine-cut pancreatic protocol.

In a significant number of patients, however, diagnostic uncertainty remains after the initial CT. This may be either because a "typical" mass in the head of the pancreas is not seen, which is the case in bile duct, ampullary, and duodenal cancers, or because of inherent limitations of the CT study, such as not performing it with a pancreatic protocol. Several options exist in that setting (Figure 8-2). One is to obtain indirect cholangiopancreatography using MRI. The technique of MRCP is noninvasive and does not expose the patient to the ERCP risk of pancreatitis and cholangitis. A second option is to clarify any indeterminate CT findings in the pancreas through EUS. This modality is performed by placing the tip of an ultrasound-emitting endoscope adjacent to the head of the pancreas in the second portion of the duodenum. It uses high ultrasound frequencies to obtain high resolution images of the pancreatic parenchyma and is a highly

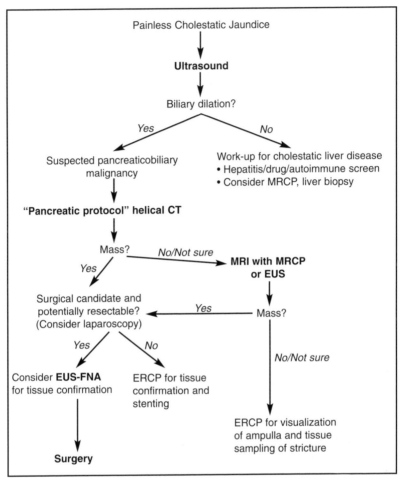

Figure 8-2. An algorithm for the evaluation of a patient with painless jaundice.

sensitive means of detecting neoplastic lesions in the pancreas. EUS can be coupled with FNA of a suspicious lesion, with a reported sensitivity of 93% and a specificity of 100% in the detection of pancreatic malignancy[2] (Figure 8-3). EUS is thus evolving as a procedure of choice in the investigation of atypical presentations of pancreatic malignancy.

For many reasons, however, ERCP remains an important diagnostic tool in pancreaticobiliary malignancy. First, both MRCP and EUS of a high quality still remain the purvue of large, specialized centers and are often not available to the wider medical community. Second, ERCP offers direct visualization of the duodenum and ampulla and is the superior means of diagnosing tumors in those locations (Figure 8-4). Third, in cases of a biliary stricture, it can provide the definitive diagnosis by tissue cytology or biopsy. A final argument in support of ERCP for "atypical" presentations of malignancy is that all experienced endoscopists have been occasionally surprised by the unexpected finding

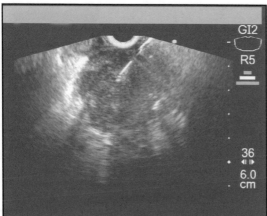

Figure 8-3. Endoscopic ultrasound-guided fine needle aspiration (EUS-FNA) of pancreatic mass. The pancreatic head is imaged from the duodenum using a specialized endoscope fitted with an ultrasound transducer at its tip. The mass is visualized as a dark, round lesion surrounded by normal pancreas, which is brighter. A needle has been advanced into the mass under ultrasound guidance in order to obtain a diagnostic specimen.

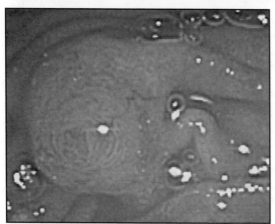

Figure 8-4A. Ampulla of Vater. Normal ampulla as seen using a side-viewing endoscope in the second portion of duodenum. A transverse duodenal fold is seen draping over the upper margin of the papillary mound. *For a full-color version, see page CA-IV of the Color Atlas.*

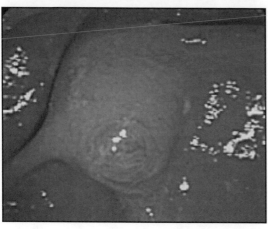

Figure 8-4B. Bulging ampulla. This was found to harbor an adenocarcinoma arising in the very distal portion of the pancreatic duct. *For full-color version, see page CA-V of the Colar Atlas.*

Table 8-2

CAUSES OF BENIGN BILIARY STRICTURES

1. Postoperative, as after cholecystectomy
2. Chronic pancreatitis
3. Primary sclerosing cholangitis
4. Extrinsic compression by cystic duct stone (Mirizzi syndrome)
5. AIDS
6. Parasitic infection (flukes, nematodes, etc)
7. Site of biliary anastomosis
8. Radiation

---

of an impacted stone at the ampulla as the cause of painless jaundice, especially in a debilitated, noncommunicative patient. For all those reasons, the importance of ERCP as a diagnostic tool increases as one moves from typical toward atypical presentations of pancreaticobiliary malignancy.

CONFIRMATION OF MALIGNANCY

A malignant stricture on cholangiogram typically displays an abrupt transition between normal and abnormal bile duct, the so-called "shouldering" or "shelflike" appearance. The location of a stricture can also determine the likelihood of malignancy, since benign strictures are almost never found at the level of the hepatic duct bifurcation. However, the appearance of a biliary stricture on ERCP cannot be considered pathognomonic for malignancy. Even the "double-duct sign" (ie, concomitant narrowing of the bile duct and the pancreatic duct with upstream dilatation), initially proposed as a specific indicator of pancreatic cancer, may be seen in benign disease such as chronic pancreatitis. The causes of benign biliary stricture are listed in Table 8-2.

Tissue confirmation of malignancy should therefore always be sought (Figure 8-5). Techniques of tissue confirmation on ERCP include forceps biopsy, bile or pancreatic juice aspiration, and brush cytology.[3] Forceps biopsy of the stricture generally requires a sphincterotomy to allow passage of the forceps into the bile duct or pancreatic duct (Figure 8-6). Bile or pancreatic juice aspiration has unacceptably low sensitivity for the detection of malignancy, around 20%. From a practical standpoint, therefore, most endoscopists limit tissue acquisition to brush cytology, because a brushing catheter can easily be passed into the duct over a guidewire.

Brush cytology has been demonstrated to have a sensitivity of approximately 40% in cases of cancer. This may be explained by the fact that pancreatic cancer often causes bile duct obstruction by means of extrinsic compression rather than direct invasion. Brushing a concomitant pancreatic duct stricture has not been shown to improve the yield significantly, but may be a reasonable supplement if it can be performed easily. The yield of brushings is even lower if obstruction is caused by hilar lymphadenopathy, local extension from an adjacent tumor (eg, gallbladder carcinoma), or metastatic disease within the liver parenchyma. On the other hand, if obstruction is caused by a cholan-

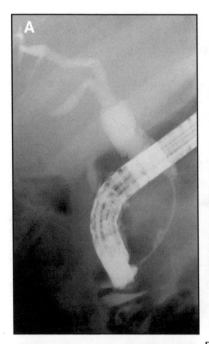

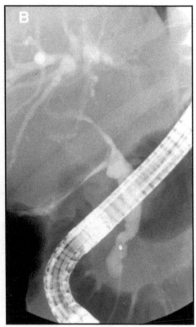

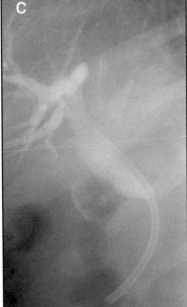

Figure 8-5. Biliary stricture. (A) Tight stricture caused by adenocarcinoma of the pancreatic head: A catheter has been placed across the stricture and contrast has been injected into a dilated proximal biliary system. (B) A benign stricture in the proximal bile duct mimicking a malignant stricture. This is in fact caused by a large stone obstructed within the cystic duct, leading to external compression of the bile duct (Mirizzi syndrome). (C) An angled plastic stent has been placed across the stricture seen in Figure 8-4A.

Figure 8-6. A forceps has been advanced into the bile duct to obtain a biopsy.

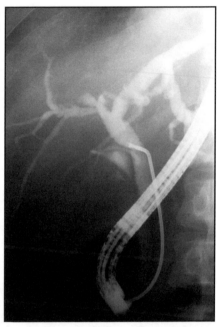

giocarcinoma, the sensitivity of brushings approaches 60%. If the cholangiocarcinoma arises in the setting of primary sclerosing cholangitis (PSC), however, the chronic inflammation of the biliary epithelium clouds the cytologic diagnosis, and the sensitivity drops to 45%.[4] For that reason, a policy of interval "surveillance" cholangiography with brush cytology has little value in patients with PSC. Instead, patients with PSC are often screened for cholangiocarcinoma with serial CEA and CA19-9 levels.

The characterization of pancreaticobiliary strictures may be improved in the future with the use of new ERCP-based techniques such as cholangiopancreatoscopy and intraductal ultrasonography.[5] Cholangiopancreatoscopy involves the advancement into the duct of a small-caliber endoscope ("baby" scope) that is passed through the channel of the regular duodenoscope ("mother" scope) (Figure 8-7). The technique allows direct visualization of the stricture. Studies from Asia report that cholangioscopy can distinguish malignant strictures by the presence of an irregular tumor vessel on their surface. However, so far cholangiopancreatoscopy has been hindered by the lack of convenient, durable, and inexpensive "baby" scopes. Intraductal ultrasonography (IDUS) involves the passage of high-frequency (12 to 30 MHz) ultrasound catheters over a guidewire into the biliary tree or pancreatic duct. Studies using criteria such as the thickness of the duct wall and symmetry of a stricture offer encouraging but still inconclusive results about the ability of IDUS to distinguish benign from malignant strictures.[6] The presence of p53 or K-*ras* mutations in cells obtained from a stricture has been shown to have little value in the diagnosis of malignancy.

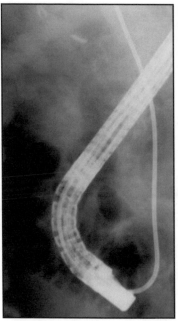

Figure 8-7. Cholangioscopy. The thin "baby" cholangioscope has been advanced into the bile duct through the "mother" duodenoscope. This allows direct evaluation and biopsy of a stricture at the bifurcation of the hepatic ducts.

Cystic Neoplasms of the Pancreas

Cystic neoplasms account for only 3% of malignant lesions of the pancreas. Mucinous cystadenocarcinomas are not ductal in origin, and their diagnosis therefore cannot be made on pancreatography. On the other hand, the rare intraductal papillary mucinous tumors (IPMT), previously termed *mucinous duct ectasia*, are often associated with the impressive and pathognomonic extrusion of mucus at the papilla of Vater. On pancreatography, diffuse filling defects of mucus are noted within a dilated main pancreatic duct and its side branches. Even if cytologic brushings in this case are not suggestive of malignancy, IPMT is almost universally a premalignant lesion, and surgical resection should be recommended if possible.

ERCP as a Staging Tool in Pancreaticobiliary Malignancy

Surgery offers the only means of potential cure in malignant tumors of the pancreas and bile duct. From the surgeon's point of view, staging of pancreaticobiliary malignancy requires answers to 2 questions. First, are there distant metastases either intra-abdominally or extra-abdominally? Second, is there local spread of tumor that precludes surgical resection?

With regard to the first question, distant metastases are usually found in the liver, lungs, and peritoneal surfaces. They are detected by CT or MRI, or laparoscopy in the case of peritoneal lesions. ERCP clearly has no role in the evaluation of these sites of distant metastases. With regard to the second question, surgery may be precluded by the invasion of vascular structures (portal vein, superior mesenteric vein, superior mesenteric artery, and hepatic artery) or lymph node metastases outside the zone of resection (such as celiac lymph node involvement). The extent of involvement with tumor of the bile duct or pancreatic duct itself is not a staging consideration because the tumors do not spread to the limit of resection of the bile duct or pancreatic duct without being unresectable for other reasons. As a result, information gleaned at ERCP has little value in the decision whether or not to operate.

One special category of tumors is that of hilar cholangiocarcinomas (also known as Klatskin tumors). These account for about two-thirds of all cholangiocarcinomas. In these lesions, the extent of bile duct involvement, especially in terms of the upper margin, is critical in determining resectability. Surgery is a reasonable option only for the rare lesions that are located below the bifurcation of the hepatic ducts (Bismuth I lesions), but not for those that extend into or above the bifucation (Bismuth II, III, or IV lesions). Cholangiography is therefore an important part of staging. This can be performed either by ERCP or MRCP. MRCP has the advantage of providing information about vascular staging and local hepatic extention as well. Furthermore, full delineation of the extent of disease in both left and right hepatic ductal systems by ERCP will result in the need for bilateral stent placement to drain the opacified ducts. For those reasons, MRCP is the preferred diagnostic method in patients with suspected hilar cholangiocarcinoma. Thus, ERCP overall has only a limited role in the staging of most pancreaticobiliary tumors.

ERCP as a Therapeutic Tool in Pancreaticobiliary Malignancy

PALLIATION OF JAUNDICE

For patients with pancreaticobiliary malignancy who are scheduled for potentially curative surgery, there is much debate on whether preoperative biliary drainage impacts on surgical morbidity and mortality. Several randomized controlled studies performed 20 years ago failed to show a benefit of preoperative biliary drainage in jaundiced patients undergoing surgery for pancreaticobiliary malignancy.[7] The majority of those patients, however, were not undergoing a Whipple pancreaticoduodenectomy, but rather palliative biliary drainage. A more recent study found that preoperative decompression increased the surgical risks due to increased infectious complications.[8] Thus, the theoretical risks of long-term biliary obstruction, such as malabsorption, malnutrition, and coagulation disorders, do not seem to be critical determinants of surgical outcome in patients with malignancy. Others have argued that stent placement in jaundiced patients may improve cardiac function by normalizing atrial natriuretic peptide (ANP) levels.[9] To this date, there is no firm consensus regarding the risks and benefit of preoperative biliary decompression by stent placement. It is fair to say that this cannot be universally recommended. If a diagnostic ERCP is performed, however, biliary decompression with stent placement is mandated once the obstructed bile duct has been instrumented.

In unresectable cases and for patients who are poor surgical candidates, long-term palliation of jaundice is an important objective, as it can ameliorate the nutritional status of the patient and the symptom of pruritus, which can be severe. Palliation of jaun-

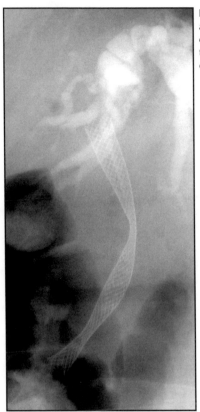

Figure 8-8. A metal stent has been placed across a malignant stricture. Its distal tip extends into the duodenal lumen, seen as the air-filled structure at the lower left side of the image.

dice can be accomplished either by endoscopic stent placement or by surgical biliary-enteric bypass, the relative merits of which have been examined in a number of studies. The most rigorous of these, published in 1994, showed that the endoscopic approach was associated with lower morbidity and mortality.[10] This study has been criticized for the unusually high number of postoperative intra-abdominal abscesses and the surgery-related mortality of 14% that it reported. On the other hand, it showed that if a patient survived surgical biliary-enteric bypass, there was rarely an episode of recurrent jaundice down the road. Superiority of the endoscopic approach shown in this study forms the basis for the current preference in most centers of endoscopic stent placement over surgical bypass in unresectable malignant biliary obstruction. As a result, most surgeons vigorously attempt to identify unresectable cases preoperatively, even employing laparoscopy to rule out occult peritoneal metastases, so as to avoid an exploratory laparotomy that would result in palliative surgical bypass.

The preference for endoscopic palliation in inoperable biliary obstruction has been strengthened by the development of SEMS, as noted earlier. These were initially designed for percutaneous deployment, but were later modified for endoscopic placement (Figure 8-8). SEMS offer the benefit of longer patency than plastic (polyethylene) stents because of their wider lumen. For distal bile duct malignant obstruction, the tip of the metal stent is left outside the papilla. For more proximal biliary tree lesions (e.g within the common hepatic duct), it is possible to place a SEMS entirely within the bile duct. In a multicenter, randomized trial of a common type of SEMS in comparison to 10 French plastic stents for the palliation of malignant biliary obstruction, overall complication rates were significantly lower in the SEMS group than the plastic stent group (20% vs 31 and p <0.05), mostly accounted for by a 2.8-fold reduction in the probability of stent occlusion.[11] The prolonged patency and reduced need for repeat endoscopic intervention translates into a cost benefit for the metallic stent, despite its initial high cost. Thus, metallic stent placement is generally recommended for inoperable patients whose life expectancy exceeds the expected patency period of 4 to 6 months of a plastic stent. A recent randomized study suggested that absence of liver metastases identifies the group of patients for whom metal stent placement is cost effective.[12] As endoscopists have increased their familiarity with SEMS, it has become possible to treat large tumors that are eroding into the duodenum by simultaneous placement of separate metal stents into the bile duct and the duodenum.[13] However, if diagnostic uncertainty exists, a plastic rather than a metal stent should be placed to avoid permanent embedding into the bile duct wall.

The palliation of jaundice in patients with hilar cholangiocarcinomas poses a special challenge. Bilateral placement of stents is technically arduous, and not always feasible even in the best endoscopic hands. The realization that only 25% of the liver needs to be drained to relieve jaundice has led to a trend toward unilateral stent placement. This has been supported by randomized studies showing no benefit for a policy of bilateral stent placement over a simpler approach of unilateral drainage.[14] One possible strategy is the use of MRCP or CT to guide unilateral stent placement into the larger of the 2 biliary systems, thus avoiding stent placement into atrophic liver segments.[15]

ERCP FOR ADJUVANT THERAPY

ERCP has been used for the delivery of adjuvant therapies for malignant biliary obstruction. Intrabiliary irradiation has been performed on an investigational basis with iridium-192 wires placed via the percutaneous or endoscopic route. Ongoing investigational work is focusing on the delivery of photodynamic therapy (PDT) to the bile duct as a means of palliation of malignant obstruction. This has been performed via an ERCP-guided catheter, using a hematoporphyrin derivative as a sensitizer, followed two days later by intraluminal photoactivation.

CONCLUSION

The most sensible approach toward pancreaticobiliary malignancy combines considerations of diagnosis, staging, and therapy. There are few evidence-based studies to prove the superiority of one single approach, and the rapid pace of change in imaging and endoscopic techniques will likely preclude any such studies from being performed. In synthesizing the available evidence, one hypothetical approach is the choice of a helical CT performed on a pancreatic protocol as the best first test for patients with suspected pancreaticobiliary malignancy. This approach will likely visualize a tumor if one is present and identify its local spread into vessels and surrounding structures, as well as hepatic metastases. Staging may then be complemented by laparoscopy for evaluation of peritoneal surfaces. If uncertainty persists, EUS or MRI with MRCP may clarify the picture. These modalities have tended to supplant the previous role of ERCP as a crucial diagnostic tool. The current trend is toward deferring possible ERCP until after a presumptive diagnosis has been made and thorough staging has been completed (see Figure 8-2). In this approach, ERCP is reserved for patients in whom a tissue diagnosis has to be confirmed preoperatively, for those who have a rare indication for preoperative decompression (such as cholangitis), and, most importantly, for palliation of biliary obstruction when the tumor is deemed unresectable. Preoperative stent placement is not universally recommended, because it does not improve surgical outcomes in malignant biliary obstruction. If a stent is placed in an unresectable tumor, the choice of stent type is determined on an individual basis and based largely on each patient's life expectancy. This approach has been endorsed in a statement issued by a conference recently convened by the National Institutes of Health regarding utilization of ERCP.[16] Nevertheless, ERCP maintains an important diagnostic role as one moves further from typical toward atypical presentations (eg, when noninvasive modalities fail to reveal a malignant-appearing mass). In that instance, ERCP offers the advantages of direct endoscopic visualization of the duodenum and ampulla as well as the ability to brush or biopsy a biliary stricture.

REFERENCES

1. Schilling D, Rink G, Arnold JC, et al. Prospective, randomized, single-center trial comparing 3 different 10F plastic stents in malignant mid- and distal bile duct strictures. *Gastrointest Endosc.* 2003;58:54-58.
2. Hunt GC, Faigel DO. Assessment of EUS for diagnosing, staging, and determining respectability of pancreatic cancer: a review. *Gastrointest Endosc.* 2002;55:232-237.
3. De Bellis M, Sherman S, Fogel EL, et al. Tissue sampling at ERCP in suspected malignant biliary strictures (part 2). *Gastrointest Endosc.* 2002;56:720-730.
4. Siqueira E, Schoen RE, Silverman W, et al. Detecting cholangiocarcinoma in patients with primary sclerosing cholangitis. *Gastrointest Endosc.* 2002;56:40-47.
5. Hawes RH. Diagnostic and therapeutic uses of ERCP in pancreatic and biliary tract malignancies. *Gastrointest Endosc.* 2002;56.
6. Vazquez-Sequeiros E, Baron TH, Clain JE, et al. Evaluation of indeterminate bile duct strictures by intraductal US. *Gastrointest Endosc.* 2002;56:372-379.
7. Strasberg SM. ERCP and surgical intervention in pancreatic and biliary malignancies. *Gastrointest Endosc.* 2002;56.
8. Povoski SP, Karpeh MS Jr, Conlon KC, Blumgart LH, Brennan MF. Preoperative biliary drainage: impact on intra-operative bile cultures and infectious morbidity and mortality after pancreaticoduodenectomy. *J Gastrointest Surg.* 1999;3:496-505.
9. Padillo J, Puente J, Gomez M, et al. Improved cardiac function in patients with obstructive jaundice after internal biliary drainage: hemodynamic and hormonal assessment. *Ann Surg.* 2001;234:652-656.
10. Smith AC, Dowsett JF, Russell RC, Hatfield AR, Cotton PB. Randomised trial of endoscopic stenting versus surgical bypass in malignant low bile duct obstruction. *Lancet.* 1994;344:1655-1660.
11. Carr-Locke DL, Ball TJ, Connors PJ et al. Multicenter randomized trial of Wallstent biliary endoprosthesis versus plastic stents. *Gastrointest Endosc.* 1993;39:310.
12. Kaassis M, Boyer J, Dumas R, et al. Plastic or metal stents for malignant stricture of the common bile duct? Results of a randomized prospective study. *Gastrointest Endosc.* 2003;57:178-182.

13. Kaw M, Singh S, Gagneja H. Clinical outcome of simultaneous self-expandable metal stent palliation of malignant biliary and duodenal obstruction. *Surg Endosc.* 2003;17:457-61.

14. De Palma GD, Galloro G, Iovino P, Catanzaro C. Unilateral versus bilateral endoscopic hepatic duct drainage in patients with malignant hilar obstruction: results of a prospective, randomized, and controlled study. *Gastrointest Endosc.* 2001;53:547-53.

15. Freeman ML, Overby C. Selective MRCP and CT-targeted drainage of malignant hilar biliary obstruction with self-expanding metallic stents. *Gastrointest Endosc.* 2003;58:41-9.

16. Cohen S, Bacon BR, Berlin JA, et al. National Institutes of Health State-of-the-Science Conference Statement: ERCP for diagnosis and therapy, January 14-16, 2002. *Gastrointest Endosc.* 2002;56:803-9.

chapter 9

Screening and Surveillance Strategies for Colorectal Cancer: Average- and Increased-Risk Individuals

Carla L. Nash, MD and Arnold J. Markowitz, MD

INTRODUCTION

Colorectal cancer is a common malignancy in the United States. The development of cancer is preceded by a premalignant precursor lesion, the adenomatous polyp, or *adenoma*. Screening for colorectal cancer provides the opportunity to detect and remove the adenoma, thus interrupting its potential progression to invasive cancer. In addition, screening also allows for the detection of colorectal cancer prior to the onset of symptoms, thus potentially allowing for cancer diagnosis at an early, more curable stage of disease. This chapter will review currently utilized screening modalities and recommended screening and surveillance guidelines for average- and increased-risk individuals.

BACKGROUND

Colorectal cancer accounts for significant morbidity and mortality in the United States. It is the fourth most common type of cancer, and the second most common cause of cancer-related death among American men and women.[1] In 2005, it is estimated that there will be approximately 145,000 new colorectal cancer cases diagnosed and about 56,000 deaths from this disease. The lifetime risk of developing colorectal cancer in the United States is approximately 6%.

Colorectal cancer is one of the few cancers that can be detected early by the presence of a premalignant lesion, the adenomatous polyp, or adenoma. Colorectal polyps are classified as either neoplastic (adenoma) or non-neoplastic. Although all adenomas have malignant potential, the majority are benign when detected. Adenomatous polyps are subcategorized histologically as tubular, villous, or tubulovillous adenomas, as well as by the degree of dysplasia. Advanced adenomas may demonstrate HGD (dysplastic cells limited to the epithelium, with no extension beyond the basement membrane) or contain invasive cancer (invasion through the muscularis mucosa into the submucosa). In contrast, non-neoplastic polyps include hyperplastic, mucosal, inflammatory, and hamartomatous polyps.

In the majority of sporadic colorectal cancers, the transformation of the adenoma into cancer is believed to occur via the adenoma-to-carcinoma pathway. Successively acquired somatic DNA mutations compound to affect the normal growth pattern of intestinal cells, resulting in the progression from normal epithelium to adenoma to invasive cancer. The presence of the adenoma is critical to cancer screening and prevention because it can be accurately identified, is relatively accessible, and can be easily removed prior to the development of cancer.

Cancer screening tests are examinations performed on asymptomatic individuals in the general population to detect premalignant lesions or early stage disease, such that the disease mortality and incidence can be reduced. In contrast, surveillance examinations are performed over time following removal of a premalignant or malignant lesion, or in a patient with an underlying predisposing disease condition. Routine screening and surveillance guidelines should not be applied to patients with symptomatic complaints, such as abdominal pain, altered bowel habits, rectal bleeding, unexplained weight loss, and iron-deficiency anemia, as these patients should instead undergo appropriate diagnostic testing as indicated.

Ideally, a screening test should be effective in identifying individuals with a premalignant lesion or early cancer (ie, highly sensitive), while also being effective in ruling out disease in those who do not in fact have such a neoplasm (ie, highly specific). The premalignant lesion or cancer must be detected early enough that intervention will reduce the mortality or incidence of the cancer within the general population. In addition, the screening test must be acceptable and easily accessible to patients, in order to reduce the burden of disease. Furthermore, the screening test should be cost-effective, and its benefits should outweigh its risks.

Screening in Average-Risk Individuals

Average-risk individuals are asymptomatic men and women over 50 years of age, with no personal or family history of colorectal cancer or polyps, and no personal history of inflammatory bowel disease (IBD). Routine screening for colorectal cancer is indicated in all appropriate average-risk individuals starting at age 50. Currently-used screening tests include the fecal occult blood test (FOBT), sigmoidoscopy, barium enema, and colonoscopy. Following are reviews these tests and the recommended screening strategies.

Fecal Occult Blood Test

The detection of occult blood within the stool may be an indicator of an underlying colorectal cancer or polyps. Commercially-available guaiac-impregnated cards may be used to detect microscopic blood in a fecal smear. In its designed use, FOBT is a self-administered outpatient test in which the patient collects 2 samples from each of 3 consecutive stools. Dietary restriction from consumption of red meat, certain vegetables and fruits (eg, turnips, horseradish), and avoidance of aspirin and other nonsteroidal anti-inflammatory drug (NSAID) use for 3 to 5 days prior to and during testing may decrease false-positive test results, whereas avoidance of vitamin C use may decrease false-negative test results. Specimen cards with fecal smears are submitted for testing. If any specimen is positive for occult blood, the patient should proceed to colonoscopy for further evaluation of the large bowel.

Table 9-1

FECAL OCCULT BLOOD TEST SCREENING TRIALS

	Minnesota[2,3] (US)	Nottingham[4] (UK)	Funen[5] (Denmark)
N	46,551	152,850	140,000
Age of subjects	50 to 80	45 to 74	45 to 75
Test frequency	Annual or biennial	Biennial	Biennial
Compliance	75%	53%	67%
Positive tests	2.4%	2.3%	1%
Follow-up	13 to 18 years	7.8 years	10 years
Test rehydration	Rehydrated	Nonrehydrated	Nonrehydrated
Mortality reduction	21% to 33%	15%	18%
PPV	31%	53%	NR
Sensitivity	80% to 92%	72%	NR
Specificity	90% to 98%	98%	NR

PPV=positive predictive value; NR=not reported

Three large prospective randomized controlled trials demonstrate that FOBT screening reduces mortality from colorectal cancer[2-5] (Table 9-1). Individuals with a positive FOBT were followed up with colonoscopy. The Minnesota trial examined over 46,000 patients 50 to 80 years of age with annual or biennial FOB testing, as compared to a control group with no screening. After 13 years of patient follow-up, the cumulative mortality from colorectal cancer was reduced by 33%. Eighteen-year follow up data showed a persistent 33% mortality reduction with annual FOB testing, and a 21% mortality reduction with biennial testing, as well as a reduction in the incidence of advanced colorectal cancer.[2,3]

Similar results have been seen worldwide. A British study of over 152,000 patients aged 45 to 74 years randomized to biennial screening reduced colorectal cancer mortality by 15% over a median follow-up of almost 8 years. Tumors were also detected at earlier stages as compared with the control group not offered screening.[4,6] A study from Denmark of 140,000 patients aged 45 to 75 years demonstrated an 18% reduction in colorectal cancer mortality using biennial screening.[5] In addition to decreasing mortality, FOBT screening has also been shown to reduce the incidence of colorectal cancer.[7]

FOBT attempts to detect blood loss from colorectal cancers and premalignant polyps; however, these neoplastic lesions may bleed intermittently. The sensitivity of FOBT has been estimated to range from approximately 30% to 50%.[8] The positive predictive value of a positive FOBT for a colorectal cancer has been estimated to be 5% to 18%, and for early stage cancer 3% to 14%.[8] Thus when used as a screening modality, FOBT must be performed on multiple stool samples, and repeated on an annual basis to maximize chance of detection of blood loss from colorectal neoplasia. Rehydration of FOBT specimens is not recommended in general practice because although it increases the sensitivity of the test, it also substantially increases false positive rates, thus reducing test specificity.

Advantages of FOBT include its low cost, ready availability, and noninvasive nature. Disadvantages include need for annual testing, relatively low sensitivity and positive predictive value for detecting colorectal cancer, high false positive rates that lead to unnecessary invasive investigations and their associated risks, and need for dietary restrictions during testing.

New immunohistochemical FOBTs have been developed that utilize monoclonal and/or polyclonal antibodies to detect human hemoglobin in stool. Since these tests do not react with nonhuman hemoglobin in red meat and certain vegetables and fruits that contain peroxidase activity, dietary restrictions are not required, and an expected decrease in false positives should result in increased test specificity.

SIGMOIDOSCOPY

Flexible sigmoidoscopy, typically performed utilizing a 60 cm scope, allows for direct visualization of the distal segments of the large bowel, up to about the distal one-third of the colorectum. Sigmoidoscopy provides a very sensitive examination of the distal colorectal mucosa and allows for biopsy of polyps or mass lesions identified within the segments of distal large bowel evaluated during this examination. Screening sigmoidoscopy is performed as an outpatient procedure by gastroenterologists, surgeons, and some primary care physicians. The procedure requires preparation of the distal large bowel, generally with an enema or laxative. It is performed without sedation, and generally takes about 10 minutes.

If an adenomatous polyp is detected during a screening sigmoidoscopy, the patient should proceed to colonoscopy to remove the polyp and screen the more proximal large bowel for potential additional synchronous neoplastic lesions. A finding of a distal advanced adenoma (size ≥1 cm or villous histology) or multiple adenomas, patient age >65 years, and a family history of colorectal cancer are factors associated with an increased risk of identifying an advanced neoplasm (adenoma ≥1 cm, villous histology, severe dysplasia, or invasive cancer) in the proximal large bowel.[9-11] In contrast, a finding of a distal hyperplastic polyp during screening sigmoidoscopy is not associated with increased risk of proximal advanced neoplasia, and thus does not require further workup.

Two case-control studies demonstrate the effectiveness of screening sigmoidoscopy in reducing distal colorectal cancer mortality.[12,13] In one study from Northern California, Selby et al. examined the records of 261 patients who had died of rectal or distal colon cancer and compared them with 868 matched controls.[12] Of the case patients, only 8.8% had undergone earlier screening with rigid sigmoidoscopy prior to cancer diagnosis, as compared to 24.2% of the control patients. Rigid sigmoidoscopy was found to be associated with a 59% reduction in rectosigmoid cancer mortality. Furthermore, this protection extended 10 years from the time of the sigmoidoscopy. In a second study from Wisconsin, Newcomb et al similarly compared a case group of 66 patients who died from colorectal cancer with 196 matched controls.[13] Case patients (10%) were less likely to have undergone prior screening sigmoidoscopy than control patients (30%). Screening sigmoidoscopy was associated with an 80% reduction in rectosigmoid cancer mortality.

Although there is currently no direct evidence from prospective randomized controlled trials to support the effectiveness of screening sigmoidoscopy, 2 studies are now in progress. Only preliminary findings have been reported to date: the National Cancer

Institute's Prostate, Lung, Colorectal and Ovarian (PLCO) Cancer Screening Trial[14] and the UK Flexible Sigmoidoscopy Screening Trial.[15]

Advantages of flexible sigmoidoscopy screening include direct visualization of up to the distal one-third of colorectum; the ability to biopsy detected polyps or masses; relatively minor bowel preparation; lack of need for sedation, thus allowing the patient to return directly to work or other daily activities, and no need for a care partner to accompany them home from the procedure; and a low risk for procedural complications. However, the procedure does remain somewhat invasive; given the lack of sedation, some patients may experience mild discomfort due to cramps and spasms related to air insufflation and scope passage.

COMBINED FECAL OCCULT BLOOD TEST AND SIGMOIDOSCOPY

The main drawback of sigmoidoscopy, however, is the lack of a complete examination of the entire large bowel. Thus, combining FOBT with flexible sigmoidoscopy has the theoretical benefit of improving detection of colorectal cancer and premalignant polyps. Although never evaluated directly in randomized trials, there is some indirect evidence to suggest that the approach of performing both FOBT and flexible sigmoidoscopy in combination is likely to be more effective than undergoing either test alone. In the large randomized FOBT trial from Denmark, screening FOBT demonstrated a lesser reduction in colorectal cancer mortality for rectal and sigmoid cancers, thus suggesting that FOBT may be less sensitive for detection of distal colorectal lesions.[16] In a controlled trial combining FOBT and rigid sigmoidoscopy vs rigid sigmoidoscopy alone, performed in approximately 12,500 patients following 5 to 11 years of follow-up, the combined screening strategy study group demonstrated a greater decrease in colorectal cancer mortality and was associated with detection of earlier stage cancers and longer survival.[17]

Thus, when selected as a choice to screen for colorectal cancer in average-risk individuals, it is preferable that flexible sigmoidoscopy every 5 years should be combined with FOBT annually to increase the effectiveness of this screening strategy.

BARIUM ENEMA

A double-contrast barium enema (DCBE) is a radiographic examination of the large bowel following administration of barium contrast followed by air per rectum. There are no randomized studies to evaluate the effectiveness of DCBE as a colorectal cancer screening test in average-risk individuals. Although DCBE is still included as an alternative option in standard screening guidelines, it has been demonstrated to be less sensitive than colonoscopy for the detection of neoplastic lesions. In a large prospective study of DCBE in the surveillance setting following polypectomy, DCBE only detected 48% of adenomatous polyps >1 cm in size and 53% of adenomatous polyps 6 to 10 mm, as compared to colonoscopy.[18]

Advantages of DCBE include its ability to evaluate the entire large bowel, its performance without sedation, and its low complication rate. Disadvantages include the potential for mild discomfort during the instillation of barium and air via a rectal catheter, the inability of some elderly or incontinent patients to hold the barium/air during the study, and the need for multiple changes in body position while on the x-ray table. Also, because DCBE is a diagnostic study, abnormal test results require further work-up by colonoscopy for polyp removal or biopsy of mass lesions. Furthermore, false positive findings on DCBE may occur due to retained fecal matter, anatomical differences, and benign mucosal abnormalities, resulting in unnecessary colonoscopy examinations.

DCBE allows for an alternative modality to examine the entire large bowel. However, because of its lower sensitivity for detection of potentially clinically important neoplastic lesions, screening guidelines recommend a 5-year interval between DCBE examinations.

COLONOSCOPY

Colonoscopy is a procedure performed by gastroenterologists and some surgeons and involves a complete direct examination of the entire colon and rectum. It is very sensitive for the detection of even small and flat neoplastic lesions. Colonoscopy allows for the removal of polyps using hot biopsy forceps or snare cautery, and for biopsy of suspicious-appearing mass lesions. It involves a somewhat more extensive bowel preparation than flexible sigmoidoscopy, and conscious sedation is used to ensure patient comfort. With an expert endoscopist, the procedure generally takes about 20 minutes to perform. Two large colonoscopy screening trials demonstrated a 97% completion rate to the cecum.[10,11] Incomplete examinations may be related to a particularly tortuous or redundant colon, adhesions related to prior abdominopelvic surgery, or patient intolerance despite sedation.

Although there are currently no prospective randomized studies in average-risk individuals to demonstrate that screening colonoscopy reduces colorectal cancer mortality or incidence, there is indirect evidence to support the effectiveness of colonoscopy as a primary screening test. Colonoscopy was utilized in the large FOBT screening trials to evaluate positive test results, and thus is felt to have played a significant role in these studies, which demonstrated a reduction in colorectal cancer mortality. Furthermore, since screening sigmoidoscopy reduces colorectal cancer mortality, it would be expected that colonoscopy would be at least as effective, if not more so, since it provides direct examination of the entire large bowel.

Particularly strong rationale to support the use of colonoscopy as a screening modality is that it allows for polyp removal, which has been demonstrated to decrease the incidence of colorectal cancer. In the United States National Polyp Study, Winawer et al followed a cohort of 1418 patients who had undergone prior colonoscopy and removal of adenomatous polyps, and demonstrated that the incidence of colorectal cancer was significantly lower in the study group as compared with the expected incidence in other reference cohorts.[19]

Recent screening colonoscopy trials have also provided evidence of added benefit of direct evaluation of the proximal large bowel, beyond the reach of the flexible sigmoidoscope. In the study by Lieberman et al, screening colonoscopy performed in over 3000 asymptomatic men (97%) aged 50 to 75 years in 13 Veterans Affairs medical centers detected colorectal neoplasms in 37.5% of patients.[10] An adenoma ≥1 cm in size or a villous adenoma was detected in 7.9%; an adenoma with HGD in 1.6%; and an invasive cancer in 1% of patients. In this cohort, 2.7% of the 1765 patients with no distal colorectal polyp (distal to the splenic flexure) had an advanced proximal neoplasm (adenoma ≥1 cm, villous histology, severe dysplasia, or invasive cancer). In addition, 52% of the 128 patients with a proximal advanced neoplasm had no distal adenoma. Similarly, in the trial by Imperiale et al, approximately 2000 asymptomatic patients, aged 50 years or older underwent screening colonoscopy as part of an employer-sponsored screening program.[11] In this cohort, 2.5% of 1564 patients with no distal polyp had an advanced proximal neoplasm (villous adenoma, severe dysplasia, or invasive cancer). In addition, 46% of the 50 patients with an advanced proximal neoplasm had no distal polyp. Thus, these 2 studies demonstrated that significant proximal colonic neoplasia may have gone undetected if patients had utilized flexible sigmoidoscopy alone as their screening strategy.

Current screening guidelines for average-risk individuals now include the option of undergoing a screening colonoscopy starting at age 50; if negative, repeat in 10 years. Although not determined by direct studies, the 10-year follow-up interval has been based on several indirect lines of support. For one, the duration of time for malignant transformation of an adenoma into a cancer has been estimated to occur, on average, over at least 10 years.[19-21] A study of 183 patients undergoing 2 back-to-back same-day colonoscopy examinations demonstrated a low 6% miss rate for advanced adenomas ≥1 cm in size.[22] In addition, the case-control study of screening rigid sigmoidoscopy demonstrated a protective effect from distal colorectal cancer mortality for up to 10 years from the last examination.[12] Further evidence is provided by a study of 154 asymptomatic average-risk patients with a previously negative colonoscopy examination that at follow-up colonoscopy 5 years later were demonstrated to have a low rate of advanced neoplasia (only 1 patient with an adenoma ≥1cm; no cancer, HGD, or villous histology).[23]

SCREENING GUIDELINES FOR AVERAGE-RISK INDIVIDUALS

Asymptomatic average-risk individuals should undergo routine colorectal cancer screening starting at age 50 years. Recently updated screening guidelines from a multidisciplinary panel of experts,[21] and endorsed by a consortium of US GI societies and various other national organizations, recommend several different screening options for the average-risk patient. One may choose any one of the following strategies: 1) FOBT annually, 2) flexible sigmoidoscopy every 5 years, 3) FOBT annually plus flexible sigmoidoscopy every 5 years, 4) DCBE every 5 years, or 5) colonoscopy every 10 years. Of note, these guidelines are also endorsed by the American Cancer Society.[24]

Of the various average-risk screening options, the authors' preference is to recommend colonoscopy every 10 years. Alternatively, they would consider FOBT annually with flexible sigmoidoscopy every 5 years, as the combination of 2 tests is preferable to only performing either test alone. With any screening strategy that utilizes FOBT or flexible sigmoidoscopy, if any one FOBT specimen is positive or if an adenomatous polyp is detected during sigmoidoscopy, then the patient should proceed to colonoscopy for further evaluation and management (Table 9-2).

SCREENING AND SURVEILLANCE IN INCREASED-RISK INDIVIDUALS

Individuals at increased risk for colorectal cancer include those with a personal or family history of colorectal cancer or adenomatous polyps and long-standing inflammatory bowel disease, such as ulcerative colitis and Crohn's colitis. Very high-risk individuals are those with hereditary colorectal cancer syndromes, such as FAP and HNPCC.

Table 9-2

SCREENING GUIDELINES: AVERAGE-RISK INDIVIDUALS[21,24]

Asymptomatic men and women ≥ age 50 with no other risk factors

Options

1. FOBT annually[A]
2. Flexible sigmoidoscopy every 5 years[B]
3. FOBT annually with flexible sigmoidoscopy every 5 years[C]
4. DCBE every 5 years[D]
5. Colonoscopy every 10 years[E]

A. Any positive FOBT should be followed up with colonoscopy.
B. Detection of an adenomatous polyp at flexible sigmoidoscopy should be followed up with colonoscopy.
C. Screening option of FOBT combined with flexible sigmoidoscopy is preferred over choosing to screen with either FOBT or flexible sigmoidsocopy alone.
D. An abnormal DCBE should be followed up with colonoscopy.
E. Authors' preferred screening strategy.

SCREENING IN INDIVIDUALS WITH A FAMILY HISTORY OF COLORECTAL CANCER OR ADENOMATOUS POLYPS

A family history of colorectal neoplasia confers an increased risk of developing colorectal cancer in an individual.[25-28] There is an approximate 2- to 3-fold increased risk of developing colorectal cancer in individuals with a first-degree relative (parent, sibling, or child) who has been affected with colorectal cancer. An individual with 2 affected first-degree relatives or one affected first-degree relative diagnosed ≤ age 50 years has an even higher 3- to 4-fold risk of developing colorectal cancer. Two affected second degree relatives confer an approximate 2- to 3-fold increased risk. An individual with a first-degree relative affected with an adenomatous polyp diagnosed at < age 60 years also has an approximate 2-fold increased risk.

Current screening guidelines from a multidisciplinary panel of experts[21] is as follows: Individuals with 2 or more first-degree relatives with colorectal cancer, or one first-degree relative with colorectal cancer or an adenomatous polyp diagnosed at age <60 years, should undergo colonoscopy screening starting at age 40, or 10 years younger than the earliest age of colorectal cancer diagnosis in the family, whichever is earlier, and if negative repeat at 5-year intervals. Individuals with one first-degree relative with colorectal cancer or adenomatous polyp diagnosed at age ≥60 years, or 2 second-degree relatives with colorectal cancer, should adhere to average-risk screening recommendations, but start earlier at age 40. Lastly, individuals with one second-degree or any third-degree relative with colorectal cancer should adhere to average-risk screening guidelines (Table 9-3).

Table 9-3

SCREENING GUIDELINES:
INCREASED FAMILIAL RISK INDIVIDUALS[21]

Family History	Screening Recommendations
≥2 FDRs with CRC, or I FDR with CRC or adenomatous polyp diagnosed age <60 years	Colonoscopy, start at age 40 (or 10 years years earlier than earliest age of CRC diagnosis in family, whichever earlier); repeat every 5 years
I FDR with CRC or adenomatous polyp diagnosed age ≥ 60 years, or 2 SDRs with CRC	Average-risk guidelines, but start at age 40
I SDR or TDR with CRC	Average-risk guidelines

FDR=first-degree relative; CRC=colorectal cancer; SDR=second-degree relative; TDR=third-degree relative

SURVEILLANCE FOLLOWING ENDOSCOPIC POLYPECTOMY OF ADENOMATOUS POLYPS

Colonoscopy is the recommended modality for surveillance in patients who have had prior endoscopic removal of a colorectal adenomatous polyp.[21] Ideally, all adenomas should be removed at the time of the initial baseline colonoscopy. Follow-up surveillance colonoscopy provides the opportunity to detect and remove any potentially missed lesions, and to identify new metachronous neoplasms. The US National Polyp Study has demonstrated that the rate of developing advanced adenomas following endoscopic removal of an adenoma is low after several years of follow-up surveillance.[29]

Current recommendations for the follow-up surveillance interval after colonoscopy with endoscopic removal of an adenoma are based on the number of polyps removed and their pathologic characteristics.[21] Following removal of multiple adenomas (≥3) or one advanced adenoma (large size ≥1 cm, villous histology, or HGD) the next follow-up colonoscopy should be in 3 years. Whereas, if only 1 to 2 small (<1 cm) tubular adenomas are removed, then the next follow-up colonoscopy should be in 5 years. Following a normal follow-up colonoscopy, the next surveillance colonoscopy examination should be repeated in 5 years (Table 9-4).

A shorter follow-up interval may be necessary after removal of numerous adenomas, excision of an adenoma with invasive cancer, incomplete or piecemeal removal of a large sessile adenoma, or a suboptimal examination due to a poor colonic preparation.

SURVEILLANCE FOLLOWING CURATIVE RESECTION OF COLORECTAL CANCER

Individuals with a history of colorectal cancer are at increased-risk for both synchronous and metachronous neoplastic lesions. Following curative resection of a colorectal cancer, if the entire colon was not completely visualized (eg, patient presented with an

Table 9-4

SURVEILLANCE GUIDELINES FOLLOWING ENDOSCOPIC REMOVAL OF ADENOMATOUS POLYPS[21]

Findings at Colonoscopy	Recommended Follow-Up
After removal of multiple (≥3) adenomas or an advanced adenoma (large ≥1 cm, villous histology, or HGD)	Repeat colonoscopy in 3 years
After removal of 1 to 2 small (<1 cm) tubular adenomas	Repeat colonoscopy in 5 years
After a negative follow-up colonoscopy	Repeat colonoscopy in 5 years

obstructing cancer) or adequately cleared of potential additional synchronous neoplasia prior to surgery, then a complete colonoscopy may be performed about 6 months following surgery. If the preoperative or 6 month postoperative colonoscopy was otherwise negative for synchronous neoplasia, then the next follow-up colonoscopy may be performed in 3 years.[21] If the postoperative 3-year follow-up colonoscopy is negative, then the patient may continue with repeat surveillance colonoscopies every 5 years.[21]

SURVEILLANCE IN INDIVIDUALS WITH INFLAMMATORY BOWEL DISEASE

The risk of colorectal cancer is increased among patients with long-standing chronic IBD, such as ulcerative colitis and Crohn's colitis. Although IBD patients may develop sporadic polyps in the same manner as people without IBD, chronic inflammation increases the risk of dysplasia in nonpolypoid areas that may not be visible macroscopically.

Ulcerative colitis patients at greatest risk for developing colorectal cancer are those with pancolitis (inflammation extending proximal to the splenic flexure), and those with duration of disease over 8 to 10 years.[30,31] Patients with pancolitis have a 15- to 19-fold increased risk of colorectal cancer when compared as a standardized incidence ratio to the rate in the general population, while those with left-sided disease have a 2- to 4-fold increased risk.[30,31] Ulcerative proctitis has a marginally increased risk, with a relative risk ratio of 1.7.[31] It is also important to recognize that disease may have been present for several years prior to diagnosis.

Surveillance recommendations for patients with chronic ulcerative colitis are tailored to the extent and duration of disease. Standard recommendations are to perform colonoscopy every 1 to 2 years starting after 8 years of disease in patients with pancolitis and after 15 years in patients with left-sided disease.[21] At the time of colonoscopy, mucosal biopsies should be taken from throughout the colon. One approach is to sample 4-quadrant biopsies every 10 cm, while another is to obtain biopsies from each region of the colon. Suspicious areas of mucosal irregularity or plaque-like lesions (dysplasia-associated lesions or masses [DALM]) should be biopsied separately.

Until recently, Crohn's disease was thought to have a lower risk of colorectal cancer development than ulcerative colitis. However, recent reports have suggested that the risk is just as great for patients with long-standing Crohn's disease, particularly those with chronic Crohn's colitis.[32,33] Current surveillance guidelines for patients with Crohn's disease are the same as those for ulcerative colitis.[21]

SCREENING INDIVIDUALS WITH A HEREDITARY COLORECTAL CANCER SYNDROME

Familial Adenomatous Polyposis

FAP accounts for about 1% of all cases of colorectal cancer. A germline mutation in the adenomatous polyposis coli (APC) gene located on chromosome 5 predisposes patients to develop hundreds to thousands of adenomatous polyps throughout the colon. FAP is inherited in an autosomal dominant fashion. In FAP, polyps typically begin to present in the second decade of life (average age 16 years), and will ultimately progress to cancer in 10 to 15 years from the onset of the polyposis (average age 39 years). An attenuated form of FAP, associated with mutations at the distal 5' and 3' ends of the APC gene, may demonstrate fewer polyps (approximately 20 to 100) and a later onset of cancer development by about 10 years; in addition, adenomas tend to be more common in the right colon.

FAP patients are also at risk for gastric, duodenal ,and periampullary adenomas. Extraintestinal manifestations of FAP (Gardner's syndrome) include osteomas (typically of the mandible and skull), soft tissue tumors (lipomas, fibromas, and epidermoid and sebaceous cysts), supernumerary teeth, desmoid tumors, mesenteric fibromatosis, and congenital hypertrophy of the retinal pigmentation epithelium (CHRPE).

For at-risk FAP family members, annual screening with flexible sigmoidoscopy is recommended beginning at puberty (age 10 to 12 years) and may be decreased in frequency to every 3 years after age 40. Once colonic polyposis has been documented, patients should consult with a surgeon regarding consideration of prophylactic colectomy, and its appropriate timing. Genetic counseling and gene testing should also be offered to at-risk members of these families. Surveillance for gastric, duodenal, and periampullary adenomas by upper GI endoscopy should begin at the time of diagnosis of colonic polyposis and continue every 1 to 3 years thereafter. At the time of endoscopy, a side-viewing endoscope should also be used to optimally assess the major papilla and periampullary region of the duodenum. In attenuated FAP, at-risk family members are recommended to undergo full colonoscopy examination to screen for polyposis likely beginning in their late teens or early 20s due to the tendency for right-sided polyp formation[21,28] (Table 9-5).

Hereditary Nonpolyposis Colorectal Cancer

HNPCC is an autosomal dominant condition that accounts for approximately 5% of colorectal cancers. The lifetime risk of developing colorectal cancer in HNPCC is approximately 80%. HNPCC is associated with a germline mutation in one of 5 DNA mismatch repair (MMR) genes; most cases are accounted for by hMLH1 and hMSH2 gene mutations. MMR gene mutations result in microsatellite instability (MSI) in the DNA of the colorectal cancers in these patients.

Table 9-5

SCREENING GUIDELINES: HEREDITY SYNDROMES[21,28]

Hereditary Syndrome	Recommendations
FAP	Flexible sigmoidoscopy annually, beginning age 10 to 12 years*; genetic counseling and gene testing
HNPCC	Colonoscopy every 1 to 2 years, beginning at age 20 to 25 (or 10 years earlier than earliest age of CRC diagnosis in family, whichever earlier); genetic counseling and gene testing

*In attenuated FAP screen with colonoscopy because of increased incidence of right colon adenomas, beginning in late teens or early 20s.

HNPCC patients are at increased risk for early onset colorectal cancer, at an average age of diagnosis of 40 to 45 years. The colon cancers are predominantly right-sided, with about 60% to 70% proximal to the splenic flexure. Patients often present with multiple primary colon cancers, and are at increased risk for metachronous cancers. In HNPCC it is believed that adenomas may progress to cancer at an accelerated rate, as compared to sporadic adenomas. HNPCC is also associated with extracolonic cancers of the endometrium, ovary, stomach, small intestine, renal pelvis and ureter (transitional cell cancer), and the pancreaticobiliary system.

The diagnosis of HNPCC has been primarily based on family history. Initial Amsterdam criteria defined an HNPCC family as one in which there are 3 or more close relatives, one a first-degree relative of the other 2, from 2 or more generations, affected with colorectal cancer, with at least one cancer diagnosed before age 50, and FAP is excluded.[34] Subsequently, updated Amsterdam II criteria expanded the definition to also include several HNPCC-associated malignancies, including endometrial, small bowel, ureter, and renal pelvis cancer.[35] Genetic testing for HNPCC is available; however, a disease causing mutation may be identified in only approximately 50% to 70% of families that meet Amsterdam criteria.

Another approach to identifying patients at risk for HNPCC is to perform testing for microsatellite instability on the colorectal cancer tissue of an affected patient who may be suspicious for possible HNPCC, but does not necessarily meet Amsterdam criteria. The Bethesda guidelines offer a set of multiple criteria that may be used to identify patients suspicious for HNPCC who should undergo MSI testing of their tumors.[36] Patients with MSI-positive tumors can then go on to germline testing for a MMR gene mutation.

A long-term Finnish study evaluated the effectiveness of screening in HNPCC patients and their families.[37] This study compared a group of 251 at-risk individuals from 22 HNPCC families who had screening examinations (colonoscopy or flexible sigmoidoscopy and barium enema) every 3 years to a control group who had no screening, and demonstrated a significant reduction in incidence (p=0.03) and a reduction in mortality (p=0.08) of colorectal cancer in the screened group. The reduction in colon cancer risk was likely due to the colonoscopic removal of adenomas.

A 15-year followup study evaluated the incidence of colorectal cancer and survival in 2 cohorts of at-risk members of the 22 Finnish HNPCC families by comparing a study group of 133 at-risk patients who underwent colorectal screening every 3 years with an unscreened control group of 119 patients.[38] Colonoscopy screening reduced the rate of colorectal cancer by 62%, prevented cancer-related death, and decreased overall mortality by 65% in HNPCC families.

Colorectal screening in HNPCC patients should be performed by colonoscopy due to the increased incidence of proximal cancers and adenomas. At-risk individuals should undergo colonoscopy screening every 1 to 2 years beginning at age 20 to 25, or 10 years earlier than the youngest family member diagnosed. Special screening for HNPCC-associated extracolonic malignancies is also recommended. In addition, HNPCC patients and their at-risk family members should also be referred for genetic counseling and possible gene testing (see Table 9-5).

FUTURE SCREENING TECHNOLOGIES

Two new emerging technologies for colorectal cancer screening include CT colonography, or virtual colonoscopy (VC), and stool testing for DNA mutations.

VC is a radiologic imaging technique that was first described by Vining, et al in 1994.[39] VC utilizes thin-cut helical CT imaging to generate two-dimensional axial images, which can then be reconstructed using specialized computer software into three-dimensional images of the colon that simulate a "virtual" image of the entire large bowel lumen. Prior to VC patients must undergo a bowel preparation similar to that for colonoscopy. During the VC procedure the colon is distended by air insufflation via a rectal catheter.

Results from early studies suggest that VC is comparable to conventional colonoscopy for the detection of lesions ≥1 cm. In a prospective study of 100 patients (60 men, 40 women; mean age 62 years) at increased risk for colorectal neoplasia who underwent same-day sequential VC followed by conventional colonoscopy, VC identified 3 of 3 cancers, 91% of polyps ≥1 cm, 82% of polyps 0.6 to 0.9, and 55% of polyps ≤0.5 cm in size.[40] There were 19 false-positive findings of polyps, and no false-positive findings of cancer. In a large prospective study of screening VC in 1233 asymptomatic individuals (728 men, 505 women; mean age 58 years), VC demonstrated a sensitivity of 93.8% and a specificity of 96% for detecting adenomas ≥1 cm.[41]

VC currently offers considerable potential as a future screening modality. Advantages include that it is a noninvasive procedure, requires no sedation, and provides an evaluation of the entire large bowel, including the ability to visualize the more proximal colon in patients with an obstructing mass lesion, or following an incomplete conventional colonoscopy due to redundant loops or patient intolerance. Disadvantages include that it is a diagnostic test, and thus abnormal findings require follow-up with colonoscopy, false-positive results may occur due to retained stool or poorly distensible segments related to significant underlying diverticular disease, and the question of its sensitivity for detection of flat adenomas.

Stool testing for DNA mutations is another exciting developing technology. It is a noninvasive test and requires minimal patient preparation. Small amounts of DNA shed from colorectal cancers and polyps can be recovered from the stool and amplified for analysis. DNA abnormalities have been detected in such genes as K-*ras*, APC, and p53. In one study, a blinded analysis of stool specimens from 33 patients with colorectal cancer or adenomas demonstrated that a multi-target assay panel was 91% sensitive in detecting cancer, and 82% sensitive for detecting adenomas ≥1 cm in size, with a specificity of 93%.[42] Another study reported similar promising results regarding the feasibility of detecting APC gene mutations utilizing a digital protein truncation assay.[43]

CONCLUSION

Colorectal cancer remains a prevalent disease in the United States, and continues to account for significant premature death and life-years lost. Currently available screening tests are effective in detecting early stage colorectal cancer and its premalignant precursor lesion, the adenoma. Evidence demonstrates that screening examinations reduce colorectal cancer mortality. Removal of adenomas by colonoscopic polypectomy has been demonstrated to significantly reduce the incidence of colorectal cancer.

Appropriate screening and surveillance recommendations should be based on the individual's colorectal cancer risk stratification. Average-risk individuals should begin screening at age 50 years. Increased-risk individuals should be identified and offered more aggressive screening recommendations beginning at an earlier age. High-risk individuals at-risk for hereditary syndromes such as FAP and HNPCC should be offered genetic counseling and specialized screening recommendations for colorectal cancer, and associated extracolonic malignancies.

At the present time, patients need to be encouraged to engage in and benefit from currently proven and available screening and surveillance strategies in order to reduce their risk of developing and dying from colorectal cancer.

REFERENCES

1. Jemal A, Tiwari RC, Murray T, et al. Cancer statistics, 2004. *CA Cancer J Clin*. 2004; 54:8-29.
2. Mandel JS, Bond JH, Church TR, et al. Reducing mortality from colorectal cancer by screening for fecal occult blood. *N Engl J Med*. 1993;328:1365-1371.
3. Mandel JS, Church TR, Ederer F, Bond JH. Colorectal cancer mortality: Effectiveness of biennial screening for fecal occult blood. *J Natl Cancer Inst*. 1999;91:434-437.
4. Hardcastle JD, Chamberlain JO, Robinson MHE, et al. Randomized controlled trial of faecal-occult-blood screening for colorectal cancer. *Lancet*. 1996;348:1472-1477.
5. Kronborg O, Fenger C, Olsen J, Jorgenson OD, Sondergaard O. Randomised study of screening for colorectal cancer with faecal-occult-blood test. *Lancet*. 1996;348:1467-1471.
6. Hardcastle JD, Chamberlain J, Sheffield J, et al. Randomised, controlled trial of faecal occult blood screening of colorectal cancer: Results for first 107 349 subjects. *Lancet*. 1989;1:1160-1164.
7. Mandel JS, Church TR, Bond JH, et al. The effect of fecal occult-blood screening on the incidence of colorectal cancer. *N Engl J Med*. 2000;343:1603-1607.
8. Ransohoff DF, Lang CA. Screening for colorectal cancer with fecal occult blood test: a background paper. *Ann Intern Med*. 1997;126:811-822.
9. Levin TR, Palitz A, Grossman S, et al. Predicting advanced proximal colonic neoplasia with screening sigmoidoscopy. *JAMA*. 1999;281:1611-1617.

10. Lieberman DA, Weiss DG, Bond JH, et al. Use of colonoscopy to screen asymptomatic adults for colorectal cancer. *N Engl J Med.* 2000;343:162-168.

11. Imperiale TF, Wagner DR, Lin CY, et al. Risk of advanced proximal neoplasms in asymptomatic adults according to the distal colorectal findings. *N Engl J Med.* 2000; 343:169-174.

12. Selby JV, Friedman GD, Quesenberry CP Jr, Weiss NS. A case-control study of screening sigmoidoscopy and mortality from colorectal cancer. *N Engl J Med.* 1992;326:653-657.

13. Newcomb PA, Norfleet RG, Storer BE, Surawicz TS, Marcus PM. Screening sigmoidoscopy and colorectal cancer mortality. *J Natl Cancer Inst.* 1992;84:1572-1575.

14. Schoen RE, Pinsky PF, Weissfeld JL, et al and the Prostate, Lung, Colorectal and Ovarian Cancer Screening Trial Group. Results of a repeat sigmoidoscopy 3 years after a negative examination. *JAMA.* 2003;290:41-48.

15. UK Flexible Sigmoidoscopy Screening Trial Investigators and Atkin WS. Single flexible sigmoidoscopy screening to prevent colorectal cancer: baseline findings of a UK multicentre randomised trial. *Lancet.* 2002;359:1291-1300.

16. Jorgensen OD, Kronborg O, Fenger C. A randomized study of screening for colorectal cancer using faecal occult blood testing: results after 13 years and seven biennial screening rounds. *Gut.* 2002;50:29-32.

17. Winawer SJ, Flehinger BJ, Schottenfeld D, Miller DG. Screening for colorectal cancer with fecal occult blood testing and sigmoidoscopy. *J Natl Cancer Inst.* 1993;85:1311-1318.

18. Winawer SJ, Stewart E, Zauber AG, et al. A comparison of colonoscopy and double-contrast barium enema for surveillance after polypectomy. *N Engl J Med.* 2000; 342:1766-1772.

19. Winawer SJ, Zauber AG, Ho MN, et al. Prevention of colorectal cancer by colonoscopic polypectomy. The National Polyp Study Workgroup. *N Engl J Med.* 1993;329:1977-1981.

20. Hofstad B, Vatn M. Growth rate of colon polyps and cancer. *Gastrointest Endosc Clin N Am.* 1997;7:345-363.

21. Winawer S, Fletcher R, Rex D, et al for the US Multisociety Task Force On Colorectal Cancer. Colorectal cancer screening and surveillance: clinical guidelines and rationale - update based on new evidence. *Gastroenterology.* 2003;124:544-560.

22. Rex DK, Cutler CS, Lemmel GT, et al. Colonoscopic miss rates of adenomas determined by back-to-back colonoscopies. *Gastroenterology.* 1997;112:24-28.

23. Rex DK, Cummings OW, Helper DJ, et al. Five-year incidence of adenomas after negative colonoscopy in asymptomatic average-risk persons. *Gastroenterology.* 1996;111:1178-1181.

24. Smith RA, Cokkinides V, Eyre HJ. American Cancer Society Guidelines for the early detection of cancer, 2004. *CA Cancer J Clin.* 2004;54:41-52.

25. St. John DJ, McDermott FT, Hopper JL, et al. Cancer risk in relatives of patients with common colorectal cancer. *Ann Intern Med.* 1993;118:785-790.

26. Slattery ML, Kerber RA. Family history of cancer and colon cancer risk: the Utah Population Database. *J Natl Cancer Inst.* 1994;86:1618-1626.

27. Winawer SJ, Zauber AG, Gerdes H, et al. Risk of colorectal cancer in the families of patients with adenomatous polyps. *N Engl J Med.* 1996;334:82-87.

28. Burt RW. Colon cancer screening. *Gastroenterology.* 2000;119:837-853.

29. Winawer SJ, Zauber AG, O'Brien MJ, et al. Randomized comparison of surveillance intervals after colonoscopic removal of newly diagnosed adenomatous polyps. *N Engl J Med.* 1993;328:901-906.

30. Gyde SN, Prior P, Allan RN, et al. Colorectal cancer in ulcerative colitis: a cohort study of primary referrals from three centres. *Gut.* 1988;29:206-217.

31. Ekbom A, Helmick C, Zack M, Adami H-O. Ulcerative colitis and colorectal cancer: a population-based study. *N Engl J Med.* 1990;232:1228-1233.

32. Sachar DB. Cancer in Crohn's disease: dispelling the myths. *Gut.* 1994;35:1507-1508.

33. Gillen CD, Walmsley RS, Prior P, Andrews HA, Allan RN. Ulcerative colitis and Crohn's disease: a comparison of the colorectal cancer risk in extensive colitis. *Gut.* 1994;35:1590-1592.

34. Vasen HF, Mecklin JP, Khan PM, et al. The International Collaborative Group on Hereditary Non-Polyposis Colorectal Cancer (ICG-HNPCC). *Dis Colon Rectum.* 1991;34:424-425.

35. Vasen HFA, Watson P, Mecklin JP, et al. New clinical criteria for hereditary non-polyposis colorectal cancer (HNPCC, Lynch syndrome) proposed by the International Collaborative Group on HNPCC. *Gastroenterology.* 1999;116:1453-1456.

36. Rodriguez-Bigas MA, Boland CR, Hamilton SR, et al. A National Cancer Institute Workshop on Hereditary Nonpolyposis Colorectal Cancer Syndrome: meeting highlights and Bethesda guidelines. *J Natl Cancer Inst.* 1997;89:1758-1762.

37. Jarvinen HJ, Mecklin JP, Sistonen P. Screening reduces colorectal cancer rate in families with hereditary nonpolyposis colorectal cancer. *Gastroenterology.* 1995;108:1405-1411.

38. Jarvinen HJ, Aarnio M, Mustonen H, et al. Controlled 15-year trial on screening for colorectal cancer in families with hereditary nonpolyposis colorectal cancer. *Gastroenterology.* 2000;118:829-834.

39. Vining DJ, Gelfand DW, Bechtold RE, et al. Technical feasibility of colon imaging with helical CT and virtual reality. *Am J Roentgenol.* 1994;62Suppl:104. abstract.

40. Fenlon HM, Nunes DP, Schroy III PC, et al. A comparison of virtual and conventional colonoscopy for the detection of colorectal polyps. *N Engl J Med.* 1999;341:1496-1503.

41. Pickhardt PJ, Choi JR, Hwang I, et al. Computed tomographic virtual colonoscopy to screen for colorectal neoplasia in asymptomatic adults. *N Engl J Med.* 2003;349:2191-2200.

42. Ahlquist DH, Skoletsky JE, Boynton KA, et al. Colorectal cancer screening by detection of altered human DNA in stool: feasibility of a multi-target assay panel. *Gastroenterology.* 2000;119:1219-1227.

43. Traverso G, Shuber AP, Levin B, et al. Detection of APC mutations in fecal DNA from patients with colorectal tumors. *N Engl J Med.* 2002;346:311-320.

chapter 10

Surgical Approach to Colorectal Neoplasia and High-Risk Conditions

Najjia N. Mahmoud, MD and J.J. Karmacharya, FRCS

INTRODUCTION

Adenocarcinoma of the colon and rectum are the third most common sites of new cancer cases and deaths in both men and women in the United States. Although surgery remains the primary treatment for this disease, surgical and medical therapy for colorectal and other cancers is currently in an exciting era of discovery. The rise of medical applications of molecular biology and the promise of new therapeutic and diagnostic modalities derived from this field necessarily requires a basic understanding of the underlying genetics of the disease. A future paradigm shift in the treatment of colorectal cancer away from intervention and toward molecular therapies seems likely, and an appreciation of the current impact of the science of colon cancer is crucial in treating the modern colorectal cancer patient and his family. The estimated incidence of new cases of colon cancer is actually stable from year to year, without appreciable increase or decrease in the last century. The American Cancer Society estimates that about 106,370 new cases of colon cancer (50,400 men and 55,970 women) and 40,570 new cases of rectal cancer (23,220 men and 17,350 women) will be diagnosed in 2004. Colorectal cancer is expected to cause about 56,730 deaths in 2004, accounting for 10% of all cancer deaths. The lifetime risk of developing colorectal cancer in the United States is 6%, with over 90% of cases occurring after the age of 50. Surgery is the critical treatment modality currently, and postoperative medical treatment is predicated on pathologic review of the surgical specimen and draining lymph nodes.

Colorectal cancer occurs in hereditary, sporadic, and familial forms. Hereditary forms of colorectal cancer have been extensively described and are characterized by family history, young age at onset, other coexisting tumors types, extraintestinal manifestations and the presence of specific germline genetic mutations. FAP and HNPCC are the 2 major hereditary colorectal cancer syndromes and are the subject of many recent investigations that continue to provide significant insights into the pathogenesis of colorectal cancer.

Figure 10-1. Distribution of causes of colorectal cancer. Causes of colorectal cancer include sporadic, familial, and HNPCC, FAP, and rare colorectal cancer (CRC) syndromes such as juvenile polyposis syndrome (JPS), Peutz-Jeghers syndrome (PJS), and the APC I1307K mutation. (Adapted from Trimbath JD, Giardiello FM. Genetic testing and counseling for hereditary colorectal cancer. *Aliment Pharmacol Ther.* 2002;16:1843-1857.)

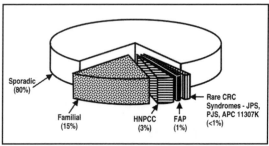

Sporadic colorectal cancer occurs in the absence of family history, generally affects an older population (60 to 80 years of age), and usually presents as an isolated colon or rectal lesion. Seventy percent to 80% of all colorectal cancers are sporadic (Figure 10-1). Genetic mutations associated with the cancer are limited to the tumor itself, unlike hereditary disease where the specific mutation is present in all cells of the affected individual. Nevertheless, the genetics of colorectal cancer initiation and progression proceed along very similar pathways in both hereditary and sporadic forms of the disease. Studies of the relatively rare inherited models of the disease have greatly enhanced the understanding of the genetics of the far more common sporadic form of the cancer.

The concept of "familial" colorectal cancer is relatively new. Lifetime risk of colorectal cancer increases for members in families in which the index case is young (less than 50 years of age) and the relative is close (first degree) (Table 10-1). The risk increases as the number of family members with colorectal cancer rises. An individual who is a first-degree relative of a patient diagnosed with colorectal cancer under the age of 50 is twice as likely as the general population to develop the cancer. This more subtle form of inheritance is currently the subject of much investigation. Genetic polymorphisms, gene modifiers, and defects in tyrosine kinases have all been implicated in various forms of familial colorectal cancer.

COLORECTAL CANCER GENETICS

TUMOR SUPPRESSORS, MISMATCH REPAIR GENES, AND ONCOGENES

Tumor suppressor genes produce proteins that inhibit tumor formation by regulating mitotic activity and providing inhibitory cell cycle control. Tumor formation occurs when these inhibitory controls are deregulated by mutation. Point mutations, loss of heterozygosity (LOH), frame shift mutations, and promoter hypermethylation are all types of genetic changes that can cause failure of a tumor suppressor gene. These genes are often referred to as "gatekeeper" genes because they provide cell cycle inhibition and regulatory control at specific checkpoints in cell division and their loss is permissive for further mutational damage. The failure of regulation of normal cellular function by tumor suppressor genes is appropriately described by the term loss of function (LOF). Both alleles of the gene must be nonfunctional to initiate tumor formation.

Table 10-1

FAMILIAL RISK AND COLON CANCER

Familial Setting	Approximate Lifetime Risk of Colon Cancer
General US Population	6%
One first-degree relative with colon cancer[1]	2- to 3-fold increased
Two first-degree relatives with colon cancer[1]	3- to 4-fold increased
First-degree relative with colon cancer diagnosed at <50	3- to 4-fold increased
One second- or third-degree relative with colon cancer[2,3]	1.5-fold increased
Two second-degree relatives with colon cancer[2]	2- to 3-fold increased
One first-degree relative with an adenomatous polyp[1]	2-fold increased

[1]First-degree relatives include parents, siblings, and children.

[2]Second-degree relatives include grandparents, aunts, and uncles.

[3]Third-degree relatives include great-grandparents and cousins.

Adapted from Burt RW. Colon cancer screening. *Gastroenterology.* 2000;119:837-53.

Mismatch repair genes (MMR) are called "caretaker" genes because of their important role in policing the integrity of the genome and correcting DNA replication errors. MMR genes that undergo a loss of function contribute to carcinogenesis by accelerating tumor progression. Mutations in MMR genes (including hMLH1, hMSH2, hMSH3, hPMS1, hPMS2, and hMSH6) result in the syndrome HNPCC. Approximately 3% of colorectal cancers in the United States are caused by HNPCC. Mutations in MMR genes produce microsatellite instability (MSI)—a measurable characteristic of tumors considered a marker for MMR gene mutations. Microsatellites are repetitive sequences of DNA that seem randomly distributed throughout the genome. Stability of these sequences is a good measure of the general integrity of the genome. MSI exists in 10% to 15% of sporadic tumors and in 95% of tumors in patients with HNPCC. Even so, only 50% of patients diagnosed with HNPCC have readily identifiable MMR mutations. For additional discussion and screening and surveillance recommendations, please see Chapter 9.

Proto-oncogenes are genes that produce proteins that promote cellular growth and proliferation. Mutations in proto-oncogenes typically produce a "gain-of-function" and can be caused by mutation in only one of the 2 alleles. Following mutation, the gene is called an oncogene. Overexpression of these growth-oriented genes contributes to the uncontrolled proliferation of cells associated with cancer. The products of oncogenes can be divided into categories. For example, growth factors (TGFß, EGF, insulin-like growth factor); growth factor receptors (*erbB2*), signal transducers (*src, abl, ras*); and nuclear

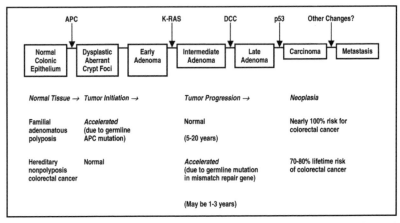

Figure 10-2. The adenoma-carcinoma sequence in sporadic and hereditary colorectal cancer. (Reprinted from Ivanovich JL, Read TE, Ciske DJ, Kodner IJ, Whelan AJ. A Practical Approach to Familial and Hereditary Colorectal Cancer. *Am J Med.* 1999;107:68-77.)

proto-oncogenes and transcription factors (*myc*) are all oncogene products that appear to have a role in the development of colorectal neoplasia. The *ras* protooncogene is located on chromosome 12 and mutations are believed to occur very early in the adenoma-carcinoma sequence. Mutated *ras* has been found to be present in adenomatous polyps. Activated *ras* leads to constitutive activity of a protein that stimulates cellular growth. Fifty percent of sporadic colon cancers possess *ras* mutations, and current trials of far-nesyl transferase inhibitors, which block a step in *ras* post-translational modification, may hold therapeutic promise.[1]

THE ADENOMA-CARCINOMA SEQUENCE

The field of colorectal cancer genetics was revolutionized in 1988 by the description of the genetic changes involved in the progression of a benign adenomatous polyp to invasive carcinoma (Figure 10-2). Since then, there has been an explosion of additional information about the molecular and genetic pathways resulting in colorectal cancer. Tumor suppressor genes, DNA mismatch repair genes, and protooncogenes all contribute to colorectal neoplasia, both in sporadic and inherited forms. The "adenoma-carcinoma" multistep model of colorectal neoplasia represents one of the best-known models of carcinogenesis and may serve as a template to illustrate how early mutations produce accumulated defects resulting in neoplasia. This sequence of tumor progression involves damage to protooncogenes and tumor suppressor genes. The specific contributing mutations in genes such as APC have been intensely investigated.

The earliest mutations in the adenoma-carcinoma sequence occur in the APC gene. The earliest phenotypic change present is known as "aberrant crypt formation" and the most consistent genetic aberrations within these cells are abnormally short proteins known as APC truncations. Most clinically relevant derangements in APC are truncation mutations created by inappropriate transcription of premature termination codons.[2,3]

Table 10-2

COLON AND RECTAL POLYPS: RISK

Type	<1 cm	1 to 2 cm	>2 cm	% Total
Tubular	1%	10%	35%	5
Tubulovillous	4%	7%	46%	23
Villous	10%	10%	53%	41

On average, only 5% of polyps <1cm in size harbor an invasive cancer. Size, rather than histology, is the major risk factor for cancer.

Adapted from Chang AE. Colorectal cancer. In: Greenfield LJ, ed. *Surgery: Scientific Principles and Practice.* Philadelphia, Pa JB Lippincott; 1993:1007.

PATHOGENESIS OF COLORECTAL CARCINOMA—FROM POLYPS TO CANCER

The adenoma-carcinoma sequence is now recognized as the process through which most colorectal carcinomas develop. Clinical and epidemiological observations have long been cited to support the hypothesis that colorectal carcinomas evolve through a progression of benign polyps to invasive carcinoma, and the elucidation of the genetic pathways to cancer described above have confirmed the validity of this hypothesis. However, before the molecular genesis of colorectal cancer was appreciated, there was considerable controversy as to whether colorectal cancer arises *de novo,* or evolved from a polyp that was initially a benign precursor. Although there have been a few documented instances of tiny colonic cancers arising *de novo* from normal mucosa, these instances are rare, and the validity of the adenoma-carcinoma sequence is now accepted by virtually all authorities. The historical observations that lead to the hypothesis are of interest because of the therapeutic implications implicit in an understanding of the adenoma-carcinoma sequence. Observations that provide support for the hypothesis include all of the following:

- Larger adenomas are found to harbor cancers more often than smaller ones—the larger the polyp, the higher the risk of cancer. While the cellular characteristics of the polyp are important, with villous adenomas carrying a higher risk than tubular adenomas, the size of the polyp is most important. The risk of cancer in a tubular adenoma smaller than 1 cm in diameter is less than 5%, whereas the risk of cancer in a tubular adenoma larger than 2 cm is 35%. A villous adenoma larger than 2 cm in size carries a 50% chance of containing a cancer (Table 10-2).

- Residual benign adenomatous tissue is found in the majority of invasive colorectal cancers, suggesting progression of the cancer from the remaining benign cells to the predominant malignant ones.

- Benign polyps have been observed to develop into cancers. There have been reports of the direct observation of benign polyps that were not removed progressing over time into malignancies.

- Colonic adenomas occur more frequently in patients who have colorectal cancer. Nearly a third of all patients with colorectal cancer will also have a benign colorectal polyp.

- Patients who develop adenomas have an increased lifetime risk of developing colorectal cancer.

- Removal of polyps decreases the incidence of cancer. Patients with small adenomas have a 2.3-increased risk of cancer after the polyp is removed, compared with an 8-fold increased incidence of colorectal cancer in patients with polyps who do not undergo polypectomy.

- Populations with a high risk of colorectal cancer also have a high prevalence of colorectal polyps.

- Patients with familial adenomatous polyposis will develop colorectal cancer virtually 100% of the time in the absence of surgical intervention. The adenomas that characterize this syndrome are genetically identical to sporadic adenomas.

- The peak incidence for the discovery of benign colorectal polyps is 50 years of age. The peak incidence for the development of colorectal cancer is 60 years of age. This suggests a 10-year time span for the progression of an adenomatous polyp to a cancer.[4] These observations and studies by molecular biologists document that colonic mucosa progresses through stages to the eventual development of an invasive cancer. Colonic epithelial cells lose "epithelial homeostasis," the balance between proliferation and apoptosis, or programmed cell death, that produces normal regeneration. With more proliferation and increasing cellular disorganization, the cells extend through the muscularis mucosae to become invasive carcinoma. The process of colorectal carcinogenesis generally follows the predictable sequence of invasion of the muscularis mucosa, pericolic tissue, lymph nodes, and finally, distant metastasis.

SPORADIC COLORECTAL CANCER

It is important to recognize the increased risk of cancer in patients with hereditary cancer syndromes, but by far the most common form of colorectal cancer is sporadic in nature, without an associated strong family history.

Although the cause and pathogenesis of adenocarcinoma are similar throughout the large bowel, significant differences in the use of diagnostic and therapeutic modalities separate colonic from rectal cancers. This distinction is largely due to the confinement of the rectum by the bony pelvis. The limited mobility of the rectum allows MRI to generate better images and increases its sensitivity. In addition, the proximity of the rectum to the anus permits easy access of ultrasound probes for more accurate assessment of the extent of penetration of the bowel wall and the involvement of adjacent lymph nodes. The limited accessibility of the rectum, the proximity to the anal sphincter, and the close association with the autonomic nerves supplying the bladder and genitalia require special and unique consideration when planning treatment for cancer of the rectum. Therefore, colon and rectal adenocarcinomas are discussed separately.

DIAGNOSIS AND PREOPERATIVE EVALUATION

The progression of colorectal cancer from a benign polyp to invasive cancer is a notoriously silent process, producing few symptoms reliably, and thus often resulting in a diagnosis at an advanced stage. Although awareness of colorectal cancer screening is increasing, greater than 50% of patients who present have advanced (Stage IV) disease. The signs and symptoms of colon cancer are varied, nonspecific, and dependent upon the location and relative diameter of the tumor in the colon or rectum. Colonoscopic inspection of the colon prompted by anemia, hematochezia, a change in bowel habits, or simply routine screening most frequently leads to the diagnosis of colorectal cancer. Biopsies taken at the time of endoscopy reveal invasive adenocarcinoma. Depth of invasion can seldom be established on the basis of these minute biopsies, however. A complete surgical specimen is required. Thus, an essential aspect of treatment is the surgical procurement of the cancer, the associated bowel, and the packet of draining lymph nodes. Before this, however, patients with nonobstructing tumors should undergo an "extent of disease" evaluation. This includes a thorough physical examination, chest x-ray, ECG, basic laboratory evaluation including hemoglobin and electrolytes, carcinoembryonic antigen level (CEA), and abdominal imaging study such as a CT or MRI to inspect the liver for metastases and to search for other intra-abdominal pathology. In addition, *complete colonoscopy* is essential once the diagnosis of colon or rectal cancer is made, in a search for synchronous neoplasms and to clear the colon of benign polyps. Most patients with colorectal cancer will eventually require operation, and, depending upon the nature of their co-morbidities, a thorough medical evaluation focused on cardiopulmonary issues may be warranted to stratify operative risk. Recommendations regarding intraoperative ß-blockers, strategies for optimizing pulmonary function, and suggestions for fluid management can then be made.[5]

The two most controversial aspects of the preoperative work-up remain the issues of CT scanning and CEA levels and bear further discussion. CEA is a fairly nonspecific tumor marker and has never been advocated as a screening strategy. Although it can be elevated in a variety of tumors and conditions such as lung and breast cancers, smoking, and benign inflammatory disorders of the GI tract, obtaining a CEA prior to and following resection of colorectal cancer is advocated for its value as a prognostic indicator postoperatively. In patients with an elevated preoperative CEA, return to normal levels complete resection, while persistently elevated values indicate presence of residual disease. In addition, a high preoperative CEA level is both independently associated with a poor outcome and correlates with a shorter disease-free survival. An initially-elevated CEA is associated with a 37% 5-year distant recurrence rate vs 7.5% of those with normal CEA. On the strength of these data, obtaining a CEA routinely is advocated.[6]

The routine use of CT scanning continues to be an area of some controversy. Although most surgeons advocate preoperative CT as an adjunct for operative planning, and oncologists appreciate an opportunity to obtain staging information, the sensitivity of CT for the detection of pathologic lymphadenopathy is fairly low, ranging from 19% to 67%.[6] For hepatic metastases greater than 1 cm in size, accuracy in the range of 90% to 95% has been documented.[6] Even so, it is widely recognized that the data obtained rarely influence the operation or result in a different surgical approach. In cases where a palpable mass is present or extension into adjacent organs is suspected, imaging may help in the operative planning and in a minority of cases (eg, where the cancer is inextricably invading retroperitoneal structures like the porta hepatis) may help the surgeon make the rare decision to treat nonoperatively first with diversion and adjuvant

Table 10-3

PREOPERATIVE ASSESSMENT REQUIREMENTS FOR COLON AND RECTAL CANCER SURGERY

Test	Colon Cancer	Rectal Cancer
Colonoscopy to the cecum with biopsies for tissue diagnosis	Yes	Yes
Cardiopulmonary risk assessment	Yes	Yes
Family history/pedigree analysis	Yes	Yes
Electrolytes/hemoglobin	Yes	Yes
ECG	Yes	Yes
CXR	Yes	Yes
Preoperative CEA	Yes	Yes
CT scan abdomen and pelvis with intravenous and oral contrast*	Maybe	Maybe
EUS	No	Yes

*Although no Level I or Level II evidence supports routine use of CT scan in the preoperative evaluation of colorectal cancer, it is recognized that it is a commonly ordered test and may affect the care of a small subset of patients. Please see text for further discussion.

chemotherapy. Preoperative CT scanning is not universally accepted but may be helpful in specific situations such as local invasion, and when additional pathology is suspected from the medical workup[6] (Table 10-3).

Colorectal cancers can bleed, causing blood to appear in the stool (hematochezia). Bleeding from right-sided colon tumors can cause dark, tarry stools (melena). Often the bleeding may be asymptomatic and detected only when anemia is discovered by a routine hemoglobin determination. Iron deficiency anemia in any male or postmenopausal female should lead to a search for a source of bleeding from the GI tract. Bleeding is often associated with colon cancer, but in approximately one-third of patients with a proven colon cancer, the hemoglobin will be normal and the stool will test negative for occult blood.

Cancers located in the left colon are often constrictive in nature. Patients with left-sided colon cancers may notice a change in bowel habit, most often reported as increasing constipation or thin stools. Frank hematochezia or blood-streaked stools are possible, but more commonly associated with rectal cancers. Sigmoid cancers can mimic diverticulitis, presenting with pain, fever, and obstructive symptoms. At least 20% of patients with sigmoid cancer will also have diverticular disease, making the correct diagnosis difficult at times. Sigmoid cancers can also cause colovesical or colovaginal fistulas. Such fistulas are more commonly caused by diverticulitis, but it is imperative that the correct diagnosis be established, because the treatment of colon cancer is substantially different than the treatment for diverticulitis. CT scan, colonoscopy with biopsy, CEA testing, and Gastrografin or barium enema can help distinguish these entities.

Cancers in the right colon more often present with melena, fatigue associated with anemia, or, if the tumor is advanced, abdominal pain. Although obstructive symptoms are more commonly associated with cancers of the left colon, any advanced colorectal cancer can cause a change in bowel habits and intestinal obstruction. Colonoscopy is the gold standard for establishing the diagnosis of colon cancer. It permits biopsy of the tumor to verify the diagnosis, while allowing inspection of the entire colon to exclude the synchronous polyps or cancers that occur in 3% to 5% of cases.

SURGICAL MANAGEMENT OF COLON CANCERS

The surgical therapy of colorectal cancer has not significantly changed in many years. Technical innovations such as laparoscopy follow the same basic principles of resection that traditional methods do. The objective of surgery for colon adenocarcinoma is still the removal of the primary cancer with adequate margins, regional lymphadenectomy, and restoration of the continuity of the GI tract. The extent of resection is determined by the location of the cancer, its blood supply and draining lymphatic system, and the presence or absence of direct extension into adjacent organs. Ligation of the vessel feeding the affected bowel segment close to its origin insures resection of the apical lymph nodes—those nodes located close to the origin of the feeding vessel. In one study, patients with involved apical lymph nodes had a 2.5-fold increase in mortality, a finding confirmed by a larger Australian series demonstrating a reduction in survival from 54% to 26% at 5 years for those with involvement. Although high ligation helps prevent local recurrence, aids in postoperative staging, and affects postoperative medical therapy, it does not affect survival.[7-9]

Likewise, performing extended bowel resections in order to improve survival has not been an effective strategy, with the possible exception of tumors occurring in the "border" or "watershed" regions of the large bowel—especially at the splenic flexure and in the midtransverse colon. The recommendation that these cancers be resected in both vascular and lymphatic drainage distributions is well taken. Although studies have not confirmed that disease-specific survival is improved, the technical benefit of creating a reliable blood supply to the anastomosis outside the tenuous watershed area is manifest in lower anastomotic leak rates[10] (Figure 10-3).

To restore the continuity of the GI tract, an anastomosis is fashioned with either sutures or staples, joining the ends of the intestine. It is important that both segments of the intestine used for the anastomosis have excellent blood supply and that there be no tension on the anastomosis. For lesions involving the cecum, ascending colon, and hepatic flexure, a *right hemicolectomy* is the procedure of choice. This involves removal of the bowel from 4 to 6 cm proximal to the ileocecal valve to the portion of the transverse colon supplied by the right branch of the middle colic artery. An anastomosis is created between the terminal ileum and the transverse colon. The ileocolic artery is routinely taken. An extended *right hemicolectomy* is the procedure of choice for most transverse colon lesions and involves division of the ileocolic and middle colic arteries at their origin, with removal of the right and transverse colon supplied by these vessels. The anastomosis is fashioned between the terminal ileum and the distal left colon. A *left hemicolectomy* (ie, resection from the splenic flexure to the rectosigmoid junction) is done for tumors of the descending colon, whereas a *sigmoidectomy* alone is appropriate for tumors of the sigmoid colon. In these approaches, the inferior mesenteric artery is taken near it's origin from the aorta. Most surgeons prefer to avoid incorporating the proximal sigmoid colon into an anastomosis because of the often-tenuous blood supply

Figure 10-3. Operative strategies for colon tumors according to location. (Reprinted with permission from Chang AE. Colorectal cancer. In: Greenfield LJ, Mulholland MW, Oldham KT, Zele-nock GB, eds. *Surgery: Scientific Principles and Practice.* Philadelp-hia, PA: JB Lippincott Company; 1993: 1024.)

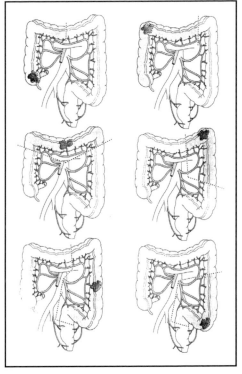

from the inferior mesenteric artery and the frequent involvement of the sigmoid with diverticular disease.

Synchronous Colon Cancer

Synchronous lesions occur in 3% to 5% of cases. Depending on the site of the tumors, a resection can be accomplished with either one or two separate resections. In general, separate tumors in close proximity sharing blood supply may be resected with a single anastomosis. Those that are separated by distance and blood supply such as a cecal and a sigmoid lesion may be resected with the formation of 2 separate anastomoses without additional morbidity. The presence of additional lesions in a patient less than 50 years of age must raise the question of familial or hereditary colorectal cancer. Those patients with either a suggestive family history or a positive genetic test for MMR gene mutations (HNPCC) will require a subtotal colectomy with an ileorectal anastomosis.

The Role of Laparoscopy in the Management of Colorectal Cancer

It has been over a decade since the first description of the use of laparoscopy for colorectal cancer. Since then, the technique has not achieved the same universal acceptance that laparoscopic cholecystectomy has, and, in the case of colorectal cancer, its early history was dogged by reports of port site metastases and inadequate lymph node dissection for pathologic staging. Today, the advantages of laparoscopic surgery are becoming clearer as more and better data become available. The specter of port site metastases has largely been banished by surgeon experience, technology that allows safer specimen delivery, and examination of the tissue through studies with large patient numbers. Through a number of studies examining lymph node harvest, we know that oncologic standards are being met, operative times for these complicated procedures are reduced, and complication rates are comparable to open procedures. What remains to be definitively clarified, however, is a decisive patient benefit. While it is clear that many patients do gain an advantage from the minimally invasive approach in general, many of the studies designed to explore this in colorectal disease have been statistically underpowered, and answers have not been easily forthcoming. Laparoscopic colorectal surgery is technically demanding and time consuming—especially for the low-volume surgeon. In the near future, prospective studies from major, high volume centers will undoubtedly demonstrate that laparoscopic colorectal surgery is at least as effective and well tolerated as traditional open techniques. Future challenges will center on the widespread incorporation of this technology into the repertoire of surgeons everywhere and definitively address issues directly impacting patient benefit such as length of stay, postoperative pain, and return to work.[11,12]

EMERGENT PRESENTATIONS

Obstructing Cancers

Patients who are obstructed commonly present emergently, without the benefit of a thorough preoperative evaluation. Dehydration and physiological stress complicates surgical treatment, and fluid resuscitation with close monitoring is advisable even in the completely obstructed patient prior to operative intervention if possible. Because of the relatively small sigmoid colon caliber, most obstructing colon cancers occur in this area, and a plain film of the abdomen reveals a distal large bowel obstruction with a dilated, distended proximal colon. The presence of free air under the diaphragm is a grave sign, indicating free perforation of the colon, usually in the thin-walled cecum.

In patients with left-sided tumors causing complete obstruction, a water-soluble contrast enema is often useful to establish the anatomic level of the obstruction. Primary anastomosis between the proximal colon and the colon distal to the tumor is usually avoided in the presence of obstruction because of a perceived high risk of anastomotic leak or infection associated with such an approach. Thus, such patients are usually treated by resection of the segment of colon containing the obstructing cancer, closure of the distal sigmoid or rectum, and contruction of a colostomy (Hartmann's operation). Intestinal continuity can be re-established later after the colon has been prepped by taking down the colostomy and fashioning a colorectal anastomosis.

One alternative to this approach is to resect the segment of left colon containing the cancer, and then cleanse the remaining colon with saline lavage by inserting a catheter through the appendix or ileum into the cecum and irrigating the contents from the colon. A primary anastomosis between the prepared colon and the rectum can then be fashioned without the need for a temporary colostomy. A loop ileostomy, easily closed a few months later, can be used to "protect" the newly formed anastomosis by diverting the fecal stream if necessary. A third approach occasionally used for obstructing cancers of the sigmoid colon, particularly when obstruction is complicated by proximal ischemia or perforation, is to resect the tumor and the entire colon proximal to the tumor and fashion an anastomosis between the ileum and the distal sigmoid colon or rectum (subtotal colectomy with ileosigmoid or ileorectal anastomosis). This approach has the advantage of avoiding a temporary colostomy and eliminating the need to search for synchronous lesions in the colon proximal to the cancer. Due to loss of the absorptive and storage capacity of the colon, however, this procedure causes an increase in stool frequency. Patients under the age of 60 years generally tolerate this well, with gradual adaptation of the small bowel mucosa, increased water absorption, and an acceptable stool frequency of 1 to 3 movements daily. In older individuals though, subtotal colectomy may result in significant chronic diarrhea.

Patients with obstructing right-sided tumors are rare, and present as distal small bowel obstruction. Right hemicolectomy with primary anastomosis, even in an unprepared colon, is the usual treatment of choice. This approach, however, is predicated on the patient's presenting hemodynamic status, with resection and end ileostomy being the most expedient, and at times, the safest alternative.

Perforated Colon Cancer

Perforated right-sided colon cancer should be resected emergently—the amount of fecal or purulent contamination from the perforation dictates whether or not a primary anastomosis can be made. An end ileostomy is a reasonable option if peritonitis with contamination and inflammation is an issue. On the other hand, a left colon cancer perforation usually results in a resection with a Hartmann's pouch. Subtotal colectomy is the safest option and indicated if proximal obstruction from a distal tumor results in ischemia or cecal perforation. Depending on the degree of contamination and the patient's clinical status, a loop ileostomy can be fashioned to protect the anastomosis. A Hartmann's pouch and end ileostomy are indicated in clinically unstable patients and preserve future reconstruction options.

STAGING

Tumor staging describes the process by which information concerning the size, location, and extraintestinal spread of the cancer is assimilated into an overall description of the state of the disease at the moment. The most significant data, however, arise from the postoperative inspection of the specimen. Tumor depth, nodal metastases, and the presence of tumor metastasis are most significant in determining prognosis. At the present time, the stage of the tumor is assessed by indicating the depth of penetration of the tumor into the bowel wall, the extent of lymph node involvement, and the presence or absence of distant metastases. For most of the last half century, the standard staging system was based on a system developed and modified by Cuthbert Dukes, a pathologist at St. Mark's Hospital in London.[13] The Dukes classification is simple to remember, and still frequently used. Dukes Stage A cancer is confined to the bowel wall; Stage B cancer penetrates the bowel wall, and Stage C cancer indicates lymph node metastases. Astler and Coller further separated the tumors that had invaded lymph nodes but did not penetrate the entire bowel wall (C1) from tumors that invaded lymph nodes and did penetrate the entire wall (C2). Turnbull and associates from the Cleveland Clinic added Stage D for tumors with distant metastasis. All of these modifications in various combinations are still in use and often called "modified Dukes classifications."

The classification in use by most hospitals in the United States was developed by the AJCC and was approved by the International Union Against Cancer (UICC). This classification, known as the TNM system, combines clinical information obtained preoperatively with data obtained during surgery and after histological examination of the specimen. There have been some modifications in the system since its introduction in 1987.

The surgeon is now encouraged to score the completeness of the resection as follows: R0 for complete tumor resection with all margins negative, R1 for incomplete tumor resection with microscopic involvement of a margin, and R2 for incomplete tumor resection with gross residual tumor not resected (see Appendix D).

There are 4 possible stages of colorectal cancer within the AJCC system. In Stage I, there is no lymph node metastasis and the tumor is either T1 or T2 (up to muscularis propria). Patients who undergo appropriate resection of T Stage 1 colon cancer have a 5-year survival rate of approximately 90%. Stage II is now subdivided into IIA (if the primary tumor is T3) and IIB (for T4 lesions), with no lymph node metastasis. The 5-year survival rate for patients with Stage II colon cancer treated by appropriate surgical resection is approximately 75%. Stage III cancer is characterized by lymph node metastasis and is now subdivided into IIIA (T1 to T2, N1, M0), IIIB (T3 to T4, N1, M0), and IIIC (any T, N2, M0). In the current version of the staging system, smooth metastatic nodules in the pericolic or perirectal fat are considered lymph node metastasis and should be included in N staging. The estimated survival for Stage III cancer treated by surgery alone is approximately 50%. With the presence of distant metastasis (Stage IV), the 5-year survival rate is less than 5%.[14]

The survival rates described above do not reflect the use of adjuvant chemotherapy following curative resection of colon cancer. There is a clearly demonstrated benefit for patients with Stage III disease treated postoperatively with 5-fluorouracil/leukovorin (67% 5-year survival). The benefits of adjuvant chemotherapy for patients with Stage II colon cancer have not been clearly demonstrated, and several ongoing clinical trials are now studying chemotherapy in this group of patients. There has been no demonstrated efficacy for adjuvant chemotherapy for patients with Stage I colon cancer.[15]

The presence of hepatic metastatic disease does not preclude the surgical excision of the primary tumor. Unless the hepatic metastatic disease is extensive, excising the primary cancer can provide excellent palliation. Bleeding and obstruction caused by the tumor can be avoided, and if the metastatic hepatic disease is resectable, the cure rate approaches 25%.

SURGICAL MANAGEMENT OF RECTAL CANCER

The preoperative assessment of patients with rectal cancer is similar to that described for patients with colon cancer with some significant differences: the requirement for precise characterization of the cancer with respect to proximity to the anal sphincters, and the extent of invasion as determined by depth of penetration into the bowel wall and spread to adjacent lymph nodes. The location of the tumor is best determined by examination with a rigid proctosigmoidoscope. Rigid proctosigmoidoscopy should be done even if the tumor has been diagnosed with a colonoscopic examination because the flexible scope may not accurately measure the exact distance from the tumor to the anal sphincter. The depth of penetration can be estimated by digital rectal exam (superficially invasive tumors are mobile, whereas the lesions become tethered and fixed with increasing depth of penetration), and EUS or MRI with endorectal coil can provide accurate assessment of the extent of invasion of the bowel wall.

The most common symptom of rectal cancer is hematochezia. Unfortunately, this is often attributed to hemorrhoids, and the correct diagnosis is consequently delayed until the cancer has reached an advanced stage. Other symptoms include mucus discharge, tenesmus, change in bowel habit, and weight loss.

Sphincter Sparing Surgery

The concept of "sphincter sparing" rectal cancer surgery is relatively new and has become a benchmark for surgeons and for patients. The measurement of "colostomy-free survival" has permeated the colorectal cancer outcomes literature as the goal of intestinal continuity becomes increasingly safely attainable, even for distal rectal cancers. Because of its importance to patients and physicians, this topic bears special discussion. A number of factors contribute to the possibility of "sphincter saving" surgery. Tumors located in the distal 3 to 5 cm of the rectum present the greatest challenge for the surgeon. Achieving local control of the tumor is more difficult here due to the confinement of the pelvic anatomy and the proximity of adjacent organs such as the urethra, prostate, seminal vesicles, vagina, cervix, and bladder. For tumors in this location, the surgeon must decide between wide margins of resection and preservation of the anal sphincter. Tumors that clearly invade the anal sphincters, very low tumors in incontinent patients, and large male patients with narrow pelvises and low cancers are usually not amenable to sphincter sparing surgery. Although in the past, a clear 2-cm distal margin has been the standard for oncologic tumor clearance, the advent of neoadjuvant radiation with concomitant tumor shrinkage has reduced this distal margin—provided that a concurrent total mesorectal excision is done for tumors in the low- and midrectum.[15] Preoperative radiotherapy, usually combined with chemotherapy, is often recommended to reduce the size of the rectal cancer. In the United States, it is becoming increasingly common to treat deeply penetrating (T3) rectal cancers and any rectal cancers associated with lymphadenopathy with preoperative radiation (4500 to 5040 cGy over 5 to 6 weeks) combined with chemotherapy (5-FU and leucovorin). This treatment program reduces the degree of wall invasion and of lymph node involvement in 70% of patients. There are a variety of advantages in preoperative radiation therapy, including biological (decreased tumor seeding at the time of surgery and increased cellular radiosensitivity), physical (no postsurgical small bowel fixation in the pelvis), and technical (ability to change the operation from an abdominal perineal resection to a sphincter preserving low anterior resection with a coloanal anastomosis). An increase in the resectability rate is an additional benefit in patients with locally advanced or "unresectable" rectal tumors. This reduction in tumor invasiveness by preoperative radiation is known as downstaging.

Once the location and stage of the cancer are determined, various options need to be considered for the optimal treatment of the rectal cancer. Other important considerations include the presence or absence of comorbid conditions and the patient's body habitus (an obese male with a narrow pelvis presents technical difficulties that differ from a thin woman with a wide pelvis). There is no single operation to treat all rectal cancers, and the appropriate operation should be tailored to eradicate the tumor while preserving function to the fullest extent possible. The following procedures all are useful in the circumstances described.

Abdominoperineal Resection

The complete excision of the rectum and anus by dissection through the abdomen and perineum with suture closure of the perineum and creation of a permanent colostomy was first described by Ernest Miles and is thus sometimes referred to as the "Miles procedure."[16] For many years, before the advent of neoadjuvant therapy and mechanical staplers, this procedure was considered the standard of care for tumors in the distal half of the rectum. An abdominal perineal resection (APR) is indicated when the tumor involves the anal sphincters, when the tumor is too close to the sphincters to obtain adequate margins, or in patients in whom sphincter-preserving surgery is not possible because of unfavorable body habitus or poor preoperative sphincter control. The rectum and sigmoid colon are mobilized along with the mesorectum through an abdominal incision to the level of the levator ani muscles. Careful attention to the oncologic and functional details of the resection mandates ligation of the IMA, sparing of the hypogastric nerve bundles, and resecting the mesorectum just outside its investing fascia. The perineal portion of the operation excises the anus, the anal sphincters, and the distal rectum.

Local Excision

Local excision of a rectal cancer is an excellent operation for a small cancer in the distal rectum that has not penetrated into the muscularis propria. This is usually accomplished through a transanal approach and usually involves excision of the full thickness of the rectal wall underlying the tumor. Other approaches less commonly utilized include the trans-sphincteric (York-Mason) approach and posterior proctectomy (Kraske's procedure). Local excisions do not allow complete removal of lymph nodes in the mesorectum; therefore, operative staging is limited. The operation is indicated for mobile tumors that are less than 4 cm in diameter, that involve less than 40% of the rectal wall circumference, and that are located within 6 cm of the anal verge. A good clinical indicator of a locally resectable tumor is a mobile tumor easily palpated via digital rectal exam. These tumors should be Stage T1 (depth limited to the submucosa), well or moderately differentiated histologically, and with no vascular or lymphatic invasion. There should be no evidence of nodal disease on preoperative endorectal ultrasound or MRI. Adherence to these principles results in acceptable local recurrence rates compared with treatment by abdominal perineal resection. Local excision is also used for palliation of more advanced cancer in patients with severe comorbid disease, in whom extensive surgery carries a high risk of morbidity or mortality.

Transanal excision requires the complete excision of the cancer with adequate margins of normal tissue. Unfortunately, as experience has accumulated with this approach, it has become clear that close follow-up is mandatory because approximately 8% to 18% of T1 lesions will recur, and the recurrence rate for T2 lesions has been shown in some series to exceed 20%. Local excision is not adequate treatment for a T2 rectal cancer, and radical excision (low anterior resection or abdominal perineal resection) is the procedure of choice.[17-20] Both the York-Mason and Kraske procedures approach the rectum posteriorly via a midline or slightly off-set incision. The York-Mason incision actually divides the sphincter mechanism to approach the low rectum. The sphincters must be carefully sewn back together at the end of the case. The Kraske procedure is used for slightly higher tumors and is suprasphincteric. The coccyx is usually removed using this approach since it impedes visualization. Both of these approaches are far less commonly used today than in the past. Technology has not only allowed us to achieve safer lower anastomoses while using good oncologic technique, it has also allowed us to operate on older, more medically challenging patients with more confidence in their ability to tolerate the surgery.

Fulguration

This technique, which eradicates the cancer by using an electrocautery device that destroys the tumor by creating a full-thickness eschar at the tumor site, requires extension of the eschar into the perirectal fat, thus destroying both the tumor and the rectal wall. The procedure is reserved for patients with a prohibitive operative risk for radical surgery and a limited life expectancy. The procedure is used only for lesions below the peritoneal reflection. Complications associated with this approach are postoperative fever, harm to adjacent structures such as the prostate or urethra, and significant bleeding that can occur as late as 10 days after the operation. This technique cannot provide a specimen to assess the pathological stage, because the tumor and margins are destroyed by fulguration.

Low Anterior Resection

Resection of the rectum through an abdominal approach offers the advantage of completely removing the portion of bowel containing the cancer and the mesorectum, which contains the lymphatic channels that drain the tumor bed. The term *anterior resection* indicates resection of the proximal rectum or rectosigmoid, above the peritoneal reflection. The term *low anterior resection* (LAR) indicates that the operation entails resection of the rectum below the peritoneal reflection through an abdominal approach. The sigmoid colon is almost always included with the resected specimen because diverticulosis often involves the sigmoid, and the blood supply to the sigmoid is often not adequate to sustain an anastomosis if the inferior mesenteric artery is transected. For cancers involving the lower half of the rectum, the entire mesorectum (which contains the lymph channels draining the tumor bed) should be excised in continuity with the rectum. This technique, total mesorectal excision (TME), produces the complete resection of an intact package of the rectum and its adjacent mesorectum, enveloped within the visceral pelvic fascia with uninvolved circumferential margins. The use of the technique of total mesorectal excision has resulted in a significant increase in 5-year survival rates (50% to 75%), decrease in local recurrence rate (from 30% to 5%), and a decrease in the incidence of impotence and bladder dysfunction (from 85% to less than 15%).[21]

Intestinal continuity is re-established by fashioning an anastomosis between the descending colon and the rectum, a feat that has been greatly facilitated by the introduction of the circular stapling device. After the colorectal anastomosis has been completed, it should be inspected with a proctoscope inserted through the anus. If there is concern about the integrity of the anastomosis, or *if the patient has received preoperative chemoradiation, a temporary proximal colostomy or ileostomy* should be made to permit complete healing of the anastomosis. The colostomy can be closed in approximately 10 weeks if hypaque enema verifies the integrity of the anastomosis.

An end-to-end anastomosis between the descending colon and the distal rectum or anus may result in significant alteration of bowel habits attributed to the loss of the normal rectal capacity. Patients treated with this operation often experience frequent small bowel movements ("low anterior resection syndrome" or "clustering"). Although this problem is most pronounced in the months following surgery with accommodation occurring thereafter, it is possible to alleviate some of these symptoms in the immediate postoperative period by fashioning a reservoir from the distal descending colon prior to making the anastomosis. A "coloplasty" and a "J pouch" are techniques designed to increase capacity and diminish clustering. The functional advantages of these techniques seem to be limited to the first year after surgery only.[22]

Coloanal Anastomosis

Abdominal perineal resection is at times required because a cancer in the distal rectum cannot be resected with adequate margins while preserving the anal sphincter. However, the use of preoperative radiation and chemotherapy has been shown, in some instances, to shrink the tumor to an extent that acceptable margins can be achieved. If the anal sphincters do not need to be sacrificed to achieve adequate margins based upon

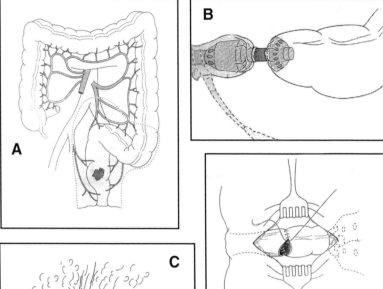

Figure 10-4. Operative strategies for rectal cancers. (A) Extent of resection for APR. (B) Stapled LAR. (C) Handsewn coloanal anastomosis. (D) Exposure for a transsacral resection. (Reprinted with permission from Chang AE. Colorectal cancer. In: Greenfield LJ, Mulholland MW, Oldham KT, Zelenock GB, eds. *Surgery: Scientific Principles and Practice*. Philadelphia, PA: JB Lippincott Company; 1993:1024.

oncologic principles, a permanent stoma may be avoided with an anastomosis between the colon and the anal canal. This operation has particular application for young patients with rectal tumors who have a favorable body habitus and good preoperative sphincter function. The operation can be conducted in a variety of ways, but all methods involve mobilizing he sigmoid colon and rectum via an abdominal approach down to the level of the anal canal. The technique may include distal dissection through the anus as well to facilitate accurate identification of the distal margin. The anastomosis is made with sutures placed through a transanal approach by the surgeon in the perineal field (Figure 10-4). Because radiated rectal tissue has a diminished rate of healing, and low pelvic anastomoses in this situation have a high leak rate (10% to 14%), a temporary diverting ileostomy is advisable for 8 to 10 weeks postsurgery.

Complications of Colorectal Surgery

Colorectal surgery has an overall morbidity rate of 8% to 15% and a mortality of 1% to 2%.[23] Serious complications specific to colon surgery include anastomotic leaks resulting in abscess formation and sepsis. This dreaded complication occurs in 5% to 8% of cases, and usually results from a technical failure stemming from inadequate blood supply to the anastomosis, tension on the anastomosis, or failure of the sutures or staples. The treatment depends upon the medical status of the patient. Peritonitis from free air and stool in the abdomen mandates immediate return to the operating room, abdominal washout, and creation of a temporary stoma. A walled-off abscess with no free air or stool in a patient without peritonitis may be percutaneously drained, and the patient may be treated with antibiotics. A resultant coloenteric fistula will usually close over time in the absence of distal obstruction or ongoing inflammation or neoplasm.

Wound infection rates for colorectal surgery are approximately 5%. Simply opening the wound to drain the infection results in cure. Antibiotics are required only when the abscess is complicated by concomitant cellulitis, and should be directed against skin flora such as *S. aureus* and *S. epidermidis,* the most common organisms involved. Emergency surgery complicated by heavy fecal loads with spillage or purulence increases the infection rate, and skin incisions are often left open above the level of the fascia to granulate and heal by secondary intention.

Complications specific to rectal surgery can be both physically and psychologically distressing. Extensive pelvic dissection can result in disruption of the autonomic nervous plexus responsible for sexual and urinary function. The reported range of impotence following radical rectal surgery varies widely in the literature from 14% to 76%.[24] In one study, age was a major factor, with 96% of patients less than 60 years old maintaining potency, compared to 50% to 75% of those greater than 60.[25] The additional insult of radiation may further degrade function. Continence can also be a problem following a low anastomosis, particularly in those who have undergone radiation. Kollmorgen studied the effects of postoperative radiation versus surgery alone in a population of patients with rectal cancer and found that the addition of radiation increased stool frequency, nighttime bowel movements, incontinence, pad wearing, and most significantly, diminished the ability to defer defecation more than 15 minutes in 78% of patients.[26] Although the colon J-pouch and coloplasty techniques were devised to address these problems and do result in short-term improvement, the functional results of "neorectum" construction do not appear to be significantly different from straight anastomosis 1 to 2 years after surgery. It is clear that the long-term consequences of neoadjuvant radiation in combination with surgery are incompletely understood. In addition, a high number of patients suffer depression following APR (32%) and LAR (10%). This may impact on ability to return to work. In a study from England, almost two-thirds of APR patients and a quarter of all LAR patients filed for permanent disability.[24]

SPECIFIC HIGH-RISK CONDITIONS

FAMILIAL ADENOMATOUS POLYPOSIS

FAP is the prototypical hereditary polyposis syndrome. A germline APC truncation mutation is responsible for this autosomal dominantly inherited disease. FAP is rare, with an estimated incidence of 1/8000 in the United States, occurring without gender predilection; however, patients who carry the mutation have a certain early death by age

44 from colorectal or duodenal cancer without appropriate surgical intervention. Unfortunately, 30% of FAP cases are *de novo* germline mutations, presenting without a family history of the disease, thus providing few clues and resulting in a delayed presentation. The average age of FAP presentation in a patient with no antecedent family history is 29 years. The average age of a patient who presents with colorectal cancer related to FAP is 39 years. Classically, greater than 100 adenomatous polyps are present, however, polyps can number in the thousands and are almost always manifest by the late second or early third decade of life. Patients with a known family history of FAP are at a great advantage. Colonoscopic screening begins at the age of 12, and proctocolectomy during adolescence results in cancer prevention. FAP is of great interest to those studying sporadic colorectal cancer because APC truncation mutations similar to those found in APC patients occur in 85% of sporadic colorectal cancers.

Classic FAP is characterized by truncation mutations occurring in the gene from codon 169 to codon 1393. This area includes the "mutational cluster region," an area responsible for beta-catenin binding. However, genotype-phenotype correlations exist with mutations in other regions of the gene. For example, mutations close to the 3' and 5' end of the gene predispose to an attenuated phenotype termed *attenuated FAP* (AFAP), a variant of the syndrome characterized by fewer than 100 colonic polyps, rectal sparing, considerable phenotypic variation within pedigrees, and delayed age of cancer onset.[22]

The FAP phenotype is also expressed by the variability of the presence of extraintestinal manifestations of disease. In the past, the term Gardner's syndrome was used to describe the coexpression of profuse colonic adenomatous polyps along with osteomas of the mandible and skull; desmoid tumors of the mesentery; gastric, duodenal, and periampullary polyps; epidermoid cysts; papillary thyroid tumors; and brain tumors. Osteomas usually present as visible and palpable prominences in the skull, mandible, and tibia of individuals with FAP. They are virtually always benign. Radiographs of the maxilla and mandible may reveal bone cysts, supernumerary and impacted molars, or congenitally absent teeth. Desmoid tumors can present in the retroperitoneum and abdominal wall of affected patients, usually following surgery. These tumors seldom metastasize, but are often locally invasive. Direct invasion of the mesenteric vessels, ureters, or walls of the small intestine may result in death. Gastric and duodenal polyps will occur in about half of affected individuals. Most of the gastric polyps represent fundic gland hyperplasia, rather than adenomatous polyps, and have limited malignant potential. However, duodenal polyps are adenomatous in nature and should be considered premalignant. Patients with FAP have an increased risk of ampullary cancer and this neoplasm constitutes, along with desmoid tumors, the leading cause of death in FAP patients who have undergone total proctocolectomy. Adenomatous polyps and cancer have also been found in the jejunum and ileum of patients with FAP. Rare extraintestinal malignancies in FAP patients include cancers of the extrahepatic bile ducts, gallbladder, pancreas, adrenals, thyroid, and liver. Congenital hypertrophy of the retinal pigmented epithelium (CHRPE), which can be detected by indirect ophthalmoscopy, will be present in about 75% of affected individuals. Turcot's syndrome describes patients who have both colorectal and concurrent central nervous system malignancies.

Surgical Management

Surgical treatment of patients with FAP is directed at removal of all affected colonic and rectal mucosa. Restorative proctocolectomy with ileal pouch anal anastomosis (IPAA) has become the most commonly recommended operation, although historically, total proctocolectomy with end ileostomy was performed for FAP. The quality of life advantages for IPAA over end ileostomy are great. Restoration of GI continuity allows these typically young patients to have a fairly normal lifestyle. While this same operation in patients with ulcerative colitis may be complicated by occasional or chronic inflammation of the pouch (pouchitis), those issues seem not to plague the FAP patient. Function is good, with good continence, and good pouch function characterized by 5 to 7 bowel movements per day typically. The ileal pouch is really a neorectum—roughly 20 cm of terminal ileum folded over and opened to create a functional reservoir that is attached directly above the anal sphincter complex at the dentate line. Either surgical stapling or hand suturing the connection is acceptable. An alternative approach, total abdominal colectomy with ileorectal anastomosis, may only be used in individuals with rectal sparing, such as patients with attenuated FAP. With this procedure, the abdominal colon is resected and an anastomosis fashioned between the ileum and top of the rectum. It is a technically simpler operation to perform, pelvic dissection is avoided, and function is often better with fewer bowel movements and improved sensation. This technique reduces the potential complication of injury to the autonomic nerves that could result in impotence. In addition, there is theoretically less risk of anastomotic leak from the relatively simple ileorectal anastomosis fashioned in the peritoneal cavity, compared to the long staple lines required to form the ileal pouch. Because the rectum remains at high risk for the formation of new precancerous polyps, a proctoscopic examination is required every 6 months to detect and destroy any new polyps, and there is a definite increased risk of cancer arising in the rectum with the passage of time. Patients who choose to be treated by abdominal colectomy with ileorectal anastomosis should realize that the risk of developing rectal cancer is real and has been shown to be 4, 5.6, 7.9, and 25% at 5, 10, 15, and 20 years after the operation, respectively. Even though sulindac and celecoxib can produce partial regression of polyps, semiannual surveillance of the rectal mucosa is required, and about one-third of patients treated by abdominal colectomy and ileorectal anastomosis will develop florid polyposis of the rectum that will require proctectomy (and either ileostomy or IPAA) within 20 years.[26]

As discussed above, polyps of the stomach and duodenum are not uncommon in patients with FAP. Gastric polyps are usually hyperplastic or fundic gland polyps and do not require surgical removal. However, duodenal and ampullary polyps are usually adenomatous and require surveillance and, if possible, excision. A reasonable surveillance program calls for upper GI surveillance every year after the age of 30, with endoscopic polypectomy to remove all large adenomas from the duodenum. If numerous polyps are identified, the endoscopy may be repeated with greater frequency dependent upon pathologic findings. If an ampullary cancer is discovered at an early stage or if duodenal polyps appear to be rapidly enlarging, endoscopic resection or pancreatoduodenectomy (Whipple's procedure) may be indicated.

Abdominal desmoid tumor can be an especially vexing and difficult extraintestinal manifestation of FAP. After surgical procedures, dense fibrous tissue forms in the mesentery of the small intestine or within the abdominal wall in some patients with FAP. If the mesentery is involved, the intestine can be tethered or invaded directly by the tumor. The locally invasive tumor can also encroach upon the vascular supply to the intestine. Small desmoid tumors confined to the abdominal wall are appropriately treated by resection, but the surgical treatment of mesenteric desmoids is dangerous and generally futile. Operation seems to stimulate them, causing them to grow more rapidly. There have been sporadic reports of regression of desmoid tumors after treatment with sulindac, tamoxifen, radiation, and various types of chemotherapy. The initial treatment is usually with sulindac or tamoxifen.

APC I1307K

The I1307K point mutation is an APC mutation implicated in up to 25% of familial colorectal cancers afflicting Ashkenazi Jewish descendants (6% of the general Ashkenazi Jewish population) and is associated with a 2-fold colorectal cancer risk increase. This mutation is now recognized as perhaps the most important cause of familial colorectal cancer in this population. It is caused by substitution of a lysine for isoleucine at codon 1307. This mutation results in an unstable polyadenine tract causing DNA replication mechanisms to fail, thus producing somatic mutations in the APC gene further downstream during cell division. Colorectal cancers in young (<50) patients of Ashkenazi Jewish descent with a positive family history should arouse suspicion of this defect. Treatment is usually limited to segmental resection of the tumor and involved lymph node basin. Close yearly surveillance in the face of a known germline defect seems reasonable, although formal surgical and screening recommendations have not yet been formulated.[27]

HEREDITARY NONPOLYPOSIS COLON CANCER

HNPCC is the most frequently occurring hereditary colorectal cancer syndrome in the United States and Western Europe. It accounts for approximately 3% of all cases of colorectal cancer, and approximately 15% of such cancers in patients with a family history of colorectal cancer. Dr. Aldred S. Warthin, chairman of pathology at the University of Michigan, initially recognized this hereditary syndrome in 1935. Dr. Warthin's seamstress prophesied that she would die of cancer because of her strong family history of endometrial, gastric, and colon cancer. Dr. Warthin's investigations of her family's medical records revealed a pattern of autosomal dominant transmission of the cancer risk. This family (Cancer Family G) has been further studied and characterized by Dr. Henry Lynch, who described the prominent features of the syndrome, including onset of cancer at a relatively young age (mean of 44 years), proximal distribution (70% of cancers located in the right colon), predominance of mucinous or poorly differentiated adenocarcinoma, an increased number of synchronous and metachronous cancers, and—despite all of these poor prognostic indicators—a relatively good outcome following surgery. Two hereditary syndromes were initially described. Lynch I syndrome is characterized by cancer of the proximal colon occurring at a young age, whereas Lynch II Syndrome is characterized by families at risk for both colorectal cancer and extracolonic cancers, including cancers of endometrial, ovarian, gastric, small intestinal, pancreatic, ureteral, and renal pelvic origin. Although initially called "Cancer Family Syndrome," it was renamed *hereditary nonpolyposis colon cancer* both to imply that the cancer arises in a single lesion and to distinguish it from FAP.

Before the genetic mechanisms underlying HNPCC were understood, the syndrome was defined by the Amsterdam Criteria, which has 3 requirements for diagnosis: 1) colorectal cancer in three first-degree relatives, 2) involvement of at least 2 generations, and 3) at least one affected individual under the age of 50 at the time of diagnosis. These requirements were recognized as being too restrictive, and the modified Amsterdam Criteria expanded the cancers to include not only colorectal, but also endometrial, ovarian, gastric, pancreatic, small intestinal, ureteral, and renal pelvic cancers. Further liberalization for identifying patients with HNPCC occurred with the introduction of the Bethesda criteria.

As outlined in the genetics section, molecular biologists have demonstrated that the increased cancer risk in these syndromes is due to mutations of MMR genes governing DNA repair. Mutations in hMSH2 or hMLH1 account for over 90% of identifiable mutations in patients with HNPCC. Although the difference in cancer types occurring in Lynch I and Lynch II syndromes cannot be accounted for by mutations in specific mismatch repair genes, the syndrome involving hMSH6 is characterized by an increased incidence of endometrial carcinoma.[28]

Although the mainstay of diagnosis of HNPCC is a detailed family history, it should be remembered that as many as 20% of newly discovered cases of HNPCC are caused by spontaneous germline mutations, so a family history may not accurately reflect the genetic nature of the syndrome. Colorectal cancer, or an HNPC-related cancer, arising in a person under the age of 50 should raise the suspicion of this syndrome. Genetic counseling and genetic testing can be offered. If the individual proves to have HNPCC by identification of a mutation in one of the known mismatch repair genes, then other family members can be tested after obtaining genetic counseling. However, failure to identify a causative MMR gene mutation in a patient with a suggestive history does not exclude the diagnosis of HNPCC. In as many as 50% of patients with a family history that clearly demonstrates HNPCC type transmission of cancer susceptibility, DNA testing will fail to identify the causative gene.[27]

Surgical Management

The management of patients with HNPCC is somewhat controversial, but the need for close surveillance in patients known to carry the mutation is obvious. It is usually recommended that a program of surveillance colonoscopy begin between the ages of 20 and 30, repeated every 1 to 2 years until age 40, then annually thereafter. Patients with known germline mutations should start yearly colonoscopic surveillance at age 25, or 5 years prior to the age at diagnosis of the index family member. In women, periodic vacuum curettage, as well as pelvic ultrasound and CA-125 levels, are begun at age 25 to 35. Annual tests for occult blood in the urine should also be obtained, because of the risk of ureteral and renal pelvic cancer.[27]

It has been shown that annual colonoscopy and removal of polyps when found decreases the incidence of colon cancer in patients with HNPCC. However, there have been well-documented cases of invasive colon cancers occurring 1 year after a negative colonoscopy. In fact, in patients with a known MMR gene defect and a history of colorectal cancer, the risk of metachronous and synchronous colorectal cancers is about 45% 10 years after resection. It is obvious that the slow evolution from benign polyp to invasive cancer is not a feature of pathogenesis in HNPCC patients, and this phenomenon of accelerated carcinogenesis mandates frequent (annual) colonoscopic examinations.

Based on these data, the surgical treatment of HNPCC in a patient with cancer should be subtotal colectomy with ileorectal anastomosis followed by annual sigmoidoscopic rectal surveillance. There is currently no consensus regarding prophylactic surgery of the colon, uterus, and ovaries for HNPCC. The role of prophylactic colectomy for patients with HNPCC has not received universal acceptance, and decisions regarding surgery should be made on an individual basis until better data-driven recommendations become available. Female patients with no further plans for childbearing are advised to undergo prophylactic hysterectomy and bilateral salpingo-oophorectomy if undergoing surgery for a colon cancer because the risk of endometrial and ovarian cancer reaches 39% and 9%, respectively by age 70. Other forms of cancer associated with HNPCC are treated according to nonhereditary cancer criteria.[27]

ULCERATIVE COLITIS

Colorectal cancer is one of the most devastating long-term sequelae of ulcerative colitis (UC). Duration of disease is directly correlated with development of colorectal cancer, with risk beginning to increase 8 years after diagnosis. At 10 years, the risk of cancer is 0% to 3%, but by 30 years, the risk increases to 50% and then 75% after 40 years of disease. Colonoscopic surveillance every 1 to 2 years beginning 8 years after diagnosis of UC is mandatory. This strategy is based on the premise that a dysplastic lesion or high-grade cellular dysplasia can be detected endoscopically before invasive cancer has developed.[29] Detailed pathologic studies have confirmed the patchy nature of dysplasia and have recommended 33 colonoscopic biopsies during yearly colonoscopy to provide a 90% chance of detecting dysplasia. A meta-analysis of 10 prospective studies of dysplasia surveillance, with a total of 1225 patients, shows that when colectomy is performed for HGD, carcinoma is present in 42% of patients. Less than 8% of patients undergoing colectomy with LGD or indefinite dysplasia had cancer in this and other series. Thus, HGD is an absolute indication for colectomy. LGD is far more controversial, with most surgeons opting for frequent surveillance and rebiopsy. The diagnosis of dysplasia is difficult to establish in the presence of active inflammation, and most authorities recommend that the diagnosis should be confirmed independently by two experienced GI pathologists.[30]

Surgical Management

The goal of surgical management of UC is excision of all affected mucosa and reestablishment of GI continuity, if possible. Indications for surgery may differ from patient to patient, and this greatly influences the choice of operation. Total proctocolectomy with IPAA, as previously described for familial polyposis, is the procedure of choice for patients with HGD, or who become refractory to medical management. This procedure involves removing the entire colon and rectum down to the dentate line and creating an ileal reservoir (Figure 10-5). This anastomosis is particularly vulnerable to leakage, especially in the presence of malnutrition and chronic or ongoing steroid usage. Anastomotic leak/pelvic abscess rate is in excess of 18% if not diverted when medical therapy includes steroid immunosuppression. In these cases, it is usually necessary to temporarily divert the fecal stream with a loop ileostomy, thus allowing the pouch-anal anastomosis to heal. Later closure of the ileostomy (in 8 to 10 weeks) is standard in the absence of pelvic infection. Functionally, patients with good preoperative continence can expect to have, on average, 7 bowel movements per day, and one to two per night. Stapled anastomoses are significantly less likely than hand-sewn ones to cause inadvertent fecal leakage. Patients with preoperative incontinence are therefore poor candidates for IPAA and may be good candidates for end ileostomy. Total proctocolectomy with end ileostomy removes all of the colon, rectum, and anal canal mucosa. This procedure was the operation of choice until the introduction of IPAA in the 1970s and is indicated for patients who are poor candidates for restorative proctocolectomy.

Ulcerative colitis patients diagnosed with colon cancer can have difficult surgical management and reconstruction requirements. These patients require total proctocolectomy but the need for postoperative chemotherapy and the sequelae of diarrhea or

Figure 10-5. Surgical construction of an IPAA. After removal of the colon and rectum to the level of the dentate line, an incision is made in the folded terminal ileum to admit a linear stapler which is used to create a sac-like pouch measuring 10 to 15 cm in length. The incision site is then either stapled or handsewn to the dentate line as shown in E. (Reprinted with permission from Chang AE. Colorectal cancer. In: Greenfield LJ, Mulholland MW, Oldham KT, Zelenock GB, eds. *Surgery: Scientific Principles and Practice.* Philadelphia, PA: JB Lippincott Company; 1993: 999-1000.

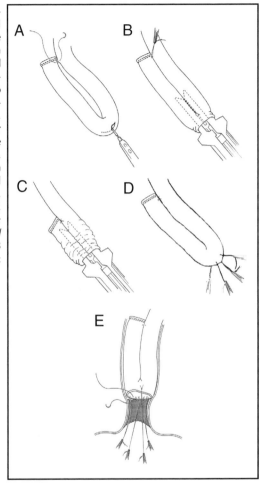

mucositis can make pouch patients miserable at best. While there are no current guidelines, it is generally felt that small cancers, likely to be early stage (T1 and T2), may be offered IPAA. Those with large bulky lesions, or distant metastatic disease facing months of chemotherapy and possible re-operation, may function better with subtotal colectomy, end ileostomy and a Hartmann's pouch (the rectum is left in place). If treatment results in cure, future reconstruction possibilities are preserved with minimal morbidity.[31]

Rectal cancer treatment in the patient with UC may present the most difficult surgical challenges of all. As discussed, the management of node positive and Stage III node negative rectal tumors require either pre- or postoperative radiation—a strategy that provides good control of local recurrence. A total proctocolectomy is required, but IPAA reconstruction in this setting is controversial. In the setting of radiation, there is an increased incidence of pelvic sepsis immediately postoperatively, diminished function, and ultimately a high rate of pouch loss. There is evidence that early stage node negative rectal tumors may safely be treated with radical resection (total proctocolectomy with total mesorectal excision) and IPAA, particularly in young patients. It is clear however, that an individualized approach sensitive to the complex oncologic, functional, and psychological issues is required.[31]

REFERENCES

1. Calvert PM, Frucht H. The genetics of colorectal cancer. *Ann Intern Med.* 2002; 137:603-612.

2. Kinzler KW, Vogelstein B. Lessons form hereditary colorectal cancer. *Cell.* 1996; 87:159-170.

3. Fearon ER, Vogelstein B. A genetic model for colorectal tumorigenesis. *Cell.* 1990; 61:759-767.

4. Haggitt RC, Glotzbach RE, Soffer EE, et al. Prognostic factors in colorectal carcinomas arising in adenomas: implications for lesions removed by endoscopic polypectomy. *Gastroenterology.*1985;89:328-336.

5. Simmang CL, Senatore P, Lowry A, et al. Practice parameters for the detection of colorectal neoplasms. *Dis Colon Rectum.* 1999;42:1123-1129.

6. Graham RA, Wang S, Catalano PJ, Haller DG. Postsurgical surveillance of colon cancer: preliminary cost analysis of physician examination, carcino-embryonic antigen testing, chest x-ray, and colonoscopy. *Ann Surg.* 1998;228(1):59-63.

7. Newland RC, Chapes PH, Smyth EJ. The prognostic value of substaging colorectal cancer. *Cancer.* 1987;60:852-857.

8. Malassagme B, Valleus P, Serra J, et al. Relationship of apical lymph node involvement to survival in resected colon carcinoma. *Dis Colon Rectum.* 1993;36:645-653.

9. Kawamura YJ, Umetani N, Sunami E. Effect of high ligation on the long-term of patients with operable colon cancer, particularly those with limited nodal involvement. *Eur J Surg.* 2000;166:803-807.

10. Rouffetto F, Jay JM, Vachas B, et al. Curative resection for left colonic carcinoma: hemicolectomy vs. segmental colectomy. A prospective, controlled, and multicenter trial. French Association for Surgical Research. *Dis Colon Rectum.* 1994;37:651-659.

11. Hartley JE, Monson JR. The role of laparoscopy in the multimodality treatment of colorectal cancer. *Surg Clin North America.* 2002;82(5):1019-1033.

12. Gerritsen van der Hoop A. Laparoscopic surgery for colorectal carcinoma: an overnight victory? *European J Cancer.* 2002;38:899-903.

13. Fisher ER, Sass R, Palekar A, Fisher B, Wolmark N. Dukes classification revisited. Findings fromt he National Surgical Adjuvant Breast and Bowel Projects (Protocol R-01). *Cancer.* 1989;64(11):2354-2360.

14. Green FL, Page DL, Fleming, et al. In: *AJCC Cancer Staging Manual.* 6th ed. New York, New York: Springer-Verlag; 2002:113-23.

15. Saltz LB, Minsky B. Adjuvant therapy of cancers of the colon and rectum. *Surg Clin North Am.* 2002;82:1035-1058.

16. Miles WE. Classic articles in colonic and rectal surgery. A method of performing abdominopherineal excision for carcinoma of the rectum and of the terminal portion of the pelvic colon. *Dis Colon Rectum.* 1980;23(3):202-205.

17. Garcia-Aguilar J, Mellgren A, Sirivongs P, Buie D, Madoff RD, Rothenberger DA. Local excision of rectal cancer without adjuvant therapy: a word of caution. *Ann Surg.* 2000;

231(3):345-351.

18. Chorost MI, Petrelli NJ, McKenna M, Kraybill WG, Rodriguez-Bigas MA. Local excision of rectal carcinoma. *Am J. Surg.* 2001;67(8):774-779.

19. Visser BC, Varma MG, Welton ML. S Local therapy for rectal cancer. *Surg Oncol.* 2001; 10(1-2):61-69.

20. Sengupta S, Tjandra JJ. Local excision of rectal cancer: what is the evidence? *Dis Colon Rectum.* 2001;44(9):1345-1361.

21. Heald RJ, Moran BJ, Ryall RDH, et al. Rectal cancer: the Basingstoke experience of total mesorectal excision, 1978-1997. *Arch Surg.* 1998;133:894-899.

22. Lazorthes F, Gamagami R, Chiotasso P, et al. Prospective, randomized study comparing clinical results between small and large colonic J-pouch following coloanal anastomosis. *Dis Colon Rectum.* 1997;40:1409-1413.

23. Brown SCW, Walsh S, Abraham JS, Sykes PA. Risk factors and operative mortality in surgery for colorectal cancer. *Am R Coll Surg Engl.* 1991;73:269-272.

24. Enker WE, Paty PB. Advances in rectal cancer surgery: the combined goals of curing cancer and reducing morbidity. In: Andersen DK, ed. *Advances in Colorectal Carcinoma Surgery.* New York, NY: World Medical Press; 1993:33.

25. Kollmorgen CF, Meagher AP, Wolff BG, Pemberton JH, Martenson JA, Illstrup DM. The long-term effect of adjuvant postoperative chemoradiotherapy for rectal carcinoma on bowel function. *Ann Surg.* 1994;220(5):676-82.

26. Heiskanen I, Jarvinen HJ. Fate of the rectal stump after colectomy and ileorectal anastomosis for familial adenomatous polyposis. *Int J Colorectal Dis.* 1997;12:9-13.

27. Trimbath JD, Giardiello FM. Review article: genetic testing and counseling for hereditary colorectal cancer. *Aliment Pharmacol Ther.* 2002;16:1843-1857.

28. Chung DC, Rustgi AK. The hereditary nonpolyposis colorectal cancer syndrome: genetics and clinical implications. *Ann Intern Med.* 2003;138(7):560-570.

29. Mayer R, Wong WD, Rothenberger DA, et al. Colorectal cancer in inflammatory bowel disease. *Dis Colon Rectum.* 1999;4:343-347.

30. Wexner SD, Rosen L, Lowry A, et al. Practice parameters for the treatment of mucosal ulcerative colitis-supporting documentation. *Dis Colon Rectum.* 1997;40:1277-1285.

31. Radice E, Nelson H, Devine RM, et al. Ileal pouch-anal anastomosis in patients with colorectal cancer: long-term functional and oncologic outcomes. *Dis Colon Rectum.* 1998;41(1):11-7.

BIBLIOGRAPHY

Lewis WG, Holdsworth PJ, Stephenson BM, Finan PJ, Johnston D. Role of the rectum in the physiological and clinical results of coloanal and colorectal anastomosis after anterior resection for rectal carcinoma. *Br J Surg.* 1992;79:1082-1062.

Neibergs HL, Hein DW, Spratt JS. Genetic profiling of colon cancer. *J Surg Oncol.* 2002;80:204-213.

Vogelstein B, Fearon ER, Hamilton SR, et al. Genetic alterations during colorectal-tumor development. *N Engl J Med.* 1988;319:525-532.

Willett CG. Sphincter preservation in rectal cancer. *Curr Treat Options Oncol.* 2000; 1(5):399-405.

chapter 11

Approach to Chemotherapy and Radiation Therapy for Colorectal Neoplasia

Weijing Sun, MD

INTRODUCTION

Colorectal cancer is the most common GI malignancy, and the second leading cause of cancer-related death in North America. There are 147,500 new cases of colorectal cancer with 57,100 deaths in 2003 based on the estimates from the American Cancer Society.[1] The overall outcome of patients with colorectal cancer has been greatly improved over the past several decades, with better understanding of the disease process, earlier diagnosis through screening, and the development of new and novel treatments. It is important for clinicians to understand that the prognosis of colorectal cancer is largely dependent on the extent of the disease at presentation, the depth of tumor penetration into the bowel wall, and the presence or absence of regional lymph node involvement and distant metastases. The goal of therapy is to improve the chance of survival and the quality of life in patients diagnosed with colorectal cancer based upon the extent of the disease and risk factors. If the disease is detected early, the prognosis is excellent and further treatment may not be needed after curative intent surgical resection. However, about two-thirds of patients have lymph node involvement or distal metastases when their disease is diagnosed. Chemotherapy or chemoradiation plays a crucial role in increasing the chance of a cure for those patients with lymph node involvement. Chemotherapy is the most important maneuver to improve the survival rate for patients with distant metastatic colorectal cancer.

THE STAGE SYSTEM OF COLORECTAL CANCER

Although the recent advances in biological and molecular characteristics of the disease have brought our understanding of the disease to a different level, pathologic staging is still the most important and reliable system for predicting the prognosis of colorectal cancer, and thereafter guiding the treatment decisions.

Two commonly-used pathological staging systems are the modified Astler-Coller system from the original Dukes classification and the TNM-based classification of the

AJCC (see Appendix D). Several modifications were included in the recently-edited AJCC classification. Smooth metastatic nodules in the pericolonic or perirectal fat are defined as *lymph node metastases*. Irregularly-contoured metastatic nodules in the peritumoral fat are considered *vascular invasion*. Stage II is subdivided into IIA (T3 lesions) and IIB (T4 lesions) based on the depth of invasion. Stage III disease is further subdivided into IIIA (T1-2N1), IIIB (T3-4N1), or IIIC (TanyN2) depending on the depth of invasion and the level of involvement of lymph node. The importance of cooperation among the different medical specialties is emphasized also by the Joint Committee. Surgeons are encouraged to score the completeness of the resection as R0 (the complete resection with all margins negative of cancer), R1 (incomplete resection with microscopic involvement of a margin), and R2 (incomplete resection with gross residual of cancer).

For stage I colorectal cancer, the cure rate exceeds 90% following surgery alone. However, once a tumor invades through the bowel wall (stage II), survival at 5 years decreases to 60% to 80%. If the pericolonic or perirectal lymph nodes are found to be involved with cancer (stage III), 5-year survival falls to 30% to 60%, with the lower survival associated with an increasing number of lymph node metastases.[3,4] The overall prognosis of patients with distant metastases is poor, although the survival rate has been improved dramatically in past several years because of the development of new cytotoxic chemotherapy agents and novel molecular oriented agents. The most frequent site of metastasis for colorectal cancer is the liver, followed by lung and intra-abdominal sites.

Other clinical and pathologic features such as perforation, obstruction, adherence or invasion of the tumor to other organs, radial (lateral) margin involvement, lymphatic and vascular invasion, and degree of tumor differentiation may also increase the risk of recurrence in those patients with localized diseases.[5] Elevation of preoperative CEA level may predict for prognosis, especially in patients with node-positive disease.[6] The change of CEA level is frequently used as a surrogate indicator of response in patients having chemotherapy for their metastatic diseases. The elevation of CEA may be an early warning sign of recurrence and/or metastasis of the disease in those patients with localized colorectal cancer with or without adjuvant therapy. A number of biological and molecular characteristics (such as mutations of p53 and p21, K-*ras* mutation, chromosome 18q loss of heterozygosity [LOH], MSI-related germline mismatch repair gene mutations, and high expression of thymidylate synthase [TS]) have been identified that may be of prognostic importance,[7-10] although none has yet been validated in prospective clinical trials.

TREATMENT OF PATIENTS WITH METASTATIC DISEASES

The chemotherapy of metastatic colorectal cancer has greatly advanced in the past several years because of the development of new cytotoxic and novel molecular-oriented agents. The paradigm of treatment has changed. Physicians should encourage all suitable patients to enter clinical studies for understanding the disease better, improving the treatment further, and achieving potentially the best outcome for enrolled patients.

For some selected patients with metastatic colorectal cancer (mainly those with limited hepatic and pulmonary lesions), there is a potential of having their diseases cured after surgical resection (metastasectomy). It is important to evaluate the resectability first for patients with metastatic colorectal cancer (Figure 11-1). The data have shown that surgical resection is safe and may achieve a long-time survival depending on the size and number of the metastases, the disease-free interval, the lymph node status of the primary

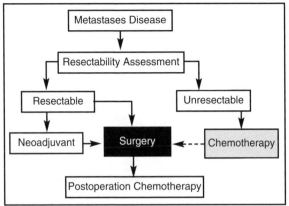

Figure 11-1. Strategies for advanced/metastatic colorectal cancer (stage IV).

Table 11-1

SURVIVAL AFTER RESECTION OF HEAPTIC METASTASES

Clinical Risk Score (Points)	5-Year Overall Survival
0 to 1	52%
2 to 3	23%
4 to 5	11%

Each of the following factors is assigned as 1 point:
1. The largest tumor is >5 cm.
2. Number of tumors in liver is >1.
3. The disease-free interval <12 months.
4. Node-positive in the primary tumor.
5. CEA >200 ng/mL.

tumor, and the level of CEA[11] (Table 11-1). The advantage of systemic chemotherapy with 5-FU/LV after resection of metastases has been demonstrated in both 5-year disease free survival (DFS) and 5-year overall survival (OS).[12] Until now, surgical resection of metastatic lesions followed by further chemotherapy for those with respectable diseases was accepted at most situations (see Figure 11-1). Preoperative chemotherapy with new agents has been investigated lately. This approach may help to select patients who will benefit from curative resection if they have good responses to the systemic chemotherapy and to avoid unnecessary surgical procedure for those patients with no response to chemotherapy or even with their diseases progressed during treatment. Successful down-staging of the disease, even with complete histologic response, has been achieved in some patients with initially unresectable metastases.[13,14] It has been reported that the postmetastasectomy outcome in patients whose disease responded to neoadjuvant chemotherapy is much better than those whose disease did not.[15]

Majority of patients with metastatic colorectal cancer are not candidates for metastasectomy, and surgical procedures are performed only for bypassing obstructive and hemorrhagic lesions. The palliative systemic chemotherapy is the only maneuver for their treatment. The median survival (MS) of individuals with metastatic disease has dramatically improved in the past several years. As a main component of chemotherapy, 5-FU is administered intravenously either with LV as bolus fashions or as continuous infusion. The combinations of 5-FU with oxaliplatin (a diaminocyclohexane platin that inhibits DNA replication and transcription through the formation of intra- and interstrand DNA adducts) or irinotecan (a topoisomerase I inhibitor) are the new standard treatments for metastatic colorectal cancer.[16-19] Various regimens are available with different doses and schedules (Figure 11-2). The question of which combination (irinotecan with 5-FU/LV or oxaliplatin with 5-FU/LV) is more effective is unknown, but preliminary data suggest a rough equivalency in efficacy of each combination in first- or second-line treatment, with differences in toxicity patterns.[20] It appears that the combination of irinotecan with bolus 5-FU may be more toxic, particularly in the elderly and patients with poor performance status. It is important for physicians to realize that patients with reasonable good performance should be treated with all 3 effective medications during their treatment courses. Capecitabine, an oral fluoropyrimidine carbamate derivative, has also been approved by the FDA as first-line therapy for patients with metastatic colorectal cancer who are not candidates for combination therapy. Capecitabine was shown to be as effective as a standard bolus 5-FU/LV regimen in 2 randomized trials.[21,22] Based on continuous dosing, capecitabine may hold the potential to replace infusional 5-FU in combination with irinotecan and oxaliplatin. Although phase II trials of capecitabine in combination with irinotecan and oxaliplatin appear promising, equivalence to standard intravenous infusional therapy needs to be proven by ongoing phase III studies.

Many novel biological agents are now being tested. These new agents target the EGFR, VEGF, and other molecular markers. Significant improvements in median survival, progression-free survival, and overall response rates have been demonstrated when bevacizumab, a recombinant humanized monoclonal antibody against VEGF, is added to irinotecan/5-FU/LV (IFL)[23] (Table 11-2). The results of the combination of bevacizumab with oxaliplatin/5-FU/LV are expected in 2005. Encouraging results have also been shown from phase II studies with cetuximab (C225), a monoclonal humanized antibody directly against EGFR in previous-treated metastatic colorectal cancer patients.[24]

Postmetastectomy hepatic artery infusion (HAI) of floxuridine (FUDR) with systemic 5-FU/LV chemotherapy may improve survival compared with systemic 5-FU/LV alone[25] (Table 11-3). However, with more effective systemic chemotherapy regimens available, the potential contribution of HAI needs to be tested further. Many other hepatic-directed treatments have been proposed for metastases of colorectal cancer, including radiofrequency ablation (RFA), hepatic artery chemoembolization (HACE), cryotherapy, and percutaneous ethanol injection.[26-28] All of these procedures have their limits, and local availability and expertise vary widely. While no survival benefit has been proven to date, trials are underway comparing chemotherapy alone to chemotherapy plus either HACE or RFA.

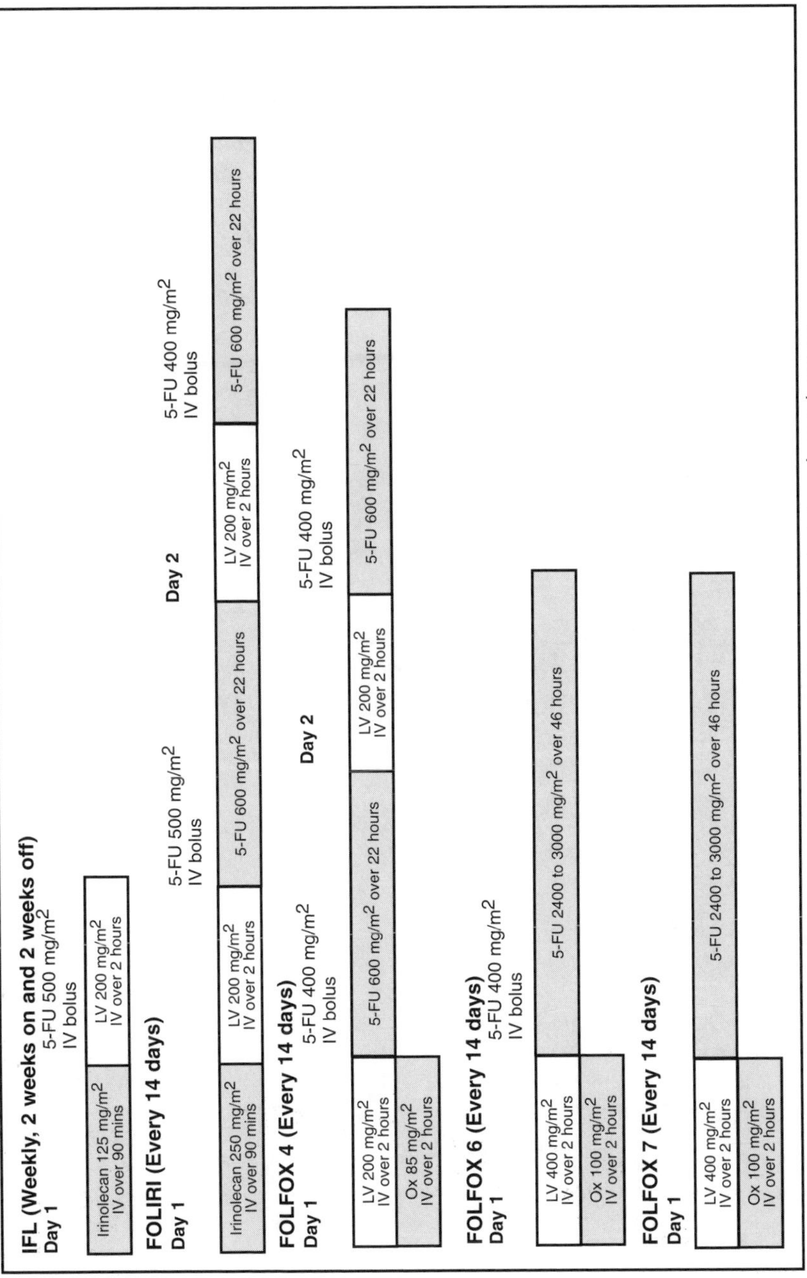

Figure 11-2. Schema of common chemotherapy regimens in treatment of metastatic colorectal cancer.

Table 11-2

EFFICACY AND TOXICITY OF IFL/BEVACIZUMAB

	IFL/Placebo (N=412)	IFL/BV (N=403)	p-value
Median survival (months)	15.6	20.3	0.00003
Progression-free survival (months)	6.24	10.6	<0.00001
Overall response rate (CR+PR, %)	35	45	0.0029
Duration of response (months)	7.1	10.4	0.0014
Grade 3/4 bleeding (%)	2.5	3.1	NS
Thromboembolism (%)	16.1 1	9.3	NS
Grade 3 proteinuria (%)	0.8	0.8	NS
Grade 3 hypertension (%)	2.3	10.9	

IFL=irinotecan, 5-FU (fluorouracil), LV (leucovorin); BV=bevacizumab

Table 11-3

BENEFIT OF SYSTEMIC CHEMOTHERAPY WITH AND WITHOUT HEPATIC ARTERY INFUSION (HAI) POST LIVER METASTASECTOMY

	No. of Patients	5-Year DFS	5-Year OS
5-FU/LV (5-FU: 370 mg/m², LV: 200 mg/m²) daily, 5 days/4 weeks for 6 cycles	82	34%	49%
5-FU/LV (5-FU: 325 mg/m², LV: 200 mg/m²) daily, 5 days/4 weeks *plus* HAI (FUDR 0.25 mg/kg/day, 20 mg dexamethasone, and 50,000 U heparin through pump), 14 days/ 3 weeks for 6 cycles	74	40%	61%

FUDR=floxuridine, or fludeoxyuridine

Table 11-4

COMMON 5-FU-BASED REGIMENS

Regimen	Dosing	Schedule
Roswell Park	**LV** 500mg/m² IV over 2 hours **5-FU** 500mg/m² IV push I hour after LV infusion started	Weekly for 6 weeks, repeated every 8 weeks
Mayo Clinic	**LV** 20mg/m² IV push **5-FU** 425mg/m² IV push	Daily for 5 consecutive days, repeated every 4 weeks
de Gramont (LV5FU2)	**LV** 200 mg/m² 2 hours IV infusion; followed by **5-FU** IV bolus of 400 mg/m²; then **5-FU** 600 mg/m² IV 22-hour continuous infusion	Two consecutive days every 14 days

LV=leucovorin; 5-FU=fluorouracil

ADJUVANT CHEMOTHERAPY FOR COLON CANCER

The benefit of adjuvant chemotherapy for colorectal cancer has become well established over the past 2 decades.[29-33] The final results of Intergroup 0089 and National Surgical Adjuvant Breast and Bowel Project (NSABP) C-04 studies confirmed that 5-FU-based therapy significantly improves disease-free and overall survival for patients with stage III colon cancer.[33,34] Neither study showed the addition of levamisole (LEV) to 5-FU/LV providing any additional benefits. The combination of 5-FU with LV for 6 to 8 months is still the "standard therapy" for stage III (Dukes C) colon cancer as adjuvant setting by the time this article was written, given by a variety of different doses and schedules that have demonstrated comparable efficacy (Table 11-4). In the United States, the Roswell Park regimen and the Mayo Clinic regimen are commonly used with somewhat different toxicity profiles. More leukopenia and stomatitis are associated with the Mayo regimen, and more grade 3 to 4 diarrhea is seen in the Roswell Park regimen, which is usually manageable with aggressive antidiarrhea medications. The infusional regimen, LV5FU2 (also called 'de Gramont regimen) was compared with a bolus regime for toxicity and efficacy in patients with stage II and III colorectal cancer.[35] There was no significant difference in disease-free or overall survival between the treatment arms; however, toxicities were significantly lower in the infusion group (p<0.001). Capecitabine, as an oral fluoropyrimidine, has been studied as an adjuvant treatment for patients with resected Dukes C colon cancer (the X-ACT trial). Preliminary safety data showed 60-day all-cause and treatment-related mortality was similar to the Mayo Clinic Regimen at ~0.5%. Capecitabine causes significantly less diarrhea, nausea, vomiting, stomatitis, and alopecia compared to bolus 5-FU/LV, but more hand-foot syndrome.[36] The efficacy data are expected soon.

Newer studies have been designed to prove whether the survival advantage of the combination of 5-FU/LV with oxaliplatin or irinotecan in metastatic colorectal cancer can be transferred to the adjuvant setting. A European study (MOSAIC) compared LV5FU2 and the combination of oxaliplatin with infusional 5-FU/LV (FOLFOX) in patients with stage II/III colon cancer after complete resection of the primary colon cancer.[38] The results showed that the 3-years DFS in the intent-to-treat population was 77.8% in the FOLFOX arm vs 72.9% in the LV5FU2 arm (p<0.01) with a risk reduction of 23% in the FOLFOX arm. This is the first study to demonstrate the combination of oxaliplatin with 5-FU/LV superior to the current standard 5-FU/LV in adjuvant therapy of colon cancer. The result also confirmed that FOLFOX is feasible and safe for use in the adjuvant setting. Although there was 12.4% of grade 3 peripheral sensory neuropathy reported that was secondary to oxaliplatin, only 1% of patients had residual neuropathy at 1 year. Other grade 3/4 toxicities were neutropenia (41%), diarrhea (10.8%), and vomiting (5.9%). It is expected that adjuvant therapy with FOLFOX in stage I colon cancer will be accepted as "new standard." An interim analysis of the study (C89803) comparing the combination of irinotecan with bolus 5-FU/LV (IFL) with 5-FU/LV alone as adjuvant setting in patients with stage III colon cancer showed the 60-day all-cause mortality was higher in patients who received the combination therapy. Although the main causes have been identified as vascular events and GI syndromes, the relationship of these events and the given medication is still not clear. More data from other studies are anticipated soon. There are more studies designed to investigate the benefits of traditional cytotoxic chemotherapy combined with molecular-oriented agents such as bevacizumab and cetuximab as adjuvant setting in stage II/III colorectal cancer patients.

Adjuvant treatment with monoclonal antibody 17-1A (Edrecolomab, Mab 17-1A), a murine IgG2a monoclonal antibody that recognizes the human tumor-associated antigen Ep-CAM, has been examined extensively. However, no obvious benefit has been shown from the available data.[39,40]

Adjuvant chemotherapy with 5-FU/LV in localized, node-negative disease (stage II or Dukes B) remains controversial, even though the benefit is considered to be real, especially for those patients with high risk factors (eg, bowel obstruction, perforation, and poorly differentiated cancer) for recurrence.[41-43] However, with the availability of more effective chemotherapy agents, significant and meaningful benefits of adjuvant chemotherapy in the treatment of stage II colon patients are possible and very likely. Furthermore, accurate molecular characteristic colon cancers may define those patients with high risk, so therefore these subset stage II colon cancer patients may truly benefit from adjuvant therapy.

ADJUVANT TREATMENT OF RECTAL CANCER

The goal of perioperative therapy in patients with localized rectal cancer is to decrease both the risk of distant metastases and the incidence of local recurrence. In contrast to colon cancer, there is a significant risk of local-regional failure as the only or first site of recurrence in patients with curative resected rectal cancer. The locoregional recurrent rate is about 25% (stage II) to 50% (stage III).[44,45] Since surgical technique plays a key role in success of tumor control of rectal cancer, standardization of surgery (TME) in patients with respectable rectal cancer is important for comparing combination therapy vs surgery alone. A large prospective, randomized trial investigated the efficacy of preoperative radiation with standardized TME.[46] The results showed the advantage of combined modality compared to TME alone in the 2-year local recurrent rate (2.4% vs 8.2%, p<0.001). However, the impact of radiation on overall survival has been minimal. The significant improvement of overall survival with protracted venous infusion (PVI) of 5-FU (225 mg/m²/day) during pelvic radiation (50.4 Gy) was demonstrated from an intergroup trial.[47] Although infusional 5-FU concurrent with radiation is the commonly accepted regimen as adjuvant therapy for rectal cancer, a recent published intergroup study compared bolus 5-FU to continuous infusion 5-FU before, during, and after pelvic radiation. The study found no significant differences between the treatment arms in DFS, OS, or significant toxicities.[48] It appeared that both bolus and infusional 5-FU could be combined with radiation with equal efficacy and toxicity for post-operative adjuvant therapy. The overall OS and DFS were dependent on TN stage and treatment method.[49,50] For patients with intermediate risk lesions (T1-2N1, T3N0) adjuvant chemotherapy had equivalent results with chemoradiation therapy, which suggested that the use of trimodality with postoperative chemoradiation for intermediate risk patients may be excessive. For those patients with high risk (TanyN2, T3-4N1) of recurrence, adding a new cytotoxic medication (eg, oxaliplatin to 5-FU) and radiation therapy may decrease the risk of both locoregional and distant recurrence and metastases based on the data from several phase II studies.[51] With the advantage of more convenient than infusional 5-FU, and potential synergistic effect with radiation therapy, capecitabine has been studied in combination with radiation, and the preliminary results are encouraging.[52] Novel targeted biologic agents, including celecoxib and bevacizumab, are being explored in combination with standard chemotherapy and radiation therapy.[51] Preoperative neoadjuvant chemoradiation of localized rectal cancer may hold potential benefit of down-staging the disease; therefore, it improves the respectability and increases the rate of salvage of the sphincter muscle. Large intergroup studies are designed to delineate the advantage of pre- versus postoperative chemoradiation therapy in rectal cancer.

REFERENCES

1. Jemal A, Murray T, Samuels A, et al. Cancer statistics, 2003. *CA Cancer J Clin.* 2003; 53:5-26.
2. Greene FL, Page DL, Fleming ID, Fritz A, Balch CM, eds. *AJCC Cancer Staging Manual.* 6th ed. New York, NY: Springer-Verlag; 2002:113-118.
3. Macdonald JS. Adjuvant therapy of colon cancer. *CA Cancer J Clin.* 1999;49(4):202-219.
4. Bokey EL, Ojerskog B, Cahpuis PH, et al. Local recurrence after curative excision of the rectum for cancer without adjuvant therapy: role of total anatomical dissection. *Br J Surg.* 1999;86(9):1164-1170.
5. Sun W, Haller DG. Chemotherapy for colorectal cancer. *Hematol Oncol Clin N Am.* 2002;16:969-994.
6. Harrison LE, Guillem JG, Paty P, et al. Preoperative carcinoembryonic antigen predicts outcomes in node-negative colon cancer patients: a multivariate analysis of 572 patients. *J Am Coll Surg.* 1997;185:55-59.
7. Jen J, Kim H, Piantadosi S, et al. Allelic loss of chromosome 18Q and prognosis in colorectal cancer. *N Engl J Med.* 1994;331:213-221.
8. Allegra CJ, Paik S, et al. Prognostic value of thymidylate synthase, Ki-67, and p53 in patients with Dukes' B and C colon cancer: a National Cancer Institute-National Surgical Adjuvant Breast and Bowel Project collaborative study. *J Clin Oncol.* 2003; 21(2):241-250.

9. Allegra CJ, Parr AL, Wold LE, et al. Investigation of the prognostic and predictive value of thymidylate synthetase, p53, and Ki-67 in patients with locally advanced colon cancer. *J Clin Oncol.* 2002;20(7):1735–43.

10. Gonen M, Hummer A, Zervoudakis A, et al. Thymidylate synthase expression in hepatic tumors is a predictor of survival and progression in patients with resectable metastatic colorectal cancer. *J Clin Oncol.* 2003;21(3):406-412.

11. Fong Y, Cohen AM, Fortner JG, et al. Liver resection for colorectal metastases. *J Clin Oncol.* 1997;15:938-946.

12. Portier G, Rougier Ph, Milan C, et al. Adjuvant systemic chemotherapy (CT) using 5-fluorouracil (FU) and folinic acid (FA) after resection of liver metastases (LM) from colorectal origin. Results of an Intergroup phase III study (trial FFCD-ACHBTH-AURC 9002). *Proc Am Soc Clin Oncol.* 2002;21:133a(A528).

13. Giacchetti S, Itzhaki M, Gruia G et al. Longterm survival of patients with unresectable colorectal cancer liver metastases following infusional chemotherapy with 5-flurouracial, leucovorin, oxaliplatin and surgery. *Ann Oncol.* 1999;10:663–669.

14. Alberts SR, Donohue JH, Mahoney MR, et al. Liver resection after 5-fluorouracil, leucovorin and oxaliplatin for patients with metastatic colorectal cancer (MCRC) limited to the liver: A North Central Cancer Treatment Group (NCCTG) phase II study. *Pro Am Soc Clin Oncol.* 2003;22:a263 (A1053).

15. Adam R, Pascal G, Castaing D, et al. Liver resection for multiple colorectal metastases: influence of preoperative chemotherapy. *Pro Am Soc Clin Oncol.* 2003;22:a296 (A1188).

16. Saltz LB, Cox JV, Blanke CB, et al. Irinotecan plus fluorouracil and leucovorin for metastatic colorectal cancer. *New Eng J Med.* 2000;343:905-914.

17. Douillard JY, Cunningham D, Roth AD, et al. Irinotecan combined with fluorouracil compared with fluorouracil alone as first-line treatment for metastatic colorectal cancer: a multicenter randomized trial. *Lancet.* 2000;355:1041-1047.

18. Rothenberg ML, Oza AM, Burger B, et al. Final results of a phase III trial of 5-FU/leucovorin versus oxaliplatin versus the combination in patients with metastatic colorectal cancer following irinotecan, 5-FU, and leucovorin. *Proc Am Soc Clin Oncol.* 2003; 22:a252 (A1011).

19. Goldberg RM, Morton RF, Sargent DJ, et al. N9741: oxaliplatin (Oxal) or CPT-11 + 5-fluorouracil (5FU)/leucovorin (LV) or oxal + CPT-11 in advanced colorectal cancer (CRC). Updated efficacy and quality of life (QOL) data from an Intergroup study. *Proc Am Soc Clin Oncol.* 2003;22:a252 (A 1009).

20. Tournigand C, Louvet C, Quinaux E, et al. FOLFIRI followed by FOLFOX versus FOLFOX followed by FOLFIRI in metastatic colorectal cancer (MCRC): final results of a phase III study. *Proc Am Clin Oncol.* 2002;21:a124 (A494).

21. Hoff PM, Ansari R, Bastist G, et al. Comparison of oral capecitabine versus intravenous fluorouracil plus leucovorin as first-line treatment in 605 patients with metastatic colorectal cancer: results of a randomized phase III study. *J Clin Oncol.* 2001;19(8):2282-2292.

22. Van Cutsem E, Twelves C, Cassidy J, et al. Oral capecitabine compared with intravenous fluorouracil plus leucovorin in patients with metastatic colorectal cancer: results of a large phase III study. *J Clin Oncol.* 2001;19(21):4097-4106.

23. Hurwitz H, Fehrenbacher L, Cartwright T, et al. Bevacizumab (a monoclonal antibody to vascular endothelial growth factor) prolongs survival in first-line colorectal cancer (CRC): results of a phase III trial of bevacizumab in combination with bolus IFL (irinotecan, 5-fluorouracil, leucovorin) as first-line therapy in subjects with metastatic CRC. *Proc Am Soc Clin Oncol.* 2003;22:(A 3646).

24. Cunningham D, Humblet Y, Siena S et al. Cetuximab (C225) alone or in combination with irinotecan (CPT-11) in patients with epidermal growth factor receptor (EGFR)-positive, irinotecan-refractory metastatic colorectal cancer (MCRC). *Proc Am Soc Clin Oncol.* 2003;22:(A1012).

25. Kemeny MM, Adak S, Gray B, et al. Combined-modality treatment for resectable metastatic colorectal carcinoma to the liver: surgical resection of hepatic metastases in combination with continuous infusion of chemotherapy – an Intergroup study. *J Clin Oncol.* 2002;20:1499-1505.

26. Sanz-Altamira PM, Spence LD, Huberman MS et al. Selective chemoembolization in the management of hepatic metastases in refractory colorectal carcinoma: a phase II trial. *Dis Colon Rectum.* 1997;40:770–775.

27. Leichman CG, Jacobson J, Modiano M et al. Hepatic chemoembolization combined with systemic infusion of 5-fluorouracil and bolus leucovorin for patients with metastatic colorectal carcinoma: a Southwest Oncology Group pilot trial. *Cancer.* 1999;86: 775–781.

28. Giovannini M, Seitz JF. Ultrasound-guided percutaneous alcohol injection of small liver metastases. Result in 40 patients. *Cancer.* 1994;73:294–297.

29. Moertel CG, Fleming TR, McDonald TS, et al. Levamisole and fluorouracil for adjuvant therapy of resected colon carcinoma. *N Engl J Med.* 1990;322:352–358.

30. Moertel CG, Fleming TR, Macdonald JS et al. Fluorouracil plus levamisole as effective adjuvant therapy after resection of stage III colon carcinoma: a final report. *Ann Intern Med.* 1995;122:321–326.

31. National Institute of Health Consensus Conference Adjuvant therapy for patients with colon and rectal cancer. *JAMA.* 1990;264:1444–1450.

32. Wolmark N, Rockette H, Fisher B et al. The benefit of leucovorin-modulated fluorouracil as postoperative adjuvant therapy for primary colon cancer: results from National Surgical Adjuvant Breast and Bowel Project Protocol C-03. *J Clin Oncol.* 1993; 11:1879–1887.

33. Haller D, Catalano P, Macdonald J, et al. Fluorouracil (FU), leucovorin (LV) and levamisole (LEV) adjuvant therapy for colon cancer: five year final report of INT-0089. *Proc Am Soc Clin Oncol.* 1998;17:256a (A982).

34. Wolmark N, Rockette H, Mamounas E, et al. Clinical trial to assess the relative efficacy of fluorouracil and leucovorin, fluorouracil and levamisole, and fluorouracil, leucovorin, and levamisole in patients with Dukes' B and C carcinoma of the colon: results from the National Surgical Adjuvant Breast and Bowel Project C-04. *J Clin Oncol.* 1999;17:3553-3559.

35. Andre T, Colin P, Louvet C, et al. Semimonthly versus monthly regimen of fluorouracil and leucovorin administered for 24 or 36 weeks as adjuvant therapy in stage II and III colon cancer: results of a randomized trial. *J Clin Oncol.* 2003;21(15):2896-2903.

36. Twelves C, Wong A, Nowacki MP, et al. Improved safety results of a ph III trial of capecitabine vs. bolus 5-FU/leucovorin (LV) as adjuvant therapy for colon cancer (the X-ACT Study). *Proc Am Soc Clin Oncol.* 2003;22:a294 (A1182).

37. de Gramont A, Vanzi N, Navarro M, et al. Oxaliplatin/5-FU/LV in adjuvant colon cancer, Results of the international randomized mosaic trial. *Proc Am Soc Clin Oncol.* 2003; 22:a253 (A 1015).

38. Rothenberg ML, Meropol NJ, Poplin EA, et al. Mortality associated with irinotecan plus bolus fluorouracil/leucovorin: summary finding of an independent panel. *J Clin Oncol.* 2001;19(18):3801–3807.

39. Punt CJ, Nagy A, Douillard JY, et al. Edrecolomab alone or in combination with fluo-rouracil and folinic acid in the adjuvant treatment of stage III colon cancer: a ran-domised study. *Lancet.* 2002;360(9334):671-677.

40. Fields AL, Keller AM, Schwartzberg L, et al. Edrecolomab (17-1A antibody) (EDR) in combination with 5-fluorouracil (FU) based chemotherapy in the adjuvant treatment of stage III colon cancer: results of a randomized North American phase III study. *Proc Am Soc Clin Oncol.* 2002;21:128a (A508).

41. Mamounas E, Wieand S, Wolmark N, et al. Comparative efficacy of adjuvant chemotherapy in patients with Dukes B versus Dukes colon cancer: results from four national surgical adjuvant breast and bowel project adjuvant studies (C-01, C-02, C-03, and C-04). *J Clin Oncol.* 1999;17:1349-1355.

42. Efficacy of Adjuvant Fluorouracil and Folinic Acid in B2 Colon Cancer. International Multicentre Pooled Analysis of B2 Colon Cancer Trials (IMPACT B2) Investigators. *J Clin Oncol.* 1999;17:1356-1363.

43. Marsoni S for IMPACT investigators. Efficacy of adjuvant fluorouracil and leucovorin in Stage B2 and C colon cancer. *Semin Oncol.* 2001;28 (suppl 1):14-19.

44. Fisher B, Wolmark N, Rockette H, et al. Postoperative adjuvant chemotherapy or radi-ation therapy for rectal cancer: Results from NSABP protocol R-01. *J Natl Cancer Inst.* 1988;80:21-29.

45. Swedish Rectal Cancer Trial. Improved survival with preoperative radiotherapy in resectable rectal cancer. *N Eng J Med.* 1997;336:980-987.

46. Kapitijin E, Marijnen CAM, Magtegaal, ID, et al. Preoperative radiotherapy combined with total mesorectal excision for respectable rectal cancer. *N Engl J Med.* 2001;345: 638-646.

47. O'Connell MJ, Martenson JA, Weiand HS, et al. Improving adjuvant therapy for rec-tal cancer by combining protracted-infusion fluorouracil with radiation therapy after curative surgery. *N Engl J Med.* 1994; 331(8):502–507.

48. Smalley SR, Benedetti J, Williamson S, et al. Intergroup 0144 - phase III trial of 5-FU based chemotherapy regimens plus radiotherapy (XRT) in postoperative adjuvant rectal cancer. Bolus 5-FU vs. prolonged venous infusion (PVI) before and after XRT + PVI vs. bolus 5-FU + leucovorin (LV) + levamisole (LEV) before and after XRT + bolus 5-FU + LV. *Proc Am Soc Clin Oncol.* 2003;22:(A1006).

49. Tepper JE, O'Connell M, Niedzwiecki D, et al. Adjuvant therapy in rectal cancer: analysis of stage, sex, and local control—final report of Intergroup 0114. *J Clin Oncol.* 2002;20(7):1744–1750.

50. Gunderson LL, Sargent D, Tepper J, et al. Impact of TN stage and treatment on sur-vival and relapse in adjuvant rectal cancer pooled analysis. *Pro Am Soc Clin Oncol.* 2003; 22:a251(A1008).

51. Zhu AX, Willett CG. Chemotherapeutic and biologic agents as radiosensitizers in rec-tal cancer. *Semin Radiat Oncol.* 2003;13(4):454-68.

52. Rodel C, Grabenbauer GG, Papadopoulos T, et al. Phase I/II trial of capecitabine, oxali-platin, and radiation for rectal cancer. *J Clin Oncol.* 2003;21(16):3098-104.

chapter 12

The Assessment and Management of Acute and Chronic Cancer Pain

Rosemary C. Polomano, PhD, RN, FAAN; Allen W. Burton, MD; Niraja Rajan, MD; and Patrick M. McQuillan, MD

INTRODUCTION

Despite recent national attention on the assessment and treatment of cancer pain, unrelieved pain from cancer treatment and disease progression continues to be alarming high. The complexity of cancer pain and its undertreatment are major factors attributed to poor pain control. Pain experiences that span from diagnosis to the end of life are highly influenced by primary tumor site, stage, treatment-related factors, physiological sources of pain (somatic, visceral, and neuropathic), and psychosocial determinants. While pain represents only one dimension of the multiple symptoms experienced by cancer patients, it is clearly a problem that has the most profound impact on health-related quality of life (HrQOL).

More than 70% of patients with cancer have significant pain during their course of their illness.[1] Worldwide estimates of the prevalence of cancer pain show that some 30% to 40% of patients undergoing cancer therapy and, more discouraging, about 70% to 90% of those with advanced disease report pain.[2] Other global appraisals of pain indicate that one-third to one-half of patients undergoing active treatment experience pain and that some cancer-specific sites are associated with more severe pain. Specific data that are available for pain associated with GI malignancies show variations in its prevalence by the primary cancer site. Through an international collaborative study of patients with advanced cancer, moderate to severe pain was found in 51% of those with esophageal cancer, 59% with colorectal cancer, and 43% with cancer of the stomach.[3] At diagnosis, almost 75% of patients with pancreatic cancer experience pain,[4] which may persist in the later stages of the disease without aggressive interventions. Locally recurrent rectal cancer, which occurs in up to one-third of patients, can be controlled in about a third of these patients, but not without significant morbidity and mortality. Whether this progression is managed with nonsurgical palliation or resection, it is associated with a significant degree of pain.[5]

BARRIERS TO EFFECTIVE PAIN MANAGEMENT

Pain management practices are highly influenced by both practitioner- and health system-related barriers. Frequently mentioned reasons for untreated pain are inadequate pain assessment, lack of knowledge and training in pain management, attitudes, beliefs and biases, concern and fear over regulatory scrutiny, and health care disparities in the treatment of vulnerable populations (eg, elderly and culturally diverse populations). Discouraging accounts of pain were noted in a national study of over 1300 outpatients across 54 Eastern Oncology Cooperative Group practice sites, with 36% of patients experiencing pain so severe that it interfered with function.[6] Even though a significant number of patients reported high pain interference, over 50% of physicians treating these patients felt that pain control in their practice was "good" to "very good."[7] They also acknowledged their reluctance to aggressively treat pain with opioid analgesics until patients were in the later stages of their disease.

Confusion regarding the terminology associated with opioid use continues to negatively affect prescribing patterns.[8,9] *Physical dependence,* which is a state of physiological adaptation that occurs from repeated exposure to a drug, is manifested by a drug class specific withdrawal syndrome resulting from abrupt cessation of the drug, rapid dose reduction, or administration of a reversal agent. Physical dependence inevitably develops with chronic opioid use. Abrupt withdrawal of therapy often results in physical symptoms such as nervousness, sweating, nausea, vomiting, abdominal cramping, diarrhea, and, more seriously, seizures. Concerns about physical dependence should not deter physicians from prescribing adequate doses of opioid analgesics because doses can always be decreased slowly to prevent acute withdrawal. More importantly, physical dependence is a separate entity—not to be confused with *addiction* or psychological dependence, which is a primary, chronic, neurobiological disease with genetic, psychosocial, and environmental factors. Addiction is characterized by compulsive drug use behaviors such as continued craving for the substance, the need to use the drug for effects other than relieving pain, and a preoccupation with procuring the drug to get "high," despite harmful effects. A number of studies have shown that short- and long-term use of opioids to control pain is unlikely to lead to addiction.[8] Patients also worry about becoming "addicted" and need appropriate information and reassurance that chronic opioid use for cancer pain seldom leads to abuse. *Tolerance* occurs when an increased dose is required to maintain the original analgesic effects. Tolerance is rarely a clinical problem, is unlikely to occur with short-term opioid use, and typically develops in cancer patients because of disease progression and worsening of pain.

Eliminating healthcare disparities has been a major research priority for the National Institutes of Health (NIH) and other funding agencies. Age, gender, ethnicity, and race can negatively affect pain management practices. For example, older persons with cancer may be less likely to be referred to pain specialists for interventional pain care and palliative care services.[10] Elders, females, and minorities are at greater risk for inadequate opioid analgesia.[6]

PAIN MANAGEMENT PRACTICE STANDARDS

In January 2001, the Joint Commission for Accreditation of Healthcare Organizations (JCAHO) instituted pain standards for hospital and ambulatory settings. The standards require the accredited health care facilities first and foremost recognize the rights of patients to appropriate assessment and management of pain.[11] Assessment of pain intensity is increasingly recognized as the fifth vital sign commonly used to gauge the effectiveness of pain relieving therapies. While dissemination of these standards has increased accountability for prompt attention and response to unrelieved pain, many agree that more stringent laws and regulations must be imposed to overcome the prevailing reluctance to aggressively treat cancer pain. A study of Wisconsin physicians revealed that more than 50% admitted to occasionally reducing the dose or quantity of refills, or prescribing an opioid in a lower scheduled category for fear of regulatory scrutiny.[12] To overcome these unfounded concerns, state medical boards have adopted guidelines to ensure that patients do not suffer needlessly because of misconceptions surrounding the prescribing of opioids. Moreover, compliance with published cancer pain management guidelines, diligence in documenting pain outcomes and response to therapy, and appropriate patient education regarding the safe use of opioid analgesics should alleviate these concerns. The University of Wisconsin Pain Studies Group/WHO Collaborating Center now tracks the introduction and enactment of new state laws and regulations. Recent data show a sustained increase in the number of states that define accepted pain practices and penalties under code for failure to render appropriate care to patients in pain.[13] Updated progress reports in the development of national and state pain-related health policies and legislation can be accessed from the University of Wisconsin Pain Policy Web site: www.medsch.wisc.edu/painpolicy.

Several strategies have been proposed to increase awareness of the proper approaches to assessing and managing cancer pain. Professional societies and government agencies have developed research- and evidence-based reviews and criteria for what constitutes "best practices." In July 2002, the NIH held a State-of-the-Science conference where national experts convened to establish consensus on the best approaches to treating the symptom cluster of pain, fatigue, and depression in cancer patients.[14] A summary of the panel's recommendations can be accessed from the Agency for Healthcare Research and Quality (AHRQ) evidence-based Web site: www.ahrq.gov. Other comprehensive guidelines for cancer pain are published through the AHRQ in an evidence report/technology assessment prepared by the New England Center EPC, Boston, Mass,[15] and the National Comprehensive Cancer Network (NCCN).[16] Current NCCN pain and distress management guidelines are available on their Web site: www.nccn.org.

Few studies have actually measured the benefits to patients when clinical care guidelines are consistently incorporated in routine patient care. The earliest attempts to evaluate the impact of practice guidelines focused on cancer prevention interventions in primary care by examining single outcomes such as written orders, tests obtained, and drugs prescribed.[17] Computerized systems to facilitate patient care orders were also studied in a variety of practice settings, but none of these investigations actually linked comprehensive pain guidelines to improvements in patient care. DuPen et al were among the first to test the effects of implementing cancer pain management clinical algorithms in a randomized controlled clinical trial involving 26 western Washington-area oncology outpatient sites.[18] Patients whose care was directed by clinical decision tools experienced statistically significant decreases in usual pain compared to those managed with standard practices (controls). Others found that individualized patient educational sessions and coaching techniques to promote self-management of pain for outpatients with cancer pain resulted in significant improvements in average levels.[19]

Figure 12-1. Pain intensity scales.

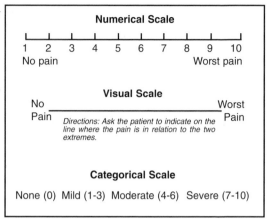

ASSESSMENT OF PAIN AND PAIN-RELATED OUTCOMES

Pain assessment begins with eliciting patient-reported data from reliable and valid measures, a physical examination, and evaluation of diagnostic criteria. Self-reports of pain intensity are most frequently obtained with the numeric rating scale (NRS) (0 to 10), 10 cm visual analogue scale (VAS) (0 no pain to 10 unbearable or worst pain imagined), and verbal rating scales (VRS) (Figure 12-1). Equally important is the ability to diagnose the physiological sources of pain (somatic, visceral, or neuropathic) through patient-reported information, physical exams, and radiological evaluations. The effectiveness of many treatment approaches is dependent on the origin of pain. Table 12-1 outlines the mechanisms for both acute and chronic cancer- and noncancer-related pain syndromes, characteristics, and an overview of treatment strategies. Somatic and visceral pain arises from activation of nociceptors in the periphery, while neuropathic pain or non-nociceptive pain results from damage to the peripheral or central nervous system. The following criteria should be a part of the clinical assessment for chronic pain:

- Etiology (cancer disease-related, cancer treatment-related, chronic nonmalignant pain, etiology unclear or unknown)
- Physiological sources of pain (somatic, visceral, neuropathic, or mixed pain)
- Mechanism (eg, inflammation, muscle spasm, visceral distention, nerve compression, or infiltration)
- Trajectory (progressive or stable)
- Severity (mild, moderate, or severe)
- Degree of physical debilitation
- Location
- Pain history (duration, temporal factors, patterns of pain)
- Confounding psychosocial (depression; anxiety; disruptions in interpersonal, family, or social relationships)
- Cognitive impairment or mental status changes (especially important in the elderly)

Table 12-1

PATHOPHYSIOLOGICAL MECHANISMS AND DIAGNOSIS OF PAIN TYPES

Pain Type	Physiological Structures	Mechanism	Clinical Evaluation of Pain Types	Examples of Syndromes
Somatic	*Cutaneous:* Skin and subcutaneous tissues. *Deep somatic:* Bone, muscle, blood vessels, connective tissues.	Activation of nociceptors.	A. Bony involvement evident by bone scans, skeletal films, CT tomography, and MRI. B. Muscle ivasion noted on CT scans or MI. C. Tumor infiltration of skin/soft tissue confirmed by physical exam and/or CT scanor MI results. D. Hiliar, retroperitoneal, axillary, inguinal, and para-aortic lymph node involvement would group as somatic sources of pain.	Bony metastases. Metastatic skin lesions. Soft tissue masses.
Visceral	Organs and the linings of body cavities.	Activation of nociceptors.	Pleural A. Pleural (thickening or effusion) and/or lung parenchymal changes noted on chest x-ray, chest CT, or MRI. Abdominal B. Visceral involvement included tumor progression affecting the peritoneum (lining of the abdominal organs and./or gynecologic structures). C. Mesenteric lymphadenopathy would be categorized as a possible source of visceral pain. D. Radiological findings from abdominal/chest CT, liver scans, and/or MRI will be used to confirm the presence of visceral involvement (ie, organ involvement or tumor studding of the pleural or peritoneum).	Liver metastases. Bowel obstruction. Acsites. Pleural effusion.

continued

Table 12-1 (continued)

PATHOPHYSIOLOGICAL MECHANISMS AND DIAGNOSIS OF PAIN TYPES

Pain Type	Physiological Structures	Mechanism	Clinical Evaluation of Pain Types	Examples of Syndromes
Neuropathic	Nerve fibers Spinal cord Central nervous system	Nonnociceptive injury to the nervous system structures.	Neuropathic pain is thought to be present if any of the following criteria is present: A. Sensory or motor impairment detected by neurological examinations and associated with the pattern of innervation such as nerve plexus involvement. B. Neurologic deficits such as sensory modality alterations or cutaneous hypersensitivity (thermal and mechanical allodynia and hyperalgesia, and dysesthesia). C. Evidence of direct nerve injury by CT tomography and/or MRI.	Cancer-related nerve injury as a result of direct tumor infiltration/compression. Epidural/spinal nerve root involvement/compression. Brachial and lumbosacral plexopathy.

Location, pain history (onset and duration), and temporal factors (precipitating factors) must also be included in a through pain assessment. Many patients with progressive cancer-related pain experience 2 or more sites of pain. A new pain location should raise suspicion for possible disease progression. Information about the patterns of pain can be useful in directing pain therapy. Patients with chronic pain often experience episodic or breakthrough pain in addition to their continuous or usual pain. In some circumstances, exacerbations of pain are predictable (such as pain with movement or activity) or occur at the end the duration of their pain medication(s). A study of 200 ambulatory patients found 90% with pain on movement.[20] On the other hand, pain episodes can be unpredictable. For example, neuropathic pain is often associated with spontaneous paroxysmal shooting pains, and cramping or stretching of hollow viscera may be sudden and unexpected. Breakthrough pains are generally a marker of more severe pain[21] and are associated with higher direct medical costs from pain-related hospitalizations and physician office visits.[22]

For chronic cancer pain, it is not enough to simply obtain pain intensity levels. Since cancer pain almost always coexists with other physical symptoms and psychosocial factors, multidimensional assessments are extremely helpful in understanding patient experiences. A critical review of the psychosocial aspects of cancer pain elucidates this strong association between pain and psychological distress.[23] Comprehensive pain assessments should be routinely incorporated into practice by including periodic or longitudinal evaluations of pain relief, symptom experiences, function, HrQOL, psychological distress, and satisfaction with pain care. Moreover, these variables may be independent of one another and outcomes from pain management.[24]

The Brief Pain Inventory (BPI) is commonly employed in outpatient settings to quantify patient-reported present, least, worst, and average pain levels; perceptions of pain relief; and pain interference[25] (Figure 12-2). The instrument is easy to administer and complete and has been tested in a variety of practice settings. The BPI has been validated with several culturally diverse populations and is translated in many languages. The 7 items measuring pain interference provide useful information on the degree to which pain interferes with function, mood, relationships, and other important aspects of daily living. Increased ratings of pain on the BPI have been associated with greater functional impairments and declines in perceptions of well-being. The Karnofsky Performance Status (KPS) Scale, which is an 11-point rating scale ranging from 0 (=dead) to 100 (=normal function), provides a unidimensional assessment of function.[26] The KPS has been traditionally a part of outcome measures in numerous clinical trials for cancer treatment.

The character and quality of pain can easily be assessed with the short form of the McGill Pain Questionnaire (SF-MPQ), which lists 11 sensory words and 4 affective words.[27] Respondents indicate whether or not they are experiencing the sensation or affective component and rank the severity on a scale of 1 (mild) to 3 (severe). Information is grouped in 3 categories: Physical Symptom Distress, Psychological Distress, and Global Distress Index. The SF-MPQ is especially useful to track the severity of sensations associated with specific pain syndromes following treatment. Since word choices such as "shooting," "hot-burning," and "stabbing" are included and often reported with nerve injury, the effectiveness of anticonvulsants and triclyic antidepressants commonly used to treat neuropathic pain can be evaluated. Patients with visceral pain often describe their pain as "cramping" or "splitting," which are also part of the SF-MPQ.

Figure 12-2. Brief pain inventory.

Symptom experiences that coexist with cancer and cancer pain can be identified and quantified with the Memorial Symptom Assessment Scale (MSAS).[28] Patients rate 32 symptoms for presence and severity and degree to which they are bothered by the symptom on a 0-to-4 Likert Scale. HrQOL while mostly measured in the context of clinical trials and outcome research studies has gained importance in routine clinical practice. Additional information on the clinical utility of HrQOL is available in an extensive review of quality of life measures and their meaningfulness in clinical care.[29]

Careful selection of pain assessment tools is needed for special populations such elders, terminally ill, cognitively impaired, culturally diverse, or those with language barriers. Pain instruments must be easily understood and administered, validated for use with these populations and capable of identifying changes in pain over time. Item burden and stress associated with responding to questions are reduced by prioritizing the most critical information and obtaining patient-reported data with short questionnaires or surveys. For specific recommendations for assessing pain in vulnerable patients, consult the American Geriatrics Society clinical care guidelines,[30,31] report from the Expert Working Group of the European Association of Palliative Care[32] and available data on the psychometric testing of instruments in culturally-based research.[13]

ACUTE PAIN MANAGEMENT

Aggressive treatment of acute pain associated with surgical intervention, procedures, and initial presentation of cancer-related pain is paramount to preventing or minimizing the physiological insults that can result in more complex chronic pain conditions. Current perspectives on the physiological mechanisms of chronic pain such as central sensitization, hyperalgesia, synaptic remodeling (plasticity), pain memory formation, and behavioral adaptation to pain are probably activated within days of acute tissue injury.[33] Central sensitization, originally described by Woolf, refers to an increased sensibility to pain stimuli that occurs at the level of the spinal cord, which can subsequently lead to ongoing disruptions in the sensing and processing of pain.[34] While acute pain generally lessens over time, there is compelling evidence to show that unresolved pain can worsen and led to a cascade of tissue and pain pathway mediated responses, which sensitize the nervous system precipitating more prolonged pain states. The onset of acute or sudden pain in patients with cancer should also raise suspicion about the likelihood for disease progression.

POSTOPERATIVE PAIN MANAGEMENT

Despite improvements in perioperative care, major abdominal and thoracic surgery is still associated with significant pain. It is believed that adquate pain control can improve post-surgical outcomes and benefits to recovery are associated with various pain management techniques.[35] However, under treatment of acute (not only chronic) pain is a prevailing problem. Untreated pain has caused serious psychological, physiological, and economic consequences. While not conclusive, a systematic review of the impact of acute pain management services showed that patients followed by pain services reported less pain at rest and on movement.[36] Primary care physicians can help patients facing surgery to have realistic expectations regarding pain control, expect pain management options to be discussed with them, and be proactive in communicating their pain.

Pain Management Strategies

Given the use of surgical intervention throughout the disease continuum, it is critical to design postoperative pain management regimens based on whether patients are opioid naive or opioid-dependent or tolerant. Further patient stratification is necessary, depending on the surgical site such as thoracic and upper vs lower abdomen. Other considerations include the appropriateness of pre-emptive analgesia, multimodal therapy or "balanced analgesia," and regional or systemic analgesia, which all have significant advantages for optimizing pain relief in selected patient populations.

Pre-Emptive Analgesia

Timing of analgesia plays an important role in the degree of effectiveness of postsurgical pain control and possibly the interruption of tissue injury responses before the surgical insult. Preemptive interventions remain controversial and the clinical benefits have been difficult to prove. Moreover, there is little consensus as to what constitutes preemptive analgesia, but most agree that preoperative and sometimes intraoperative administration of analgesics falls within the applied use of the concept.

In experimental models, antinociceptive strategies implemented prior to the time of tissue injury show a reduction in the development of postinjury central sensitization. Clinically, however, research with preemptive analgesia yields wide variations in achieving desired postoperative pain outcomes. An extensive systematic review by Moiniche, et al[37] evaluating the effects of preemptive strategies (preoperatively or intraoperatively) analyzed the results from double-blind randomized studies of analgesia initiated before or after surgical incision. For the most part, preemptive analgesia with NSAIDs, intravenous opioids or ketamine, peripheral local anesthetics and caudal analgesia offered no appreciable benefit over postsurgical treatment. The greatest benefit seemed to occur with single-dose epidural analgesia, although the same was not supported with continuous epidural infusions.

NONSTEROIDAL ANTI-INFLAMMATORY DRUGS

NSAIDs have little effect on surgical stress responses and organ dysfunction; however, in combination with opioid analgesics they provide measurable benefits for pain relief. Their opioid sparing effects have been shown to reduce opioid requirement by about 20 to 30%,[38] thereby, decreasing the incidence and severity of opioid-induced adverse effects such as constipation, nausea and vomiting, and sedation. Unlike most opioid analgesics, the analgesic potency of NSAIDs is limited by the ceiling dose effect of this class of drugs. NSAIDs can be administered as single analgesic agent therapy only after minor surgery. Randomized controlled studies involving the perioperative use of NSAIDs have included a variety of surgical procedures and a relatively small number of patients. Commonly prescribed NSAIDs and their antipyretic, analgesic, and anti-inflammatory effects are listed in Table 12-2.

INTRAVENOUS PATIENT-CONTROLLED ANALGESIA

Intravenous (IV) patient-controlled analgesia (PCA), which gives patients the opportunity to self-medicate on demand, has become the mainstay for the management of postsurgical pain. Morphine is the most common opioid administered by PCA; however, fentanyl and hydromorphone are equally as effective and are associated with less pruritus, sedation, and nausea. A meta-analysis of IV PCA studies with demand dosing only and no continuous background infusion revealed significantly greater pain relief with PCA compared to intermittent IM, IV, and subcutaneous (SC) opioid administration, and continuous IV opioid infusions alone.[39] In general, PCA is associated with higher levels of patient satisfaction with pain control.

Enormous variation in PCA opioid requirements is found with age, extent of pain, and prior opioid use. Continuous basal or background infusions should be used cautiously with elderly patient who are opioid naive. Typically, opioid naïve patients benefit from PCA demand dosing only, while opioid dependent or tolerant patients usually require a basal infusion in addition to demand dosing for PCA to be effective. Pre-existing opioid requirements must be taken into account when designing PCA regimens,

Table 12-2

COMMONLY USED NONSTEROIDAL ANTI-INFLAMMATORY DRUGS

Properties of Properties of Some Commonly Used NSAIDs

DRUG	ANALGESIC EFFECT	ANTIPYRETIC EFFECT	ANTI-INFLAMMATORY EFFECT
Salicylic Acids			
ASA	+	+	+
Propionic Acids			
Diclofenac	+	+	+
Ibuprofen	+	+	+
Naproxen	+	+	+
Carbo and Heterouyclicacetic Acids Indomethacin	+	+	++
Fenamates			
Meclofenamate Acid	+	+	±
Oxicams			
Piroxicam	+	+	+
Pyrazolines			
Phenybutazone	+	+	++
Paracetamol	+	+	+
Pyrrolo-Pyrroles			
Ketorolac	+	+	±

Adverse Effects by System

SYSTEM	EFFECTS
CNS	Headaches, nausea
Pulmonary	Asthma/bronchospasm, pulmonary edema
Gastric	Ulceration/Hemorrhage, stomatitis
Renal	ARF, Hypertension, Interstitial Nephritis
Dermatological	Photosensitivity, Erythema Multiforme, Fixed Drug Eruption, Reye's Syndrome
Hepatic	Aplastic Anemia, Hemolytic Anemia
Systemic	Anaphylactoid Reactions

especially for patients with chronic cancer or nonmalignant pain syndromes. Most opioid-dependent patients require at least 100% more opioid for pain management than their daily requirement prior to surgery. Consult Macintyre[40] for an extensive review of the safety and efficacy of PCA not only for postoperative pain, but also for other acute pain syndromes and chronic pain.

Epidural Analgesia

For major thoracic and abdominal surgical procedures, epidural analgesia is superior in its pain-relieving effects when compared to other analgesic therapy. Evidence from a recent meta-analysis on postoperative epidural analgesia confirms that better pain control is achieved compared to parenteral opioids regardless of the analgesic agent and level of the catheter.[41] The optimal approaches for this technique are often debated as epidural analgesia can involve both single agent or combination therapy and delivery of agents at different levels in the epidural space. Moreover, variations exist in reported failure rates and risk/benefit analyses. Most often therapy with continuous infusions with or without patient-controlled epidural analgesia is associated with better pain outcomes than intermittent dosing schedules alone. Studies consistently show that combinations of an opioid and local anesthetic provide significantly greater pain relief following upper and lower abdominal surgery in contrast to single agent administration. The advantages of lipophilic opioids (fentanyl and hydromorphone) alone are questionable, especially for pain management after upper and lower abdominal procedures.[42]

There is definitely a role for epidural analgesia following major abdominal surgery for GI malignancies. Despite the lack of randomized controlled trials to evaluate the effectiveness of catheter levels with abdominal procedures, the use of thoracic epidurals remains the standard for practice. The key is concordance of anatomic site and catheter location (ie, thoracic dermatome incision and thoracic epidural). With opioid and local anesthetic combinations, thoracic administration promotes the drug delivery of smaller doses of lipophilic agents at the same level of the incision and lessens chances for motor and sympathetic blockade from local anesthetics.[42] Successful placement of thoracic catheters requires technical expertise that is often present among pain management trained anesthesiologists or general anesthesiologists with extensive experience.

Along with the level of catheter placement, the selection of an opioid and local anesthetic combination solution and hourly rate of administration seem to be the most important determinants of treatment success with epidural analgesia. The mechanism of action of epidural opioids is by mu receptor activity in the spinal cord and systemic absorption. Fentanyl, because of its lipophilic pharmacological property, provides more segmental pain relief and is probably effective through absorption into the systemic circulation. Epidural doses often approximate those required for systemic administration. While fentanyl causes less pruritis and nausea compared to morphine, which has some advantage in patients with GI malignancies already experiencing preoperative nausea, its limited vertical distribution may lead to less effective pain control with extensive abdominal incisions when administered through lumbar catheters. Morphine, because of its hydrophilic properties, has greater rostral (vertical) spread in the epidural space, thus it is more appropriate for managing pain from surgical incisions that are more remote from the catheter tip. Hydromorphone, used less often, provides similar relief as morphine with limited side effects. Approximately one-fifth to one-fourth of the systemic dose is required for epidural morphine and hydromorphone administration; therefore, additional systemic opioids may be needed to abate physiological withdrawal in opioid-dependent patients.

Bupivacaine, in concentrations of 0.065% to 0.125%, is the most common local anesthetic for postoperative epidural analgesia solutions, and levobupivacaine and ropivacaine are less often used. Motor blockade is more common with bupivacaine and levobupivacaine, while ropivacaine in typical doses is selective for sensory blockade only. Patients receiving local anesthetics should be observed for sensory impairment below the catheter level including routine inspection of the skin, repositioned frequently to alleviate pressure, given range of motion exercise to improve circulation and prevent thrombophelebitis, and assisted when getting out of bed. Adjustments in infusion rates, typically a decrease of 20 to 25%, changes in the concentration of local anesthetic or switching the local anesthetic to ropivacaine can prevent moderate to dense motor blockade.

Complication rates for epidural analgesia include dural puncture (0.32% to 1.23%), direct neurological trauma (extremely rare), spinal hematoma from puncture of epidural vessels during catheter insertion (3% to 12%), catheter migration (0.15% to 0.18%), and infection (extremely rare). Respiratory depression (respiratory rate <8 per minute), while the most serious, is no greater than the incidence associated with systemic opioids.[42] Patients closely followed by acute pain management services are less likely to experience respiratory depression, and frequent monitoring of respiratory rate and cautious use with older patients >70 years of age and those with pre-existing respiratory diseases can often prevent its occurrence. Pruritis, which is a less serious adverse effect but more distressing to patients, occurs in about 40% of patients, more commonly with morphine. Small intravenous doses of naloxone (<0.1 mg) administered IV every 2 to 3 hours is the most effective treatment.

CHRONIC PAIN MANAGEMENT

CANCER PAIN SYNDROMES

Patients with cancer may also experience pain from pre-existing or new chronic nonmalignant pain syndromes. Regardless of the etiology, cancer pain can be classified as somatic, visceral or neuropathic, or mixed pain syndromes including any combination of these physiological sources. In an international study involving a sample of over 1000 patients with severe cancer pain, 71.6% were found to have a component of somatic pain, 39.7% visceral pain, and 34.7% neuropathic pain.[43]

Clinical assessment of cancer pain syndromes, whether related to cancer treatment or disease progression, begins with identifying the cause and determining the likelihood for worsening. Early aggressive intervention to gain control of the pain should always be attempted, especially for patients who present with pain as a symptom of advancing disease. In fact, palliative or supportive care should be initiated earlier rather than later so that multiple approaches to relieving pain and symptom and emotional distress have the greatest chance to ameliorate needless suffering and maximize quality of life. To help physicians' understand suffering, Chapman and Gavrin elucidate its meaning to patients and clarify that pain is not synonymous with suffering.[44] While pain is one cause, suffering is much less tangible and spans a person's entire existence. Referrals to palliative care can be difficult as this often requires confronting the realization that it may not be possible to control or reverse tumor progression and communicating this to patients. Palliative care has evolved not only as an approach to assist patients to die, but also to help them live. Unlike hospice care, fewer restrictions are placed on treatment and aggressive interventions with palliative services so patients can still receive active therapy for their cancer.

Treatment-Related Pain Syndromes

Cancer treatment-induced pain syndromes that might be associated GI malignancies include postsurgical syndromes (eg, postthoracotomy syndrome), postradiation syndromes (radiation-induced lumbosacral plexopathies, enteritis and proctitis, burning perineum, and osteoradionecrosis), and chemotherapy-induced (painful peripheral neuropathy and plexopathy associated with intraarterial infusion, and hepatic arterial infusion).

Cancer-Related Pain Syndromes

SOMATIC PAIN

Somatic pain, the most common form of cancer pain, arises from nociceptor activation in the skin, subcutaneous tissue, bones, blood vessels, and muscle. It is generally well localized; however, bone and muscle pain can be more diffuse. The bone is the most frequent site for metastasis, accounting for over 40% of pain syndromes associated with cancer progression.[43] Skeletal involvement occurs less often with advanced gastrointestinal malignancies compared to primary cancers of the breast, lung, kidney, and prostate. Tumor invasion of bone is associated with intense pain, especially on movement, which can significantly compromise mobility. Of 108 patients presenting to a multidisciplinary pain clinic for bony metastases, 79% reported moderate to severe pain on average and, after examining their treatment plans, investigators concluded that the majority required more aggressive pain therapy than what was prescribed.[45] Severe muscle spasms may occur in the areas of the lesions over unstable vertebral bodies or long bones. Serious and painful complications of bony metastases include pathological fractures, compression fractures, and nerve root compression.

Treatment approaches for bony metastases include pharmacotherapy, surgical intervention for stabilization, chemotherapy and radiation therapy, and radioisotopes; however, the indications and effectiveness of many treatment strategies are tumor-dependent. Recently, a systematic review of randomized studies showed that single fraction radiation is just as effective as multifraction radiotherapy in relieving pain; however, retreatment rates (21.5% vs 7.4%) and pathological fractures (3% vs 1.6%) were higher in patients who received single fraction treatment plans.[46] NSAIDs may be helpful initially alone or combination with opioids, but typically when patients require higher doses of opioids the added risk for adverse effects may outweigh the benefits. Flexible schedules for opioid analgesia should be prescribed to allow patients to self-medicate for episodic pains associated with activity. If long-acting opioids are used, adequate rescue medication with short-acting opioids should be prescribed for breakthrough pain.

A variety of pain-elieving agents exert their pharmacological actions by specifically targeting mechanisms of cancer-mediated pain both systemically and at the site of tumor infiltration. These include tumor necrosis alpha receptor antagonists, osteoclast inhibitors, inhibitors of glutamate release, substance P inhibitors, nitric oxide synthetase inhibitors, and other novel compounds.[28] Consult the following references for more detail on the mechanisms and treatments for bone pain.[47,48]

VISCERAL PAIN

Pain arising from nociceptors in the organs and those that line the organs and body cavities constitutes visceral pain. Tumor invasion of viscera often results in painful stimuli that cause stretching or enlargement, especially of hollow viscera, and inflammation. Cervero describes the five major characteristics of visceral pain: 1) is not evoked from all viscera, 2) in not linked to visceral injury, 3) causes referred pain, 4) is poorly localized and diffuse, and 5) is accompanied by autonomic reflexes.[49] Intense visceral pain may be associated with autonomic responses such as sweating or nausea or vomiting. With inflammation, visceral nociceptors, unlike somatic, can be sensitized to non-noxious stimuli pain. This may cause heightened pain or exaggerated pain responses during diagnostic procedures that manipulate or stretch inflamed tissues. Interventional techniques described later may be extremely helpful in controlling visceral pains.

NEUROPATHIC PAIN

Neuropathic pain is the most complex and challenging to treat. It results from direct injury to peripheral nerves or central nervous system and can also occur from a disruption in the central processing of pain caused by peripheral nerve injury (central pain). The primary mechanisms for neuropathic pain do not involve direct activation of nociceptors—hence it is often referred to as non-nociceptive mediated pain. Clinically, neuropathic pain syndromes appear to be less responsive to opioid analgesics than somatic and visceral pain. As a result, patients will often require higher doses of opioid analgesics and may still not achieve acceptable pain relief. Opioid therapy can be slowly titrated up to the point that patients get relief or experience intolerable toxicities (eg, sedation, nausea). Selection of opioid analgesics is critical, and nonopioid combinations should be avoided so that doses can be escalated without added toxicities and ceiling effects. Greater benefits may be derived from combining opioid analgesics with effective adjuvant agents such as tricyclic antidepressants and anticonvusants that have documented efficacy in the treatment of neuropathic pain. Selective interventional techniques including temporary nerve blocks, neurolysis or nerve destruction procedures, and neuraxial (epidural or subarachnoid) therapy have demonstrated significant benefits.

PRINCIPLES OF CHRONIC OPIOID ANALGESIC THERAPY

Chronic opioid analgesic therapy is indicated for mild to severe pain that has not responded to nonopioid preparations. Centrally acting opioid-agonists (eg, codeine, fentanyl, hydrocodone, oxycodone, morphine, hydromorphone) have an affinity for mu receptors and are preferred over other opioid preparations. Opioids such as meperidine (Demerol, Sanofi-Synthelabo, New York, NY) and proproxyphene (active agent in Darvocet, Eli Lilly & Co, Indianapolis, In) are weak and have toxic metabolites that accumulate with repeated dosing, and therefore should not be used for the management of chronic cancer pain. The toxic metabolite of meperidine (normeperidine) can lead to seizures; and cardiac toxicity may occur from the metabolite of proproxyphene. Even with its serious limitations, proproxphene is over prescribed; it is no better in its analgesic efficacy than acetaminophen or aspirin. The NCCN has recommendations for opioid prescribing, titration, and maintenance, as well as oral and parenteral dose equivalents.

Guidelines for Chronic Opioid Therapy

For mild to moderate pain: Begin with less potent, regularly scheduled short-acting opioids such as combination opioid products. These include codeine + acetaminophen (Tylenol #3, #4 [McNeill PPC, Milltown, NJ]), hydrocodone + acetaminophen (Vicodin, [Abbott Labs, Abbott Park, Ill]), and oxycodone + acetaminophen (Percocet, [Novartis, Cambridge, Mass]). Use caution to avoid doses of combination products containing acetaminophen that exceed the maximum daily dose of 4000 mg, especially in older persons.

For moderate to severe pain: Initiate therapy with regularly scheduled more potent short-acting opioids such as oxycodone (Oxy IR, OxyFast [Purdue, Stamford, Conn]), morphine (MSIR [Purdue]) or hydromorphone (Dilaudid [Abbott]).

FOR THE ELDERLY

Start low and go slow. Be aware of analgesic peak effects and duration. A trial of short-acting opioids at half the usual starting dose for adults should be initiated. Peak effects from the opioid may be heightened in the elderly and duration extended. Initial prescribing should allow for longer dosing intervals until the response to therapy can be evaluated. In addition, avoid initial therapy with opioids having an extended T½ (half-life) (eg, methadone) or long-acting opioid preparations in older persons who are opioid-naive.

FOR LONG-TERM PAIN CONTROL

Consider long-acting opioids when the response to shorter-acting agents can be evaluated and controlled-released morphine (MSContin [Purdue]), oxycodone (OxyContin [Purdue]), or transdermal fentanyl system (Duragesic [Abbott]). The transdermal fentanyl patch, which provides a convenient application every 72 hours, should be considered for patients who are not able to take oral medication or absorb it (eg, chronic nausea or intermittent vomiting, noncompliance with opioid use, or mechanical GI obstruction). Titration may be difficult with severe progressive pain and therefore, adequate rescue medication should be available until steady state levels are reached. The lowest available patch strength, 25 mcg/hour, should not be applied to opioid-naive patients.

RESCUE OR SUPPLEMENTAL MEDICATION

Supplemental analgesia with short-acting opioid agents can prevent and minimize intermittent painful episodes; however, rescue opioid medication is most effective if adequate doses are taken in anticipation of exacerbations of pain. Transmucosal fentanyl citrate (OTCF) (Actiq [Cephalon, West Chester, Pa]) can provide pain relief within 5 minutes.[8,50] Generally, intermittent rescue doses of oral opioids should be approximately 10 to 30% of the daily oral opioid requirement of regularly scheduled continuous opioid analgesia.

RESPONSE TO THERAPY

Subjective pain rating scales and a pain relief scale can be used to evaluate response to opioid therapy. Clinically, other parameters such as improved function, mood, and appetite may also be indicators of decreased pain.

CONCURRENT USE OF OTHER PSYCHOACTIVE DRUGS

The concurrent use of other psychoactive drugs, particularly if initiated with opioids or close to the time of starting therapy with opioids, obscures assessment of the untoward effects of opioids. If adjuvant agents for pain must be initiated, it is best to introduce agents singly and allow ample time (at least several days before giving a new agent with potential psychoactive effects.

OPIOID-RELATED SIDE EFFECTS

A major side effect of opioids is constipation. Mild laxatives such as milk of magnesia, senna preparations (Senokot [Purdue]), casanthranol and docusate (Pericolace [Purdue]), lactulose, or bisacodyl (Dulcolax [Boehringer Ingelheim, Germany]) should be started when opioids are intiated. Stool softeners alone do little or nothing to alleviate opioid-induced constipation. Unlike many other adverse effects from opioids, patients do not develop tolerance to the effects of opioids on the bowel, therefore, continued use of laxatives is necessary as long as opioid therapy is maintained.

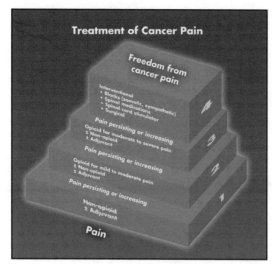

Figure 12-3. Modified WHO Analgesic Step Ladder for cancer pain management to include a fourth step of interventional pain management modalities. (Adapted from Miguel R. *Cancer Control.* 2000;7:149-156.)

INTERVENTIONAL TECHNIQUES

When optimal oral pharmacological therapy is ineffective or leads to unacceptable side effects, interventional pain management techniques should be considered. The WHO Analgesic Step Ladder for cancer pain management outlines several sequential strategies for alleviating persistent and uncontrolled pain with Step 4, the highest level, encompassing invasive procedures (Figure 12-3). Several interventional approaches such as parenteral opioid infusions, neuraxial medication infusion, neurolytic blockade, and other procedures (eg, vertebroplasty) offer effective alternatives to pain management. Substantial progress has been made over the past two decades in elucidating appropriate selection criteria and refining technology for these invasive techniques. Moreover, advances in the radiological diagnostics have provided significant advantages in precise placement of neuraxial (intraspinal) catheters and safety with the delivery of neuroablative agents (ie, phenol and alcohol). The NCCN recommendations for procedural strategies are outlined in Figures 12-4.

PARENTERAL OPIOD INFUSIONS

CONTINUOUS INTRAVENOUS INFUSION OF OPIOIDS

Parenteral opioid administration is indicated in patients who experience intolerance to oral administration because of GI obstruction, malabsorption, opioid-induced nausea/vomiting, dysphagia, or high opioid requirements necessitate large number of pills or applications of transdermal systems. Patients with severe episodic pain with movement or unpredictable spontaneous pain may benefit from self-administered demand dose or a patient-controlled analgesia (PCA) feature in addition to a continuous intravenous infusion (CII). Calculations for PCA demand doses are determined based on the hourly continuous infusion. The bolus dose should be 50 to 100% of the continuous

NCCN Practice Guidelines in Oncology—v.1.2004   CANCER PAIN

Procedural consultation[1]

Major indications for referral:

- Pain likely to be relieved with nerve block (eg, pancreas/upper abdomen with celiac plexus block, lower abdomen with superior hypogastric plexus block, intercostal nerve, or peripheral nerve
- Failure to achieve adequate analgesia with out intolerable side effects (may be handled with intraspinal agents, blocks, or destructive neurosurgical procedures

Commonly used procedures:

- Regional infusions (requires infusion pump)
  - Epidural: Easy to place, requires large volumes and an externalized catheter; for infusions of opioids, local anesthetics, clonidine
  - Intrathecal: Easy to internalize to implanted pump; for infusions of opioids, local anesthetics, clonidine
  - Regional plexus: For infusions of local anesthetics, to anesthetize single extremity
- Neurodestructive procedures for well-localized pain syndromes
  - Head and neck: Peripheral nerve block
  - Upper extremity: Brachial plexus neurolysis
  - Thoracic wall: Epidural neurolysis
  - Upper abdominal pain (visceral): Celiac plexus block, thoracic splanchnicectomy
  - Midline pelvic pain: Superior hypogastric plexus block
  - Rectal pain: Intrathecal neurolysis, midline myelotomy or superior hypogastric plexus block
  - Unilateral pain syndromes: Cordotomy
  - Consider intrathecal L/S phenol block
- Percutaneous vertebroplasty

Appropriate procedural approaches
- Nerve blocks
- Spinal opioids
- Neuroaxial analgesia

→ Evaluate which pain site can be relieved. Will interventional technique provide tangible benefit?

— YES ——→ See following page

— NO ——→ Reassess therapeutic plan. Procedural approaches not indicated at this time.

Procedural approaches are not appropriate ——→ Reassess therapeutic plan. Procedural approaches not indicated at this time.

[1]High benefits/risk ratio examples: celiac plexus, superior hypogastric plexus, and peripheral nerves

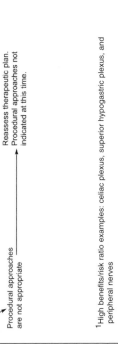

Figure 12-4A. NCCN cancer pain guidelines. (Adapted and reproduced with permission from the NCCN 1.2004 Cancer Pain Guideline, *The Complete Library of NCCN Clinical Practice Guidelines in Oncology* [CD-ROM]. Jenkintown, Pennsylvania: ©National Comprehensive Cancer Network, December 2004. To view the most recent and complete version of the guideline, go online to www.nccn.org.)

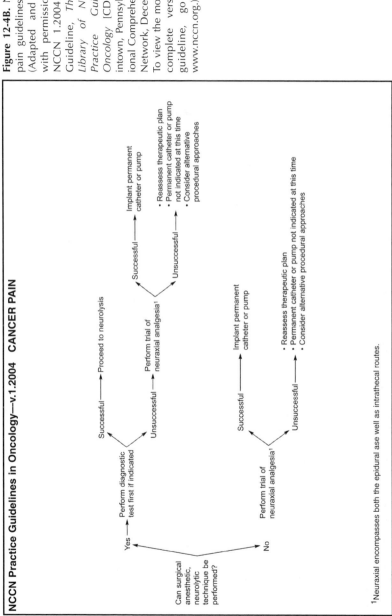

NCCN Practice Guidelines in Oncology—v.1.2004   CANCER PAIN

Can surgical anesthetic, neurolytic technique be performed?

Yes → Perform diagnostic test first if indicated

Successful → Proceed to neurolysis

Unsuccessful → Perform trial of neuraxial analgesia[1]

Successful → Implant permanent catheter or pump

Unsuccessful →
- Reassess therapeutic plan
- Permanent catheter or pump not indicated at this time
- Consider alternative procedural approaches

No → Perform trial of neuraxial analgesia[1]

Successful → Implant permanent catheter or pump

Unsuccessful →
- Reassess therapeutic plan
- Permanent catheter or pump not indicated at this time
- Consider alternative procedural approaches

[1]Neuraxial encompasses both the epidural ase well as intrathecal routes.

Figure 12-4B. NCCN cancer pain guidelines (continued). (Adapted and reproduced with permission from the NCCN 1.2004 Cancer Pain Guideline, *The Complete Library of NCCN Clinical Practice Guidelines in Oncology* [CD-ROM]. Jenkintown, Pennsylvania: ©National Comprehensive Cancer Network, December 2004. To view the most recent and complete version of the guideline, go online to www.nccn.org.)

infusion dose and the interval for patient access may vary from every 15 to 60 minutes. PCA allows patients to gain rapid control over exacerbations of pain without the need for family and home health nurse interventions. PCA technology is only effective if patients have the cognitive and functional capabilities to self-administer medication. Doses are adjusted by taking into account pain intensity, demand dose requirements and disposition of the patient. If patients are not experiencing side effects from the opioid, escalations of about 10 to 25% of the hourly rate can be safely done every 24 hours for unrelieved pain.

Continuous Subcutaneous Infusion of Opioids

Continuous subcutaneous infusion of opioids (CSCI) is often considered for the same reasons as CII, but when it is not possible to insert an intravenous access line or when venous access is limited. Starting doses are calculated based on the conversion of the 24-hour oral/transdermal to an equianalgesic intravenous dose requirement, using an opioid conversion table and dividing this dose by 24 for an hourly rate. Tissue irritation is minimized when volumes under 2 mL/hour are delivered by using the maximum concentration of the opioid. A patient-controlled demand dose feature can be programmed into the drug delivery infusion device. Demand doses should not exceed 1 to 2 mL and availability of access with a lock-out interval should be every 30 to 60 minutes. A 25- or 27-gauge butterfly needle is inserted subcutaneously anywhere with the most preferred sites including the infraclavicular fossa, chest wall, or abdomen for ease of ambulation. Absorption of subcutaneous opioids is rapid, and steady-state plasma levels are generally approached within an hour. Most parenteral opioids are suitable for CSCI, although morphine and hydromorphone are used most commonly.[51]

NEURAXIAL (INTRASPINAL) ANALGESIA

Neuraxial analgesia is achieved by the epidural or intrathecal administration of opioids alone or in combination with other agents such as local anesthetics (bupivacaine or ropivacaine) or clonidine, an alpha-2 agonist effective for the treatment of neuropathic pain. This modality is useful in basically two groups of patients: those with intolerable opioid related side-effects or pain unrelieved in spite of escalating doses of opioids and adjuvant agents. Neuraxial opioid therapy is accomplished by introducing minute quantities of opioids in close proximity to their receptors (substantia gelatinosa of the spinal cord) achieving high local concentrations. With this therapy, analgesia may be superior to what is achieved when opioids are administered systemically by other routes, and since the absolute amount of drug administered is reduced, side effects are minimized. In addition to opioids, local anesthetics and other coanalgesic medications can enhance the analgesic effect. The neuraxis can be accessed via an intrathecal, epidural, or intraventricular approach. For more long-term therapy, greater than three months, intrathecal administration with an implantable device or epidural therapy with a tunneled externalized catheter or implantable port are preferred to avoid potential infection.

The most important aspect of this therapy is its reversibility and the reliability and simplicity of advanced screening measures to confirm effectiveness. Screening is generally accomplished on an outpatient basis by observing the patient's response either to a morphine infusion via a temporary percutaneous epidural catheter or a single intrathecal injection. If improved pain control and reduced side effects are sufficiently compelling to warrant more prolonged therapy, then a temporary catheter for period of days to weeks is placed or a permanent implanted catheter along with medication reservoir

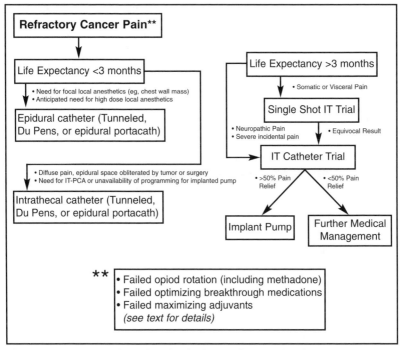

Figure 12-5. Decision-making algorithm for the use of neuraxial analgesia in treating cancer pain. (Adapted from Burton AW, Rajagopal A, Shah HN, et al. Epidural and intrathecal analgesia is effective in treating refractory cancer pain. *Pain Medicine,* 5(3);239-247, 2004.)

infusion device is surgical implanted.[52] The MD Anderson Cancer Center decision-making algorithm is shown in Figure 12-5. A recently published multi-center prospective randomized clinical trial by Smith et al compared intrathecal therapy to continued medical management, revealing a trend toward better analgesia in the intrathecal group with improved side effect profile and increased survival in the intrathecal group.[53] Neuraxial analgesia is suitable for patients at any stage of their disease, including those who are considered free of disease, but who are plagued with persistent unrelieved pain. This technique is contraindicated in patients with systemic or localized infections or those with any form of a coagulopathy.

NERVE BLOCKS

Cancer patients are often referred to pain management specialists for a "quick cure" or because systemic analgesics seem to be ineffective. Many referring physicians are under the mistaken impression that "nerve blocks" alleviate all types of pain. Some focal pain syndromes are amenable to these procedures, as outlined below, but many are not. Generally, the more focal the pain, the easier it is to locally block sensory nerves involved in pain transmission. Unfortunately, peripheral sensory blocks also cause motor impairment as both fibers are intertwined. With peripheral blocks using local anesthetic, pain relief and any motor impairment are temporary; however, permanent blocks or neurolysis with alcohol or phenol are much more risky and not possible without major morbidity. Some areas where neurolytic nerve blocks can be useful include pancreatic or upper abdominal malignancy with the celiac plexus block; lower abdominal pain with the superior hypogastric plexus block; chest wall pain with intercostal nerve blockade, and end stage lumbosacral plexopathy with intraspinal neurolysis.[54-56] Although infrequent, symptoms may arise as a result of tumor invasion of nervous system structure (eg, brachial or lumbosacral plexopathy), in which case either local anesthetic blockade of the stellate ganglion or lumbar sympathetic chain has been used with some success to relieve pain.[57]

Neurolytic blocks play an important role in the management of intractable cancer pain. This modality should only be offered when pain persists despite thorough trials of aggressive pharmacological management or when drug therapy produces undesirable and uncontrollable side effects. Patient selection is of utmost importance including some general tenets:

- Severe pain
- Pain is expected to persist
- Pain cannot be modified by less invasive means
- Pain is well-localized
- Pain is well-characterized
- Pain is not multifocal
- Pain is of somatic or visceral origin
- Limited life expectancy

Alcohol and phenol are the only agents commonly used to produce chemical neurolysis. Ethyl alcohol is a pungent, colorless solution that can be readily injected through small-bore needles and that is hypobaric with respect to CSF. For peripheral and subarachnoid blocks, alcohol is usually diluted (referred to as 100% alcohol, dehydrated alcohol, or absolute alcohol), while a 50% solution is used for celiac plexus block. With alcohol blocks, denervation and pain relief sometimes accrue over a day following injection. Phenol has a biphasic action—its initial local anesthetic action produces subjective warmth and numbness that usually give way to chronic denervation over a day's time. Hypoalgesia after phenol is typically not as dense as after alcohol, and the quality and extent of analgesia may diminish slightly within the first 24 hours of administration. The average duration of all neurolytic blocks is estimated at 3 to 6 months, with a wide variation in effectiveness. Reports of analgesia persisting 1 to 2 years are fairly common.

Subarachnoid neurolysis can be performed at any level up to the midcervical region. Above this area, increases any risk of drug diffusion to medullary centers and the potential for cardiorespiratory collapse increases. Blocks in the region of the brachial outflow are best reserved for patients with preexisting compromise of upper limb function. Similarly, lumbar injections are avoided in ambulatory patients, as are sacral injections in patients with normal bowel and bladder function.

Celiac plexus block continues to be one of the most efficacious and common nerve blocks employed in patients with pain from pancreatic cancer and liver metastases. It is most effective for relieving upper abdominal and referred back pain secondary to malignant neoplasm involving structures derived from the foregut (distal esophagus to midtransverse colon, liver, biliary tree, and adrenal glands). The most common indication

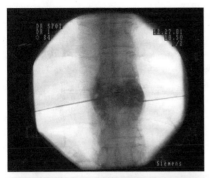

Figure 12-6A. Anteroposterior fluoroscopic view of a retrocrural celiac plexus block. (Courtesy of Allen W. Burton, MD.)

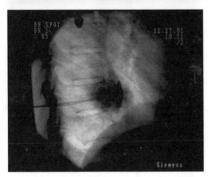

Figure 12-6B. Lateral fluoroscopic view of a retrocrural celiac plexus block. (Courtesy of Allen W. Burton, MD.)

for celiac axis block is pancreatic cancer. Celiac axis block is most frequently attempted by positioning needles bilaterally either antero- or retrocrurally via a posterior percutaneous approach (Figure 12-6). Despite the proximity of major organs (aorta, vena cava, kidneys, pleura) and requirements for a large volume of the neurolytic agent (30 to 50 mL of 50% alcohol in the anterocrural technique and much less volume in the retrocrural) complication rates are uniformly low.

More recently, radiofrequency-generated thermal lesions are another effective means of inducing therapeutic nerve injury and, when directed to the tumor itself, it can have a tumoricidal effect often with salutary effects on symptoms.[58] Peripheral cranial nerve blocks have a limited role in the management of cancer pain. Control of neoplastic-related pain from locally invasive head and neck carcinomas are challenging because of rich sensory innervations to these structures. In selected patients, blockade of involved cranial and/or upper cervical nerves is extremely helpful in treating pain. Blockade of the trigeminal nerve within the foramen ovale at the base of skull or its branches may be beneficial for facial pain. If neural blockade is not effective, intraspinal opioid therapy by means of an implanted cervical epidural catheter or intraventricular opioid therapy may be considered.

VERTEBROPLASTY

Metastatic vertebral compression fractures (VCFs) or osteoporotic VCFs are often associated with movement-related back pain. Percutaneous vertebroplasty (PV) is a minimally invasive procedure that is accomplished by injecting opacified bone cement (usually polymethymethacrylate or PMMA) into the fractured vertebral body to alleviate the pain and perhaps enhance structural stability. This procedure is performed by placing needles under fluoroscopic guidance with a uni- or bipedicular approach. PMMA is injected in a carefully controlled manner to avoid unintended cement spread into the spinal canal. The injection is stopped as soon as cement starts approaching in posterior on third of vertebral body. PV has been shown to be highly efficacious in treating VCF cancer-related pain.[59] Complications are rare but can be serious, including paralysis and death.

NEUROMODULATION

Spinal cord stimulation is a nonpharmacologic method used to treat refractory chronic neuropathic pain states. Recently, investigators at MD Anderson Cancer Center have demonstrated success in treating painful chemotherapy induced neuropathic pain with spinal cord stimulation.[60]

NEUROSURGICAL INTERVENTIONS

Neurosurgical palliative techniques are seldom performed as more aggressive, reversible, titratable, and lower risk techniques have largely replaced these procedures. Techniques such as pituitary ablation, myelotomy, and cordotomy should only be considered in patients who have not responded to more conservative pharmacological and interventional approaches aforementioned.

SUMMARY

Principles of interventional cancer pain management are in most respects similar to those that apply to "good medical practice." These procedures should only be considered in collaboration with pain experts and performed by skilled pain trained anesthesiologists, neurosurgeons or neurologists. Eligibility criteria are stringent and patients should be carefully examined prior to undertaking any procedure. A realistic, frank discussion of the risks, benefits, alternatives, and goals of care must take place with patients and family members so that they have a clear understanding of what the technique entails and the expected outcomes. After the procedure, follow-up care should be maintained as long as desired by the patient and or primary physician. While rarely eliminated altogether, pain can be controlled in the vast majority of patients, usually with the careful application of straightforward pharmacological measures combined with diagnostic acumen and conscientious follow up. In a small but significant cohort of patients whose pain is not readily controlled with noninvasive analgesics, a variety of alternative measures, when selected carefully, are also associated with a high degree of success.

An increasingly large cadre of anesthesiologists have come to recognize that far from an exercise in futility, caring for patients with advanced irreversible illness can be highly satisfying and met with considerable success. Multidisciplinary approaches to cancer pain management yield the greatest success. Recognizing that primary care physicians may benefit from criteria-based information for initiating referrals to pain management specialists, the NCCN has developed indications for specialty consultations. Thus, no patient should ever wish for death as a result of inadequate control of pain or other symptoms, or be deprived of expert evaluation for interventional procedures or other modalities. Comprehensive cancer care is best regarded as a continuum that commences with prevention and early detection, focuses intensely on curative therapy, and ideally is rendered complete by a seamless transition to palliation and attention of quality of life.

PAIN MANAGEMENT RESOURCES

Some of the most compelling data to drive clinical practice come from meta-analyses and systematic reviews. Physicians are challenged to incorporate these findings into best practices for managing pain. Unfortunately, there is a paucity of research in many areas of pain management, so often it is necessary to rely on consensus from expert panels and other professional forums. Several evidence-based guidelines, which are available from professional societies, government agencies, and private foundations, interpret and translate available information into practical approaches to managing cancer pain. Some of these clinical care guidelines, pain assessment and treatment decision algorithms, and educational materials can be accessed from the following Web site listings:

- Agency for Healthcare Research and Quality: www.ahrq.gov
- American Academy of Pain Medicine: www.painmed.org
- American Geriatrics Society www.americangeriatrics.org
- American Pain Society: www.aps.org
- International Associations for the Study of Pain: www.isap-pain.org
- National Cancer Center Network: www.nccn.org
- National Pain Educational Council: www.npecweb.org

REFERENCES

1. Ad hoc Committee on Cancer Pain of the American Society Clinical Oncology. Cancer pain assessment and treatment curriculum guidelines. *J Clin Oncol.* 1992;10:1976-1982.
2. Nicholson A, Davies A, Reid C. Methadone for cancer pain. *The Cochrane Library*. Vol. 1. Chichester, UK: John Wiley & Sons, Ltd; 2005.
3. Vainio A, Auvinen A, Members of the Symptom Prevalence Group. Prevalence of symptoms among patients with advanced cancer: an international study. *J Pain Symptom Manage.* 1996;12:3-10.
4. Grahm AL, Andren-Sandberg A. Prospective evaluation of pain in exocrine pancreatic cancer. *Digestion.* 1997;58:542-549.
5. Esnaola NF, Cantor SB, Johnson ML, et al. Pain and quality of life after treatment in patients with locally recurrent rectal cancer. *J Clin Oncol.* 2002;20:4361-4367.
6. Cleeland CS, Gonin R, Hatfield AK, et al. Pain and its treatment in outpatients with metastatic cancer. *N Engl J Med.* 1994;330:592-596.
7. Von Roenn JH, Cleeland CS, Gonin R, Hatfield AK, Pandya KJ. Physician attitudes and practice in cancer pain management: a survey from ECOG. *Ann Intern Med.* 1993;119:121-126.
8. American Pain Society. *Principles of Analgesic Use in the Treatment of Acute Pain and Cancer Pain.* 5th ed. Glenview, IL: American Pain Society; 2004.
9. American Academy of Pain Medicine, American Pain Society, and American Society of Addiction Medicine. *Definitions related to the use of opioids for the treatment of pain.* American Academy of Pain Medicine:Glenview, Ill; 2001.

10. Cleary JF, Carbone PP: Palliative medicine in the elderly. *Cancer.* 1997;80:1335-1347.

11. Berry PH, Dahl JL. The new JCAHO pain standards: implications for pain management nurses. *Pain Manage Nurs.* 2000;1:3-12.

12. Weissman, DE, Joranson DE, Hopwood MB. Wisconsin's physicians' knowledge and attitudes about opioid analgesic regulations. *Wisc Med J.* 1991;December:53-58.

13. Joranson DE, Gilson AM, Dahl JL, Haddox JD. Pain management, controlled substances, and state medical board policy: a decade of change. *J Pain Sympt Manage.* 2002;23:138-147.

14. *NIH State-of-the-Science Statements.* 2002;19:1-29.

15. Carr DB, Goudas L, Lawrence D, et al. Management of cancer symptoms: pain, depression, and fatigue. *Evidence Report/Technology Assessment, Agency for Healthcare Research and Quality.* US Department of Health and Human Services 2002; AHRQ Publication No. 02-E032.

16. Benedetti C, Brock C, Cleeland C, et al for the National Comprehensive Cancer Network. NCCN Practice Guidelines for Cancer Pain. *Oncology.* 2000;14:135-150.

17. McPhee SJ, Bird JA, Fordham D, et al. Promoting cancer prevention activities by primary care physicians: results of a randomized controlled trial. *JAMA.* 1991;266:538-544.

18. DuPen SL, DuPen AR, Polissar N, et al. Implementing guidelines for cancer pain management: results of a randomized controlled clinical trial. *J Clin Oncol.* 1999;17:361-370.

19. Oliver JW, Kravitz RL, Kaplan SH, Meyers FJ. Individualized patient education and coaching to improve pain control among cancer outpatients. *J Clin Oncol.* 2001;19:2206-2212.

20. Blanning A, Sjogren P, Henriksen H. Treatment outcome in a multidisciplinary cancer pain clinic. *Pain.* 1991;47:129-134.

21. Portenoy RK, Payne D, Jacobsen P. Breakthrough pain: characteristics and impact in patients with cancer pain. *Pain.* 1999;81:129-134.

22. Fortner BV, Okon TA, Portenoy RK. A survey of pain-related hospitalizations, emergency department visits, and physician office visits reported by cancer patients with or without history of breakthrough pain. *J Pain.* 2002;3:38-44.

23. Zara C, Baine N. Cancer pain and psychosocial factors: a critical review of the literature. *J Pain Symptom Manage.* 2002;24:526-542.

24. Hwang SS, Chang VT, Kasimins B. Dynamic cancer pain management outcomes: the relationship between pain severity, pain relief, functional interference, satisfaction and global quality of life. *J Pain Symptom Manage.* 2002;23:190-200.

25. Daut RL, Cleeland CS, Flanery RC. Development of the Wisconsin Brief Pain Inventory to assess pain in cancer and other disease. *Pain.* 1983;17:197-210.

26. Karnofsy DA, Bruchenal JH. The clinical evaluation of chemotherapeutic agents in cancer. In: Macleod CM, ed. *Evaluation of Chemotherapeutic Agents.* New York, NY: Columbia University Press; 1949:191-205.

27. Melzack, R. The short-form McGill Pain Questionnaire. *Pain.* 1987;30:191-197.

28. Portenoy RK, Thaler HT, Kornblith AB, L, et al. The Memorial Symptom Assessment Scale: an instrument for the evaluation of symptom prevalence, characteristics and distress. *Eur J Cancer.* 1994;30A(9):1326-1336.

29. Osoba D. A taxonomy of the uses of health-related quality of life instruments in cancer care and the clinical meaningfulness of the results. *Med Care.* 2002;40:III31-38.

30. American Geriatrics Society. The management of chronic pain in older persons. AGS Panel on chronic pain in older persons. *Geriatrics.* 1998;53(suppl 3):S8-24.

31. American Geriatrics Society releases persistent pain management guidelines. *J Pain Palliat Care Pharmacother.* 2002;16:127-129.

32. Caraceni A, Cherry N, Fainsinger R, Kaasa S, Poulin P, Radbruch L, DeConno F. Pain measurement tools and methods in clinical research in palliative care: recommendations of an Expert Working Group of the European Association of Palliative Care. *J Pain Symptom Manage.* 2002;23;239-255.

33. Carr DB, Goudas LC. Acute pain. *Lancet.* 1999353;2051-2058.

34. Woolf CJ. Evidence for a central component of postinjury pain hypersentivity. *Nature.* 1983;308:386-388.

35. Lewis KS, Whipple JK, Michael KA, Quebbeman EJ. Effect of analgesic treatment on the physiological consequences of acute pain. *Am J Hosp Pharm.* 1994:51:1539-1554.

36. Werner MU, et al. Does acute pain service improve postoperative outcome? *Anesth Analg.* 2002;95:1361-1372.

37. Moiniche S, Kehlet H, Dahl JB. A qualitative and quantitative systematic review of pre-emptive analgesia for postoperative pain relief. *Anesthesiology.* 2002;96:725-41.

38. Power I, Barrat S. Analgesic agents for the postoperative period. Nonopioids. *Surg Clin N Am.* 1999;79:275-95.

39. Ballantyne JC, Carr DB, Chalmers TC, et al. Postoperative patient-controlled analgesia: meta-analysis of initial randomized control trials. *J Clin Anesth.* 1999;5:182-193.

40. Macintyre PE. Safety and efficacy of patient-controlled analgesia. *Br J Anaesth.* 2001; 87:36-46.

41. Block BM, Liu SS, Rowlingson AJ, et al. Efficacy of postoperative epidural analgesia. *JAMA.* 2003;290:2455-2463.

42. Wheatley RG, Sching SA, Watson D. Safety and efficacy of postoperative epidural analgesia. *Br J Anaesth.* 2001;87:47-61.

43. Caraceni A, Portenoy RK. An international survey of cancer pain characteristics and syndromes. IASP Task Force on Cancer Pain. International Association for the Study of Pain. *Pain.* 1999;82:263-274.

44. Chapman RC, Gavrin J. Suffering: the contributions of persistent pain. *Lancet.* 1999;353:2233-2237.

45. Janjan NA, Payne R, Gillis T, et al. Presenting symptoms in patients referred to a multidisciplinary pain clinic. *J Pain Symptom Manage.* 1998;16;171-178.

46. Sze WM, Shelley MD, Held, I, Wilt TJ, Mason MD. Palliation of metastatic bone pain: single fraction versus multifraction radiotherapy—systematic review of randomised trails. *Clin Oncol.* 2003;15:342-344.

47. Clohisy DR, Mantyh PW. Bone cancer pain. *Cancer.* 2003;97:866-73S.

48. Ripamonit C, Fulfaro F. Malignant bone pain: pathophysiology and treatment. *Curr Rev Pain.* 2000;4:187-196.

49. Cervero F, Laird JMA. Visceral pain. *Lancet.* 1999;353:2145-2148.

50. Farra JT, Cleary J, Rauck R, Busch M, Norbrock E. Oral transmucosal fentanyl citrate: randomized, double-blinded, placebo-controlled trial for treatment of breakthrough pain in cancer patients. *J Natl Cancer Inst.* 1998;90:611-616.

51. Bruera E. Subcutaneous administration of opioids in the management of cancer pain. In: Foley K, Ventafridda V, eds. *Recent Advances in Pain Research.* Vol 16. New York, NY: Raven Press; 1990:203-218.

52. Burton AW, Rajagopal A, Shah HN, et al. Epidural and intrathecal analgesia is effective in treating refractory cancer pain. *Pain Medicine.* 2004;I5(3):239-47

53. Smith TJ, Staats PS, Deer T, et al. Randomized comparison of Intrathecal Drug Delivery System (IDDS) + Comprehensive Medical Management (CMM) vs. CMM alone for unrelieved cancer pain. *J Clin Oncol.* 2002;20(19):4040-9.

54. Eisenberg E, Carr DB, Chalmers TC. Neurolytic celiac plexus block for abdominal pain associated with malignancy: a meta-analysis. *Anesth Analg.* 1995;80:290-295.

55. De Leon-Casasola OA, Kent E, Lema MJ. Neurolytic superior hypogastric plexus block for chronic pelvic pain associated with cancer. *Pain.* 1993;54:145-151.

56. Swerdlow M. Intrathecal neurolysis. *Anaesth.* 1978;33:733-740.

57. Racz GB, Holubec JT. Stellate ganglion phenol neurolysis. In: Racz GB, ed. *Techniques of Neurolysis.* Boston, Mass: Kluwer, 1989;133-143.

58. Patti JW, Neerman Z, Wood BJ. Radiofrequency ablation for cancer-associated pain. *J Pain.* 2002;3(6):471-3.

59. Fourney DR, Schomer DF, Nader R, et al. Percuteneous vertebroplasty and kyphoplasty for painful vertebral body fractures in cancer patients. *J Neurosurgery.* 2003;98:21-30.

60. Cata J, Cordiella J, Burton AW, Hassenbusch SJ, Dougherty PM, Weng HR. Spinal cord stimulation relieves chemotherapy-induced pain: a clinical case report. *J Pain Symptom Manage.* 2004;27(1):72-78.

chapter 13

Endoscopic Ultrasound in the Diagnosis and Staging of Gastrointestinal Malignancy

Janak N. Shah, MD

INTRODUCTION

EUS was first introduced in the United States in the late 1980s, and has since become an important technological advance in GIs endoscopy. EUS enables the endoscopist to obtain high-resolution, detailed images of the GI luminal wall and pancreaticobiliary system. This ability has allowed EUS to make substantial contributions to the clinical management of GI malignancies. Other technological improvements, such as the ability to perform EUS-FNA, have led to expanded roles, and EUS is now increasingly utilized in patient care. This chapter will review the current clinical uses of EUS in the setting of GI malignancies.

EUS: INSTRUMENTS AND TECHNIQUE

EUS is performed using specialized endoscopes (echoendoscopes) with radial or linear array ultrasound transducers at the instrument tip (Figure 13-1). Most echoendoscopes use ultrasound frequencies ranging from 7.5 to 12 MHz. Newer instruments allow the operator to choose from a wider range of scanning frequencies while using the same echoendoscope. Smaller, high-frequency (20 to 30 MHz), catheter based probes are available to perform intraluminal and intraductal ultrasonography via the instrument channel of standard endoscopes. In general, higher frequency scanning produces more detailed, high-resolution images, but at the cost of decreased depth of penetration. Lower frequency scanning generates the opposite effect.

EUS is considered a technically demanding modality, as it calls for expert procedural skills, detailed knowledge of cross-sectional anatomy, and the ability to interpret ultrasound images. EUS is not routinely performed by most gastroenterologists, and is ideally learned under the direction of an experienced endosonographer. Although there are no formal requirements establishing EUS proficiency, it is reasonable that endoscopists performing EUS should obtain diagnostic accuracy rates similar to those in previously published series. Diagnostic EUS is a safe procedure, with types and rates of

Figure 13-1. Mechanical radial array echoendoscope (GFUM-130, Olympus America Corp, Melville, NY). *For a full-color version, see page CA-V of the Color Atlas.*

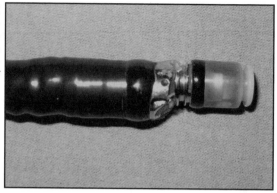

complications similar to that of standard endoscopy. The most common complications are cardiopulmonary and are related to the medications used for conscious sedation. Complications of EUS-FNA are discussed separately in this chapter (see section on EUS-FNA).

ESOPHAGEAL MALIGNANCY

Treatment recommendations for esophageal cancer are largely dependent on tumor stage. For example, patients with early, localized disease are offered immediate surgery. Patients with high operative risk superficial disease limited to the mucosa may be candidates for endoscopically-directed intraluminal therapy (eg, endoscopic mucosal resection or photodynamic therapy). The optimal management in those with locoregionally advanced disease may include chemoradiotherapy prior to surgical resection. Therefore, it is imperative to accurately stage esophageal cancer in order to guide appropriate therapy for each particular patient.

Once a histologic diagnosis of esophageal cancer is established (usually by forceps biopsies during diagnostic endoscopy), further evaluation should occur in stepwise fashion (Figure 13-2). First, the presence of metastases should be ascertained. This is usually evaluated using cross-sectional imaging. Where available, positron emission tomography (PET) may be used, and may be more accurate than computerized tomography (CT) to detect stage IV disease.[1] If metastases are present, palliative measures should be considered, and EUS examination would be unnecessary.

If there is no evidence for metastatic disease, EUS should be performed to assess locoregional staging of the primary tumor site (see Appendix A). Tumor involvement of the esophageal wall is seen endosonographically as a hypoechoic mass or thickening of the wall with disruption of the normal ultrasonic wall layer pattern. The depth of abnormality and extent of wall pattern disruption guide the endosonographer in determining T stage by EUS (Figure 13-3). For N staging, several sonographic criteria suggest malignant involvement of visualized lymph nodes: 1) homogeneous echo pattern, 2) smooth borders, 3) circular shape, and 4) size greater than 10 mm.[2] When all four features are present (in only 25%), EUS is highly accurate (>80%) in identifying malignant lymph nodes.[3]

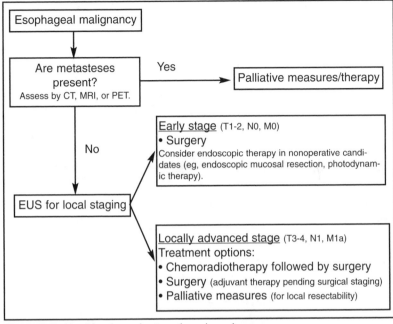

Esophageal malignancy

Are metasteses present?
Assess by CT, MRI, or PET.

Yes → Palliative measures/therapy

No

EUS for local staging

Early stage (T1-2, N0, M0)
• Surgery
Consider endoscopic therapy in nonoperative candidates (eg, endoscopic mucosal resection, photodynamic therapy).

Locally advanced stage (T3-4, N1, M1a)
Treatment options:
• Chemoradiotherapy followed by surgery
• Surgery (adjuvant therapy pending surgical staging)
• Palliative measures (for local resectability)

Figure 13-2. Algorithm for evaluation of esophageal cancer.

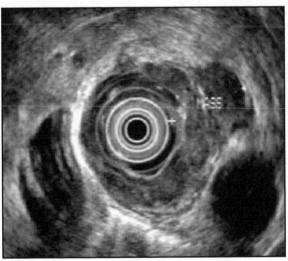

Figure 13-3. EUS image demonstrates a circumferential, hypoechoic lesion in the distal esophagus, with disruption of normal wall layer pattern and extension of mass through the esophageal wall into periesophageal tissue. By EUS criteria, the lesion is stage T3 N0 MX.

EUS has proven to be the most accurate modality to evaluate the local extent of esophageal malignancy, and is more accurate than CT, magnetic resonance imaging (MRI), or PET scanning for determining T and N stage.[1,4,5,6] The average overall accuracy of EUS for T and N staging of esophageal malignancy is about 85% and 77%, respectively.[6] For superficial tumors, high frequency EUS scanning may be required to verify the precise depth of involvement, but EUS remains an accurate staging modality for these lesions as well. EUS accuracy for determining local unresectability (T4) is about 86%,[6] and given the morbidity and mortality rates following esophagectomy, EUS can be particularly useful in identifying inappropriate surgical candidates. Overall T and N staging accuracy using CT scan is poorer, ranging 40% to 50% and 50% to 70%, respectively.[6]

EUS-FNA of periesophageal lymph nodes can be performed to confirm nodal involvement. However, this technique is only reliable when lymph nodes can be accessed without traversing the primary tumor (to avoid false positive contamination of the cytology specimen). When performed, EUS-FNA improves the assessment of lymph node staging by yielding sensitivity, specificity, and accuracy of over 90% in several series, and should be utilized when histologic confirmation of nodal involvement would alter clinical management.[7,8]

Complete EUS staging evaluation can be difficult in patients with stenotic tumors, and incomplete examinations can lead to decreased staging accuracy. One published technique that has been safely employed to allow echoendoscope passage through stenotic segments is luminal dilation. Esophageal dilation to a diameter of 14 to 16 mm permits complete EUS examination in the majority (>85%) of cases.[9,10] Other instruments that may enable the completion of EUS examination through stenoses include catheter based ultrasound probes and nonfiberoptic ("blind"), wire-guided, small diameter echoendoscopes.

Many centers treat patients with locally advanced tumors with preoperative chemoradiotherapy, with the anticipation of improved outcomes compared to surgery alone. Although it would be of interest to subsequently assess the tumor response to neoadjuvant treatment prior to surgical resection, the accuracy of EUS for restaging in this scenario is poor (about 42% and 54% for T and N stage, respectively)[11,12] This is likely due to the inability to sonographically distinguish tumor from post-treatment inflammation (both appear hypoechoic). However, a reduction in maximal cross-sectional area (≥50%) following chemoradiotherapy has been associated with longer survival, and may be a helpful sonographic prognostic criteria.[13]

In patients who have undergone resection for esophageal malignancy, locoregional recurrence is often difficult to detect with standard endoscopic and radiologic evaluation. As EUS can provide detailed images of the luminal wall and extraluminal tissue, it is particularly useful in this setting, and has reported sensitivity and specificity of over 90%.[14]

GASTRIC MALIGNANCY

GASTRIC ADENOCARCINOMA

Gastric adenocarcinomas occur in two clinico-histologic varieties: an intestinal type and a diffusely spreading type (linitis plastica). The intestinal type of gastric cancer is usually detected endoscopically as a discrete polypoid mass or ulcerated lesion, and diagnosed on endoscopic forceps biopsies. In linitis plastica, the tumor may be difficult to detect, as it infiltrates along the gastric wall and may diffusely spread to involve large portions of the stomach. EUS plays an important role in the management of patients with both clinical varieties of gastric cancer. For discrete masses or infiltrative tumors that have already been diagnosed as adenocarcinoma, EUS provides local staging information. For patients suspected of having linitis plastica but are undiagnosed, EUS offers valuable diagnostic data to help direct further evaluation and/or treatment.

As with other malignancies, accurate staging helps estimate survival and guides further treatment. Sonographic assessment of T and N staging in gastric cancer is done similar to that of esophageal cancer (see Appendix B). In those with established malignancy and no evidence for metastases, EUS should be used to determine the locoregional involvement, and has overall accuracy rates for T and N staging of about 80% and 70%, respectively.[15,16] Patients with tumors that appear resectable by imaging are usually offered gastrectomy. Anastomotic recurrences can occur after surgery, and EUS has high sensitivity (95%) and specificity (80%) for detecting recurrent tumor.[17]

Select patients with superficial, mucosal-based tumors who are poor operative candidates may be considered for endoscopic resection at expert endoscopic centers. But to even contemplate this mode of therapy, EUS examination is critical as it is the only nonsurgical means of accurately identifying the depth of wall invasion for superficial lesions. EUS (with high-frequency scanning) accurately identifies T1 gastric cancers in 80% to 90% of cases.[15]

In evaluating patients suspected of having linitis plastica, EUS can be particularly useful in diagnosis. Sonographically, the gastric wall is usually thickened (>3 mm). When tumor cells have infiltrated all wall layers, by EUS there appears to be hypoechoic thickening with complete loss of normal wall layer pattern. When the tumor has diffusely spread along intact histologic planes (eg, along the submucosa or muscularis propria), the wall layer pattern may be preserved, but the involved histologic layer is quite thickened sonographically. In this setting, mucosal forceps biopsies obtained during standard endoscopy may be nondiagnostic, and EUS findings provide crucial information to guide further evaluation.[18] When the diagnosis of linitis plastica is clinically entertained, sonographic findings are suspicious, and mucosal forceps biopsies are nondiagnostic, a full-thickness surgical biopsy should be considered.

GASTRIC LYMPHOMA

The most common site for primary non-Hodgkins extranodal lymphoma is the stomach, and accounts for about 5% of all gastric neoplasms. Gastric lymphomas often manifest as a polypoid, exophytic mass, but may also diffusely infiltrate, similar to linitis plastica. Histologically, the tumors may be high-grade lymphomas or MALT (mucosa-associated lymphoid tissue) lymphomas, which are usually low-grade but may have high-grade foci.

In patients with high-grade lymphomas, treatment considerations include radiation, chemotherapy, surgical resection, or combination multimodality therapy. EUS is useful in guiding the treatment plan by determining the local involvement of disease through assessment of depth (partial- or full-thickness) and extent (fundus, body, and/or antrum) of tumor, as well as regional lymph nodes. Sonographically, their appearance is usually similar to that of gastric adenocarcinoma, with a hypoechoic mass or thickening, and disruption of the normal wall layer pattern. EUS accurately determines the depth of infiltration (T stage) in about 90%, and accurately detects lymph node disease (N stage)

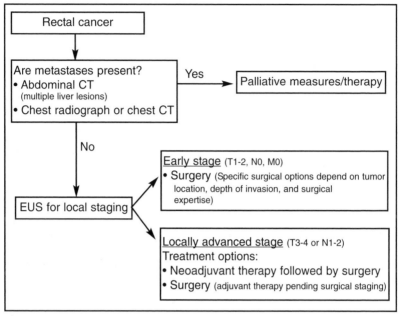

Figure 13-4. Algorithm for evaluation of rectal cancer.

in over 80%.[19] When needed, the accuracy for detecting lymph node disease can be improved by performing EUS-FNA with flow cytometry.[20]

MALT lymphomas are associated with *H. pylori* infection, and have an overall better prognosis than high-grade gastric lymphomas. Some MALT lymphomas, those limited to the mucosa or submucosa with no suspicious regional lymph nodes, may respond to antimicrobial therapy alone, without need for more extensive treatment with surgery and/or chemoradiotherapy. By determining an accurate depth of tumor extent, EUS has proven helpful in identifying patients that can be appropriately treated with *H. pylori* eradication as the sole initial therapy.[21] Moreover, interval EUS can be used to detect those that did not respond to antimicrobial therapy, so that appropriate further treatment can be administered.

RECTAL MALIGNANCY

Similar to the setting of esophageal cancers, the treatment options for rectal neoplasms are largely contingent on tumor stage. As an accurate means of determining the locoregional extent of rectal tumors, EUS plays an important role in guiding the optimal therapy for these malignancies.

Rectal tumors are usually diagnosed histologically by forceps biopsies obtained during endoscopy. Further evaluation should occur in a stepwise manner (Figure 13-4). The presence of lung and liver metastases should be excluded using a chest radiograph and/or cross-sectional imaging. The presence of distant metastases obviates the need for local staging. Patients with no evidence for metastases should undergo rectal EUS to determine the locoregional extent of tumor (see Appendix D). On EUS, tumors appear as hypoechoic masses or thickening with loss of the normal rectal wall layer pattern. The T stage is determined by assessing the depth of tumor involvement, and accuracy rates for EUS range from 80% to 95%.[22] EUS appears to be least accurate in correctly identifying T2 lesions; these are often incorrectly overstaged as T3, likely due to the inability to distinguish adjacent inflammation from tumor penetration through the muscularis propria. Comparatively, overall T stage accuracy rates for CT and MRI are lower, ranging 65% to 75% and 75% to 85%, respectively.[23]

N stage is determined by assessing perirectal lymph nodes for suspicious sonographic criteria (large size, homogenous echo pattern, circular shape, and smooth borders). Accuracy rates for EUS range from 70% to 75%.[23] Although lymph node size is considered an important feature in identifying suspicious nodes elsewhere in the GI tract, up to 50% of malignant perirectal nodes are less than 5 mm in diameter.[24] Thus, even small nodes should be regarded malignant. Given that nonmalignant perirectal lymph nodes are sonographically heterogenous, small, and rarely seen by EUS, some experts advocate that any visualized node should be considered malignant. Unlike other areas of the GI tract, EUS-FNA does not significantly increase N stage accuracy over EUS alone, and should not be routinely used.[25] EUS-FNA is likely most useful in confirming lymph node status in patients with early T stage tumors and sonographically visible nodes, in which true nodal involvement is in question and the knowledge of which would impact clinical management. Comparative N stage accuracy rates for CT and MRI are lower, about 55% to 65% and 60% to 65%, respectively.[23]

Findings on rectal EUS help determine appropriate therapy for each particular patient. For instance, individuals with locally advanced tumors (T3, T4, N1, or N2) may be offered neoadjuvant therapy. Analogous to other sites, EUS is not useful to assess response to neoadjuvant treatment due to the difficulty in sonographically differentiating tumor from therapy effect, and has lower accuracy rates for both T and N staging (about 50%) following radiation therapy.[26] Surgical planning is often guided by EUS findings. For example, those with superficial tumors (T1-2, N0) in the distal rectum may be candidates for sphincter-saving transanal excision, and sonographic evaluation provides valuable information to select the appropriate candidate (Figures 13-5 and 13-6). Those with more advanced lesions in the distal rectum would likely require more extensive surgery (abdominoperineal or mesorectal resection).

Up to 25% of patients develop local recurrence of cancer following sphincter-saving operations.[22] These can be very difficult to diagnose, as recurrences may develop extraluminally. The ability of EUS to image perirectal tissue is particularly useful in this situation, and allows better detection rates compared to CT scan.[27] EUS-FNA improves the accuracy of detecting recurrent tumor over EUS alone, from about 75% to greater than 90%, and should be utilized when needed.[28] Some advocate the routine use of postoperative rectal EUS for surveillance of recurrent cancer.

GASTROINTESTINAL STROMAL TUMORS

Gastrointestinal stromal tumors (GISTs) are mesenchymal neoplasms arising from precursors of connective tissue cells of the myenteric plexus, and can occur at any location in the GI tract. The most common anatomic sites include the stomach and small intestine, but they can also be found in the esophagus, colon, and mesentery. GISTs may be benign or malignant, and virtually all GISTs express the c-kit protein, a cell membrane receptor with tyrosine kinase activity.[29]

Figure 13-5. Endoscopic image demonstrates a polypoid mass in the distal rectum. Histology from forceps biopsies revealed adenoma with foci of adenocarcinoma. *For a full-color version, see page CA-VI of the Color Atlas.*

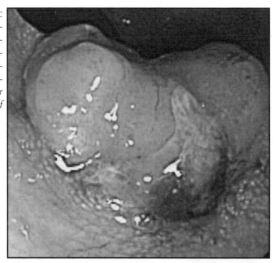

Figure 13-6. Corresponding EUS image suggests that the rectal mass is mucosal-based, without extension into muscularis propria. By EUS criteria the lesion is stage T1 N0 MX. This patient was referred to surgery for transanal excision.

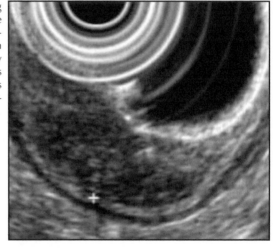

On endoscopy, GISTs are usually seen as submucosal lesions with normal appearing, overlying mucosa. Occasionally, mucosal ulcerations can be seen. Unfortunately, an accurate diagnosis is extremely difficult to make on standard endoscopy, as other submucosal lesions can produce a similar endoscopic appearance, and forceps biopsies are usually not of adequate depth to obtain histologic confirmation.

The unique ability of EUS to provide detailed images of the luminal wall makes it a particularly attractive modality in the evaluation of GISTs (Figure 13-7). Sonographically, GISTs appear as hypoechoic masses that are usually located in the muscularis propria (fourth wall layer on EUS). They may also arise from the muscularis mucosa (second wall layer). Rarely, they may appear to be in the third wall layer (sub-

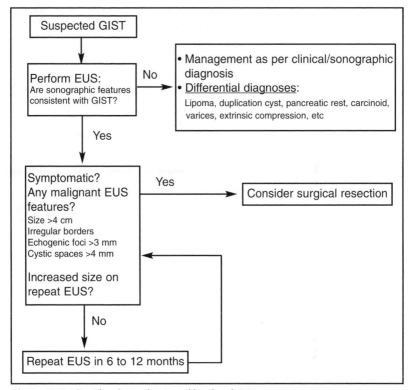

Figure 13-7. Algorithm for evaluation of localized GIST.

mucosa), in which case the tumor has likely extended into the submucosa from the muscularis propria or muscularis mucosa. EUS findings can additionally exclude other common lesions that look similar endoscopically, but differ in sonographic appearance, such as lipomas (hyperechoic), duplication cysts (anechoic), gastric varices (anechoic), and extrinsic compression from adjacent structures.

GISTs may be benign or malignant. Several EUS features appear to be helpful in identifying malignant tumors: 1) size >4 cm, 2) irregular extraluminal border, 3) echogenic foci >3 mm within lesion, and 4) cystic spaces >4 mm within lesion.[30] Symptomatic tumors or those with malignant-appearing EUS characteristics should be resected (Figure 13-8). Lesions that are suspected to be GISTs, but are asymptomatic without high-risk sonographic features may be followed by repeat EUS every 6 to 12 months. Those that develop interval increase in size, suspicious EUS criteria, or become symptomatic should undergo surgical resection. Tumors that appear unresectable or that are metastatic may be considered for therapy with imatinib mesylate, a selective tyrosine kinase inhibitor.[29]

Histologic confirmation of GISTs has been difficult short of an operation. Endoscopic forceps biopsy may be attempted using large particle forceps, with a "tunnel" or "bite-on-bite" technique. But, specimens are often nondiagnostic due to the typ-

Figure 13-8. EUS image demonstrates a hypoechoic mass arising from the muscularis propria (fourth layer) of the gastric wall. The sonographic appearance is suggestive of GIST. The irregular extraluminal border (white arrow) raised the concern for malignancy, and surgical resection was recommended.

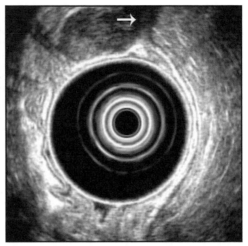

ical deep location of the tumor in the luminal wall (usually in the muscularis propria). However, EUS-FNA can be used to establish a diagnosis. Immunohistochemical analysis of FNA specimens can reveal c-kit expression, which is a highly accurate marker for GISTs.[31] One must keep in mind that the presence of c-kit identifies GISTs, but is not useful to discriminate between benign and malignant tumors. Special stains of FNA samples for other cell markers (eg, Ki-67) may prove useful in establishing malignancy.[32] Where available, newer EUS devices that allow retrieval of tissue core specimens could provide larger samples to more accurately assess mitotic activity and other pathologic features.

PANCREATICOBILIARY MALIGNANCY

PANCREATIC ADENOCARCINOMA

EUS is an important modality in the evaluation of patients with known or suspected pancreatic adenocarcinoma, but its specific role may evolve with technological advances in other, noninvasive imaging techniques (eg, helical CT and multidetector CT). The evaluation of patients with suspected pancreatic adenocarcinoma should occur in a stepwise manner (Figure 13-9). Where available, helical/multidetector CT or state-of-the-art MRI, tailored to examination of the pancreas ("pancreatic protocol"), should be requested as these provide the most detailed, cross-sectional images possible, and may improve the detection and evaluation of tumors compared to conventional CT.

As with other malignancies, assessment of metastases is of first priority. If metastases are present on cross-sectional imaging, EUS for staging purposes would be unnecessary. Where available, PET scanning may be used to clarify questionable liver lesions that are seen on cross-sectional imaging. When histologic confirmation is desired, either a CT guided biopsy or EUS-FNA can be used to establish a tissue diagnosis.

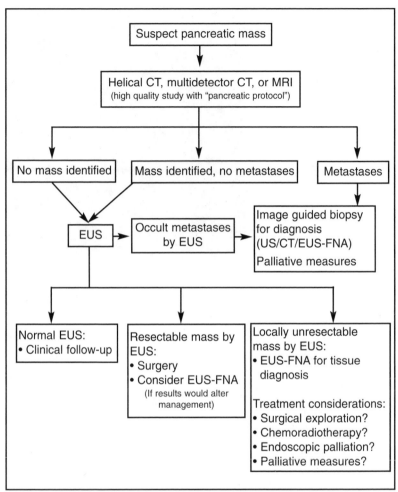

Figure 13-9. Algorithm for evaluation of suspected pancreatic mass.

If no pancreatic mass is seen on cross-sectional imaging but clinical suspicion remains, EUS is recommended, as it is currently the most sensitive modality to detect pancreatic tumors. The sensitivity of EUS to detect pancreatic tumors ranges from 94% to 100%, compared to 69% to 85% for standard CT.[33,34] Based on pooled data from four studies, EUS is also more sensitive than helical CT for the detection of pancreatic masses (97% vs 73%).[35] Where available, PET scanning may also be considered, as it may approach detection rates similar to that of EUS.[36] Endosonography is highly effective in identifying small lesions that may be missed by other imaging procedures (Figure 13-10). One study revealed higher sensitivity for EUS compared to MRI for the detection of tumors <3 cm (93% vs 67%).[37] Moreover, in patients with suspected pancreatic

Figure 13-10. EUS image demonstrates a hypoechoic mass (2.7 x 2.1 cm) in the head of the pancreas. This lesion was not identified on standard CT scan. The mass involves the common bile duct (CBD) with evidence of biliary dilation, and abuts the portal vein (PV). By EUS criteria the tumor is stage T3 N1 MX (Note: regional lymph nodes not shown in figure).

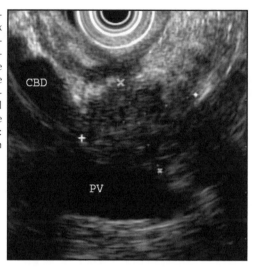

malignancy, a normal EUS is particularly useful in excluding pancreatic tumor with a high negative predictive value. In a recent investigation, none of a 76-patient cohort with suspected malignancy but normal EUS developed pancreatic cancer during a mean follow-up of nearly 2 years.[38]

When cross-sectional imaging reveals a solid pancreatic mass without evidence for metastases, EUS examination should be considered to provide more detailed anatomic information on the locoregional extent of the tumor. Certainly, the availability of expert EUS, tempered with the quality of noninvasive imaging, should be factored into the decision. Accurate imaging helps predict tumor stage (see Appendix C), and thereby guides subsequent treatment strategies. As survival rates for those diagnosed with pancreatic cancer are very poor and surgical resection offers the only potential cure, determination of resectability is the most important factor to distinguish. Accuracy in this regard will select appropriate candidates for surgical exploration while preventing unnecessary procedures in patients with locally unresectable tumors. T and N stage accuracy of EUS for pancreatic tumors ranges from 69% to 94% and 54% to 80%, respectively.[33] Although there is a wide range of staging accuracy by EUS, results are still superior to those achieved by cross-sectional imaging. Accuracy for T stage seems lower in those with larger size masses (>3 cm), likely due to peritumoral inflammation and artifact effect of increased tumor size on ultrasound attenuation.[39] EUS is more accurate than helical CT in predicting resectability (91% vs 83%) based on pooled data from four studies.[35] Using findings from multiple imaging modalities may be the most accurate means of estimating resectability. One recent study suggested that when both EUS and MRI findings concur on lesions being either resectable or unresectable, the positive and negative predictive values are 89% and 76%, respectively.[40]

Histologic diagnosis of pancreatic masses may be needed for a variety of scenarios. For individuals with locally advanced lesions, tissue confirmation may identify candidates for preoperative chemoradiotherapy. For those who appear to have resectable lesions but are poor operative candidates, a tissue diagnosis may be requested prior to committing the patient to a major operation. In the setting of obvious metastatic disease, tissue acquisition may provide the patient the satisfaction of a definite diagnosis. Occasionally, cross-sectional imaging and/or EUS demonstrate lesions that are atypical for pancreatic adenocarcinoma, and histologic confirmation is desirable to confirm malignancy, exclude other types of lesions (eg, lymphoma, neuroendocrine tumor), and guide appropriate therapy.

EUS-FNA has emerged as an important means of obtaining tissue diagnosis of pancreatic tumors, with high sensitivity for establishing malignancy (75% to 90%) and high accuracy rates (85% to 96%).[33] False negative results can occur in up to 15% to 20%, thus EUS-FNA should not be used to preclude operative resection in an otherwise appropriate surgical candidate with high suspicion for pancreatic cancer.[35] EUS-FNA of the pancreas is performed transgastrically or transduodenally, and can be used to target the primary mass, lymph nodes, liver metastases, and even small areas of ascites (suggestive of peritoneal involvement). For patients with nonmetastatic, potentially resectable tumors that require histologic confirmation, EUS-FNA is preferred to percutaneous FNA (ultrasound or CT guided), as one recent study reveals a significantly increased association of peritoneal carcinomatosis with the latter.[41]

PANCREATIC CYSTIC NEOPLASMS

About 1% of all pancreatic malignancies arise from cystic neoplasms. Malignant and premalignant cystic lesions of the pancreas include mucinous cystadenomas, cystadenocarcinomas, and intraductal papillary mucinous tumors (IPMT). Nonmalignant cystic lesions of the pancreas include pseudocysts and serous cystadenomas.[42] Unfortunately, distinguishing the specific type of cystic lesion can be difficult using standard imaging (CT or MRI). With its ability to provide high-resolution images of the pancreas and to interrogate internal cystic architecture, EUS has emerged as an important modality in the evaluation of pancreatic cysts.

In general, cysts that are sonographically well-defined, simple, and thin-walled are likely benign in nature. Those that seem more complex with thick walls, septae, mural nodules, or have solid components, should be considered malignant or premalignant. Clinical history and presentation are important considerations to help distinguish cystic neoplasms from pseudocysts (which may also appear complex). Mucinous cystadenomas typically appear macrocystic with few (if any) septations. Any localized wall-thickening or associated mass component should raise the concern for cystadenocarcinoma. Serous cystadenomas are typically microcystic, composed of numerous small compartments with thin septations. IPMTs have a wide range of appearances, which may include cystic abnormalities that represent dilated main pancreatic ducts or dilated side branches. Although there has been much interest in using EUS to characterize pancreatic cysts, recent data suggests poor interobserver agreement among experienced endosonographers in discriminating neoplastic versus non-neoplastic cystic lesions based on EUS features.[43] Nevertheless, EUS remains an unique means of acquiring detailed images of the pancreas and internal cyst structure, and EUS findings should be used in conjunction with other imaging and clinical data to help differentiate cystic abnormalities and thereby guide appropriate management.

EUS-FNA has been used to provide further diagnostic information in the evaluation of cystic lesions. As false negative findings do occur, this technique should only be used when results would potentially alter the management plan. A variety of biochemical and histologic analyses can be performed on aspirated contents.[42] The presence of mucin in aspirated cyst fluid is very suggestive of a mucinous cystic neoplasm. Glycogen containing cells in FNA specimens are diagnostic of serous cystadenomas. Histiocytes and elevated amylase concentrations are associated with pseudocysts. Any solid component of cysts should be considered for EUS-FNA to assess for malignancy. There has been recent interest in analyzing cyst fluid for tumor markers. Higher concentrations of CEA and CA 72-4 have been found in mucinous neoplasms compared to serous cystadenomas.[44] However, at this time tumor marker analysis should be interpreted with caution and within the overall clinical context, as one recent investigation revealed poor sensitivity (28%) and specificity (25%) for the use of CEA fluid analysis in classifying cystic lesions.[45]

PANCREATIC NEUROENDOCRINE TUMORS

EUS can play an important role in the evaluation of pancreatic neuroendocrine tumors. Endosonography should be considered for tumor localization when an endocrinologic diagnosis of a hypersecreting tumor has been established, but standard imaging (CT/MRI) has failed to reveal the tumor location (occurs in 60% to 80% of patients). EUS has high sensitivity and accuracy (80% to 90%) in detecting pancreatic neuroendocrine neoplasms.[46,47] However, it is not reliable for extrapancreatic disease. Performance characteristics of somatostatin receptor scintigraphy may approach that of EUS for locating tumors in the pancreas, but are superior for detecting distant disease.[48] For the localization of insulinomas (which may have decreased, high-affinity somatostatin receptors), EUS is the imaging modality of choice, with a sensitivity approaching 90%.[48] When needed, EUS-FNA can be used to establish a preoperative histologic diagnosis with high accuracy (90%).[49]

CHOLANGIOCARCINOMA

There are limited data on the utility of EUS for biliary tract cancers. Nevertheless, endosonography is used at many centers to provide additional diagnostic information for biliary neoplasms, and particularly for those tumors that are small and not well characterized by other imaging techniques. On EUS, cholangiocarcinoma typically appears as a hypoechoic lesion or thickening that arises from or surrounds the bile duct wall, with disruption of the normal three-layer biliary wall pattern. Sonographic images are obtained using either echoendoscopes or ultrasound miniprobes placed into the bile duct during ERCP (intraductal ultrasonography). For detecting extrahepatic cholangiocarcinomas, EUS appears to be as sensitive as ERCP (95%), and more sensitive than CT (79%) or angiography (42%).[50] The local staging accuracy of EUS for cholangiocarcinomas is about 86%.[51] Perhaps of greater importance, one study found higher accuracy of determining portal venous invasion by EUS (100%), compared to CT (84%) or angiography (89%).[50]

Establishing a preoperative diagnosis of a biliary tract malignancy can be difficult. Conclusive results from cytology brushings obtained at ERCP have been disappointing and are not consistent. Although EUS is highly sensitive at identifying bile duct abnormalities, it is not useful at discriminating benign from malignant processes. EUS-FNA has recently emerged as a useful tool in confirming biliary malignancy. An accuracy, sensitivity, and specificity of 91%, 89%, and 100% has been reported for EUS-FNA in evaluating patients with suspected hilar cholangiocarcinoma, but negative brush cytology.[52]

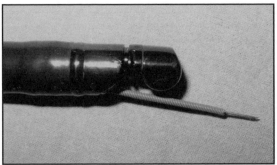

Figure 13-11. Electronic curvilinear array echoendoscope (GFUC-30P, Olympus America Corp., Melville, NY) with FNA device (Echotip ultrasound needle, Wilson-Cook Medical, Winston-Salem, NC) exiting the instrument channel. *For a full-color version, see page CA-VI of the Color Atlas.*

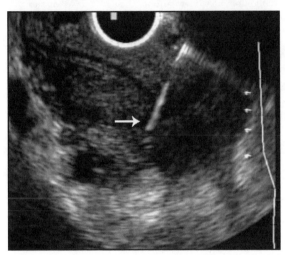

Figure 13-12. Sonographic image demonstrates EUS-FNA of a pancreatic mass. The ultrasound needle is the hyperechoic linear structure (white arrow) within the hypoechoic mass.

EUS-GUIDED FINE NEEDLE ASPIRATION AND FINE NEEDLE INJECTION

EUS-FNA is performed using hollow needle devices placed through the instrument channel of linear array echoendoscopes (Figure 13-11). The orientation of the imaging plane permits the real-time sonographic visualization of the needle as it is being advanced (Figure 13-12). Frequently used needles range from 19- to 22-gauge, and may be advanced to a depth of 10 cm. Large bore needles, which allow the acquisition of tissue core specimens, should become widely available in the near future.

Specifics regarding EUS-FNA by tumor site have been discussed on page 222. In general, EUS-FNA should only be employed when the result would potentially alter the management plan. As false negative results do occur, cytology results should be interpreted in the overall clinical context, and should not prevent definitive therapy. For instance, negative EUS-FNA results would not likely alter the plan to proceed with surgery in a middle-aged, low surgical risk patient presenting with painless jaundice, weight loss, biliary obstruction, and a visible pancreatic lesion that appears resectable on EUS and cross-sectional imaging. On the other hand, FNA may be useful in an elderly, high surgical risk patient, as cytology results may influence the treatment plan.

When EUS-FNA is performed, the lesion that would have the greatest impact on subsequent management (lesion that confirms the most advanced stage) should be targeted first. In descending order of importance, these would include: suspicious metastasis (ascites/pleural fluid, peritoneal nodule, or liver mass), distant lymph node, peritumoral lymph node, and primary mass. Multiple FNA passes may be required to obtain an adequate specimen, with pancreatic tumors generally requiring the greatest number (3 to 5).[53] Where available, on-site cytologic interpretation should be performed, as recent data suggest improved diagnostic yield and decreased need for repeat procedures using intraprocedural evaluation as compared to postprocedure cytology analysis.[54]

EUS-FNA is generally a safe procedure with complications similar to those of diagnostic EUS. Additional complications that may be unique to EUS-FNA due to the advancement of needles extraluminally include infections, hemorrhage, and pancreatitis. Based on a large multicenter study, infectious and hemorrhagic complications seem particularly associated with EUS-FNA for cystic lesions (14%) as compared to solid masses (0.5%).[55] Antibiotic prophylaxis is recommended for procedures involving cystic or perirectal lesions.[53] Acute pancreatitis may complicate EUS-FNA of pancreatic masses in up to 2%, and appears to be associated with FNA performance after a recent history of pancreatitis (within 2 months).[56] Malignant seeding is a concern, but EUS-FNA appears to be safer for this potential risk as compared to percutaneous, image-guided biopsy techniques.[41]

The same needle devices that are used for EUS-FNA can be used to perform EUS-guided fine needle injection (EUS-FNI), and inject pharmaceuticals into specific locations under "real-time" image guidance. For the management of pain due to advanced intra-abdominal malignancies, EUS-FNI techniques have been used to perform celiac plexus neurolysis using absolute alcohol, with significant reduction of pain scores for at least 12 weeks.[57] There has also been recent interest in using EUS-FNI to deliver anticancer drugs or direct other anticancer therapies (eg, radiofrequency ablation, photodynamic therapy) with precision targeting into tumors.[58,59] Increasing applications will likely be seen in the coming years.

REFERENCES

1. Flamen P, Lerut A, Van Cutsem E, et al. Utility of positron emission tomography for the staging of patients with potentially operable esophageal carcinoma. *J Clin Oncol.* 2000;18:3202-3210.

2. Catalano MF, Sivak MV, Rice T, et al. Endosonographic features predictive of lymph node metastasis. *Gastrointest Endosc.* 1994;40:442-446.

3. Bhutani MS, Hawes RH, Hoffman BJ. A comparison of the accuracy of echo features during endoscopic ultrasound (EUS) and EUS-guided fine needle aspiration for diagnosis of malignant lymph node invasion. *Gastrointest Endosc.* 1997;45:474-479.

4. Kelly S, Harris K, Berry E, et al. A systematic review of the staging performance of endoscopic ultrasound in gastro-esophageal carcinoma. *Gut.* 2001;49:534-539.

5. Koch J, Halvorsen RA. Staging of esophageal cancer: computed tomography, magnetic resonance imaging, and endoscopic ultrasound. *Semin Roentgenol.* 1994;29:364-372.

6. Rosch T. Endosonographic staging of esophageal cancer: a review of literature results. *Gastrointest Endosc Clin N Am.* 1995;5:537-547.

7. Eloubeidi MA, Wallace MB, Reed CE, et al. The utility of EUS and EUS-guided fine needle aspiration in detecting celiac lymph node metastasis in patients with esophageal cancer: a single center experience. *Gastrointest Endosc.* 2001;54:714-719.

8. Vazquez-Sequerios E, Norton ID, Clain JE, et al. Impact of EUS-guided fine needle aspiration on lymph node staging in patients with esophageal carcinoma. *Gastrointest Endosc.* 2001;53:751-757.

9. Pfau PR, Ginsberg GG, Lew RJ, et al. Esophageal dilation for endosonographic evaluation of malignant esophageal strictures is safe and effective. *Am J Gastroenterol.* 2000; 95:2813-2815.

10. Wallace MB, Hawes RH, Sahai AV, et al. Dilation of malignant esophageal stenosis to allow EUS guided fine needle aspiration: Safety and effect on patient management. *Gastrointest Endosc.* 2000:51:309-313.

11. Zuccaro G, Rice TW, Goldblum J, et al. Endoscopic ultrasound cannot determine suitability for esophagectomy after aggressive chemoradiotherapy for esophageal cancer. *Am J Gastroenterol.* 1999;94:906-912.

12. Laterza E, de Manzoni G, Guglielmi A, et al. Endoscopic ultrasonography in the staging of esophageal carcinoma after preoperative radiotherapy and chemotherapy. *Ann Thorac Surg.* 1999;67:1466-1469.

13. Chak A, Canto MI, Cooper GS, et al. Endosonographic assessment of multimodality therapy predicts survival of esophageal cancer patients. *Cancer.* 2000;88:1788-1795.

14. Fockens P, Manshanden CG, van Lanschott JJ, et al. Prospective study on the value of endosonographic follow-up after surgery for esophageal carcinoma. *Gastrointest Endosc.* 1997;46:487-491.

15. Rosch T. Endosonographic staging of gastric cancer: A review of literature results. *Gastrointest Endosc Clin N Am.* 1995;5:549-557.

16. Rosch T, Lorenz R, Zenker K, et al., Local staging and assessment of resectability in carcinoma of the esophagus, stomach, and duodenum by endoscopic ultrasound. *Gastrointest Endosc.* 1992;38:460-467.

17. Lightdale CJ, Botet JF, Kelson DP, et al. Diagnosis of recurrent upper gastrointestinal cancer at the surgical anastomosis by endoscopic ultrasound. *Gastrointest Endosc.* 1989; 35:407-412.

18. Mendis RE, Gerdes H, Lightdale CJ, et al. Large gastric folds: A diagnostic approach using endoscopic ultrasonography. *Gastrointest Endosc.* 1994;40:437-441.

19. Palazzo L, Roseau G, Ruskone-Fourmestraux A, et al. Endoscopic ultrasonography in the local staging of primary gastric lymphoma. *Endoscopy.* 1993;25:502-508.

20. Wiersema MJ, Gatzimos K, Nisi R, et al. Staging of non-Hodgkin's gastric lymphoma with endosonography-guided fine-needle aspiration biopsy and flow cytometry. *Gastrointest Endosc.* 1996;44:734-736.

21. Caletti G, Fusaroli P, Togliani T. EUS in MALT lymphoma. *Gastrointest Endosc.* 2002; 56:S21-S26.

22. Savides T, Master SS. EUS in rectal cancer. *Gastrointest Endosc.* 2002;56:S12-S18.

23. Schwartz DA, Harewood GC, Wiersema MJ. EUS for rectal disease. *Gastrointest Endosc.* 2002;56:100-109.

24. Spinelli P, Schiavo M, Meroni E, et al. Results of EUS in detecting perirectal lymph node metastases of rectal cancer: the pathologist makes the difference. *Gastrointest Endosc.* 1999;49:754-758.

25. Harewood GC, Wiersema MJ, Nelson H, et al. A prospective, blinded assessment of the impact of preoperative staging on the management of rectal cancer. *Gastroenterol.* 2002; 123:24-32.

26. Rau B, Hunerbein M, Barth C, et al. Accuracy of endorectal ultrasound after preoperative radiochemotherapy in locally advanced rectal cancer. *Surg Endosc.* 1991;78:785-788.

27. Rotondano G, Esposito P, Pellecchia L, et al. Early detection of locally recurrent rectal cancer by endosonography. *Br J Radiol.* 1997;70:567-571.

28. Hunerbein M, Totkas S, Moesta KT, et al. The role of transrectal ultrasound-guided biopsy in the postoperative follow-up of patients with rectal cancer. *Surgery.* 2001;129: 164-169.

29. Davila RE, Faigel DO. GI stromal tumors. *Gastrointest Endosc.* 2003;58:80-88.

30. Chak A, Canto MI, Rosch T, et al. Endosonographic differentiation of benign and malignant stromal cell tumors. *Gastrointest Endosc.* 1997;45:468-473.

31. Gu M, Ghafari S, Nguyen PT, et al. Cytologic diagnosis of gastrointestinal stromal tumors of the stomach by endoscopic ultrasound-guided fine-needle aspiration biopsy: cytomorphologic and immunohistochemical study of 12 cases. *Diagn Cytopathol.* 2001; 25:343-350.

32. Ando N, Goto H, Niwa Y, et al. The diagnosis of GI stromal tumors with EUS-guided fine needle aspiration and immunohistochemical analysis. *Gastrointest Endosc.* 2002; 55: 37-43.

33. Ahmad NA, Shah JN, Kochman ML. Endoscopic ultrasonography and endoscopic retrograde cholangiopancreatography imaging for pancreaticobiliary pathology: The gastroenterologist's perspective. *Radiol Clin N Am.* 2002;40:1377-1395.

34. Kochman ML. EUS in pancreatic cancer. *Gastrointest Endosc.* 2002;56:S6-S12.

35. Hunt GC, Faigel DO. Assessment of EUS for diagnosing, staging, and determining resectability of pancreatic cancer: a review. *Gastrointest Endosc.* 2002;55:232-237.

36. Mertz HR, Sechopolous P. Delbeke D, et al. EUS, PET, and CT scanning for evaluation of pancreatic adenocarcinoma. *Gastrointest Endosc.* 2000;52:367-371.

37. Muller MF, Meyenberger C, Bertschinger P, et al. Pancreatic tumors: Evaluation with endoscopic US, CT, and MR imaging. *Radiology.* 1994;190:745-751.

38. Catanzaro A, Richardson S, Veloso H, et al. Long-term follow-up of patients with clinically indeterminate suspicion of pancreatic cancer and normal EUS. *Gastrointest Endosc.* 2003;58:836-840.

39. Ahmad NA, Lewis JD, Ginsberg GG, et al. EUS in preoperative staging of pancreatic cancer. *Gastrointest Endosc.* 2000;52:578-582.

40. Ahmad NA, Lewis JD, Siegelman ES, et al. Role of endoscopic ultrasound and magnetic resonance imaging in the preoperative staging of pancreatic adenocarcinoma. *Am J Gastroenterol.* 2000;95:1926-1931.

41. Micames C, Jowell PS, White R, et al. Lower frequency of peritoneal carcinomatosis in patients with pancreatic cancer diagnosed by EUS-guided FNA vs. percutaneous FNA. *Gastrointest Endosc.* 2003;58:690-695.

42. Van Dam J. EUS in cystic lesions of the pancreas. *Gastrointest Endosc* 2002;56:S91-S93.

43. Ahmad NA, Kochman ML, Brensinger C, et al. Interobserver agreement among endosonographers for the diagnosis of neoplastic versus non-neoplastic pancreatic cystic lesions. *Gastrointest Endosc.* 2003;58:59-64.

44. Hammel P, Voitot H, Vilgrain V, et al. Diagnostic value of CA72-4 and carcinoembryonic antigen determination in the fluid of pancreatic cystic lesions. *Eur J Gastroenterol Hepatol.* 1998;10:345-348.

45. Sedlack R, Affi A, Vazquez-Sequeiros E, et al. Utility of EUS in the evaluation of cystic pancreatic lesions. *Gastrointest Endosc.* 2002;56:543-547.

46. Anderson MA, Carpenter S, Thompson NW, et al. Endoscopic ultrasound is highly accurate and directs management in patients with neuroendocrine tumors of the pancreas. *Am J Gastroenterol.* 2000;95:2271-2277.

47. Rosch T, Lightdale CJ, Botet JF, et al. Localization of pancreatic endocrine tumors by endoscopic ultrasonography. *N Engl J Med.* 1992;326:1770-1772.

48. Zimmer T, Stolzel U, Bader M, et al. Endoscopic ultrasonography and somatostatin receptor scintigraphy in the preoperative localization of insulinomas and gastrinomas. *Gut.* 1996;39:562-568.

49. Gines A, Vazquez-Sequeiros E, Soria MT, et al. Usefulness of EUS-guided fine needle aspiration (EUS-FNA) in the diagnosis of functioning neuroendocrine tumors. *Gastrointest Endosc.* 2002;56:291-296.

50. Sugiyama M, Hagi H, Atomi Y, et al. Diagnosis of portal venous invasion by pancreatobiliary carcinoma: value of endoscopic ultrasonography. *Abdom Imaging.* 1997; 22:434-438.

51. Tio TL, Reeders JW, Sie LH, et al. Endosonography in the clinical staging of Klatskin tumor. *Endoscopy.* 1993;25:81-85.

52. Fritscher-Ravens A, Broering DC, Knoefel WT, et al. EUS-guided fine-needle aspiration of suspected hilar cholangiocarcinoma in potentially operable patients with negative brush cytology. *Am J Gastroenterol.* 2004;99:45-51.

53. Chang KJ. Maximizing the yield of EUS-guided fine-needle aspiration. *Gastrointest Endosc.* 2002;56:S28-S34.

54. Klapman JB, Logrono R, Dye CE, et al. Clinical impact of on-site cytopathology interpretation on endoscopic ultrasound-guided fine needle aspiration. *Am J Gastroenterol.* 2003;98:1289-1294.

55. Wiersema MJ, Vilmann P, Giovannini M, et al. Endosonography-guided fine-needle aspiration biopsy: diagnostic accuracy and complication assessment. *Gastroenterology.* 1997;112:1087-1095.

56. Gress F, Michael H, Gelrud D, et al. EUS-guided fine-needle aspiration of the pancreas: evaluation of pancreatitis as a complication. *Gastrointest Endosc.* 2002;56:864-867.

57. Wiersema MJ, Wiersema LM. Endosonography-guided celiac plexus neurolysis. *Gastrointest Endosc.* 1996;44:656-662.

58. Chan HH, Nishioka NS, Mino M, et al. EUS-guided photodynamic therapy of the pancreas: a pilot study. *Gastrointest Endosc.* 2004;59:95-99.

59. Chang KJ, Nguyen PT, Thompson JA, et al. Phase I clinical trial of allogeneic mixed lymphocyte culture (cytoimplant) delivered by endoscopic ultrasound-guided fine-needle injection in patients with advanced pancreatic cancer. *Cancer.* 2000;88:1325-1335.

Color Atlas

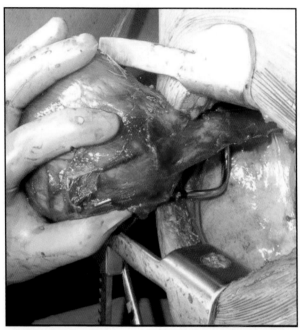

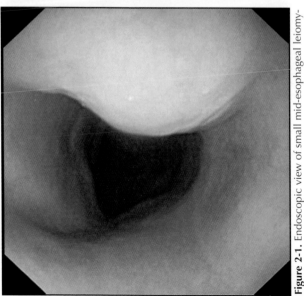

Figure 2-1. Endoscopic view of small mid-esophageal leiomyoma. (Photo courtesy of Michael Kochman, MD, University of Pennsylvania Medical Center.) *Also shown on page 12.*

Figure 2-2C. Intraoperative photo through right thoracotomy showing massive leiomyoma and resected esophagus. This patient required a complete esophagectomy via right thoracotomy, upper midline abdominal incision and left neck incision. Continuity was restored by creation of a gastric tube with cervical anastomosis. (Photo from personal collection.) *Also shown on page 13.*

Figure 2-3A. Typical small esophageal leiomyoma appropriate for extramucosal enucleation. (Reprinted from *Atlas of Surgery,* 2e, Cameron JL, pp 73-75, Copyright 1994 with permission from Elsevier.) *Also shown on page 14.*

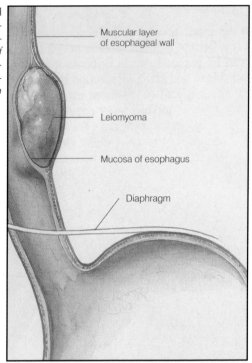

Muscular layer of esophageal wall

Leiomyoma

Mucosa of esophagus

Diaphragm

Figure 2-3B. A longitudinal myotomy is performed exposing the leiomyoma. (Reprinted from *Atlas of Surgery,* 2e, Cameron JL, pp 73-75, Copyright 1994 with permission from Elsevier.) *Also shown on page 14.*

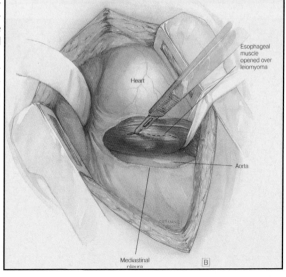

Esophageal muscle opened over leiomyoma

Heart

Aorta

Mediastinal pleura

B

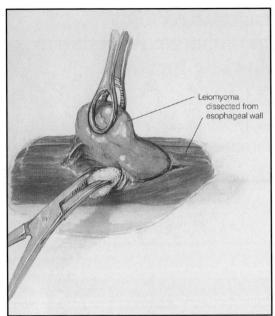

Figure 2-3C. The leiomyoma is gently dissected away from the esophageal mucosa. (Reprinted from *Atlas of Surgery*, 2e, Cameron JL, pp 73-75, Copyright 1994 with permission from Elsevier.) *Also shown on page 14.*

Leiomyoma dissected from esophageal wall

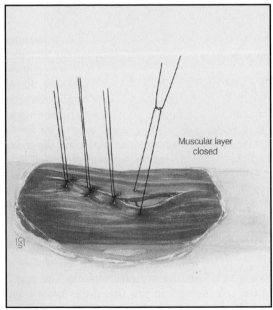

Figure 2-3D. The myotomy is closed to prevent pseudodiverticulum formation. (Reprinted from *Atlas of Surgery*, 2e, Cameron JL, pp 73-75, Copyright 1994 with permission from Elsevier.) *Also shown on page 14.*

Muscular layer closed

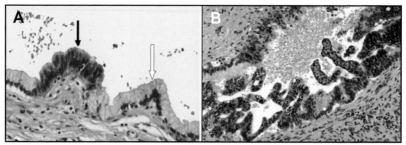

Figure 5-2. Histology of pancreatic intraepithelial neoplasia (PanIN). (A) PanIN 1 (open arrow) is characterized by elongation of epithelial cells with abundant supranuclear mucin and PanIN 2 (solid arrow) is defined by nuclear abnormalities including enlargement and crowding, hyperchromatism, and stratification. (B) In PanIN 3, there are lush papillary projections, loss of nuclear polarity, and nuclear atypia with mitoses. (Photomicrographs courtesy of Dr. Teresa Brentnall.) *Also shown on page 76.*

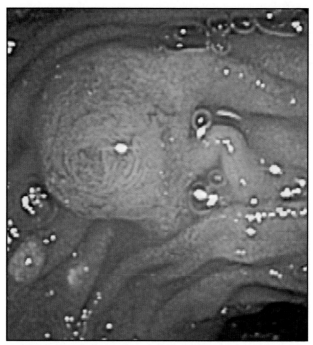

Figure 8-4A. Ampulla of Vater. Normal ampulla as seen using a side-viewing endoscope in the second portion of duodenum. A transverse duodenal fold is seen draping over the upper margin of the papillary mound. *Also shown on page 131.*

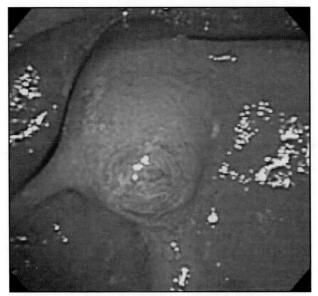

Figure 8-4B. Bulging ampulla. This was found to harbor an adeno-carcinoma arising in the very distal portion of the pancreatic duct. *Also shown on page 131.*

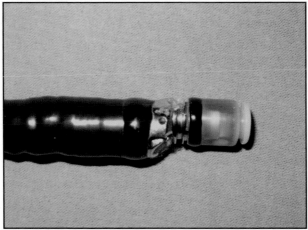

Figure 13-1. Mechanical radial array echoendoscope (GFUM-130, Olympus America Corp, Melville, NY). *Also shown on page 224.*

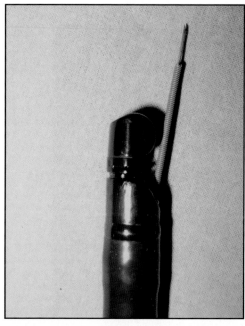

Figure 13-11. Electronic curvilinear array echoendoscope (GFUC-30P, Olympus America Corp., Melville, NY) with FNA device (Echotip ultrasound needle, Wilson-Cook Medical, Winston-Salem, NC) exiting the instrument channel. *Also shown on page 237.*

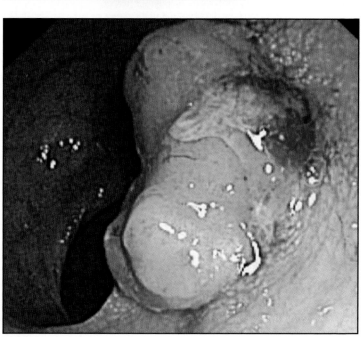

Figure 13-5. Endoscopic image demonstrates a polypoid mass in the distal rectum. Histology from forceps biopsies revealed adenoma with foci of adenocarcinoma. *Also shown on page 230.*

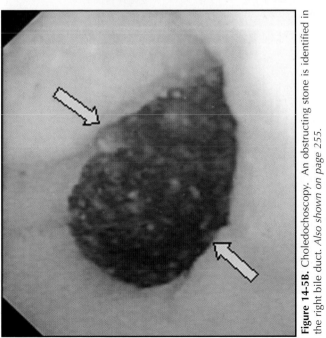

Figure 14-5C. A basket was advanced through the instrument channel and used to remove the stone. *Also shown on page 255.*

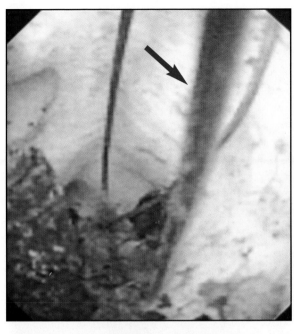

Figure 14-5B. Choledochoscopy. An obstructing stone is identified in the right bile duct. *Also shown on page 255.*

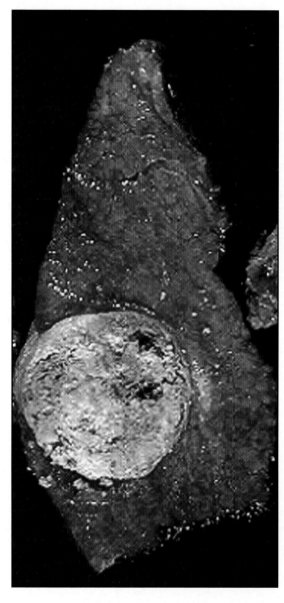

Figure 14-6D. Following resection 6 weeks later, no viable tumor was present, and hepatic vessels containing microspheres were identified in the background of necrosis. *Also shown on page 258.*

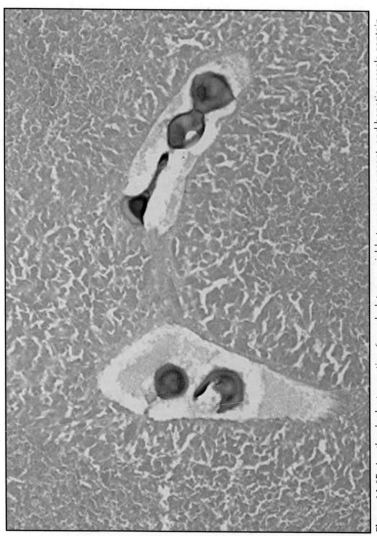

Figure 14-6E. Another look at resection 6 weeks later, no viable tumor was present, and hepatic vessels containing microspheres were identified in the background of necrosis. *Also shown on page 258.*

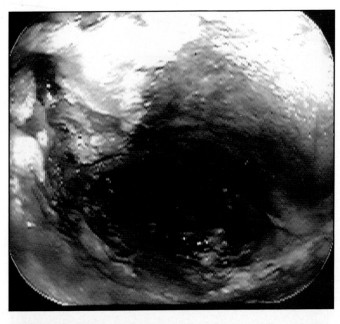

Figure 15-2B Endoscopic visualization of same patient 48 hours after application of photodynamic therapy showing extensive tissue necrosis and tumor debris. *Also shown on page 289.*

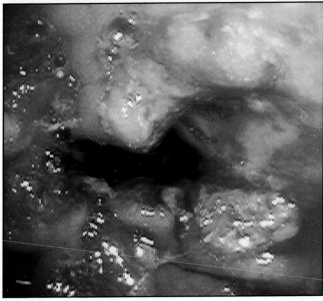

Figure 15-2A. Endoscopic appearance of an obstructing esophageal cancer. *Also shown on page 289.*

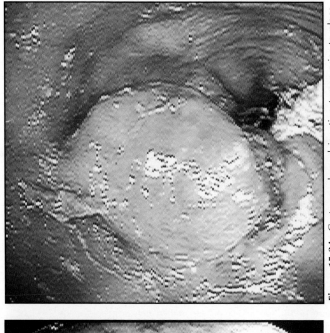

Figure 15-3A. Gastroesophageal junction tumor prior to placement of esophageal stent. *Also shown on page 292.*

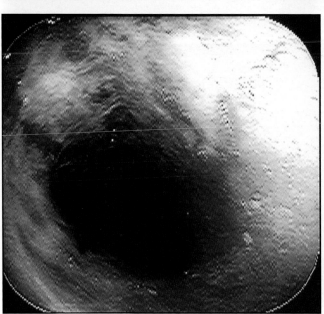

Figure 15-2C. Post-treatment image demonstrating no endoscopic evidence of tumor with restoration of the esophageal lumen. *Also shown on page 290.*

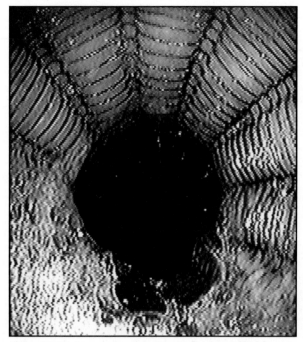

Figure 15-3B. Appearance of stent immediately postdeployment, which shows a recreated lumen. *Also shown on page 292.*

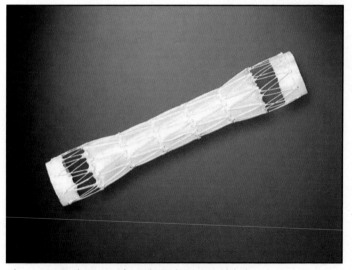

Figure 15-5B. The covered esophageal Z-stent. *Also shown on page 294.*

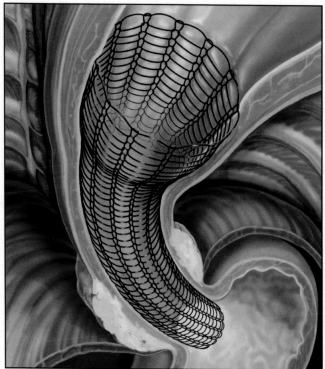

Figure 15-6. Illustration of an esophageal Flamingo stent bridging a distal esophageal tumor. *Also shown on page 294.*

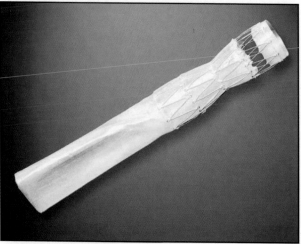

Figure 15-7. Covered Dua stent with distal sleeve to prevent acid reflux into esophagus post-stent deployment. *Also shown on page 295.*

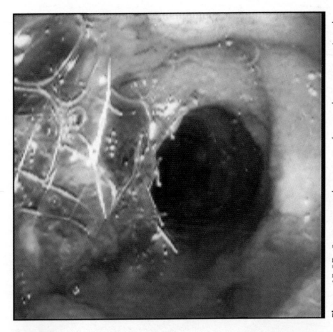

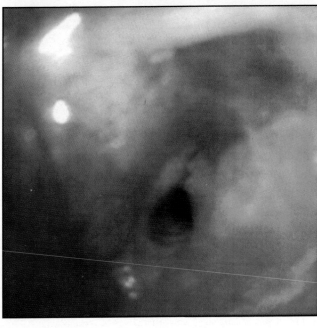

Figure 15-9A. Endoscopic visualization of narrowed duodenal lumen secondary to metastatic cancer. *Also shown on page 298.*

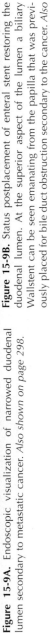

Figure 15-9B. Status postplacement of enteral stent restoring the duodenal lumen. At the superior aspect of the lumen a biliary Wallstent can be seen emanating from the papilla that was previously placed for bile duct obstruction secondary to the cancer. *Also shown on page 298.*

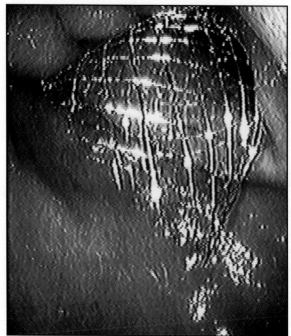

Figure 15-10. Enteral Wallstent seen extending proximally through the pylorus into the stomach. Stent was placed through pylorus into duodenum for malignant gastric outlet obstruction. *Also shown on page 298.*

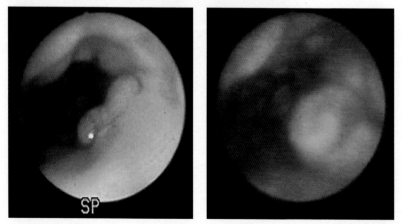

Figure 18-2. Endoscopic image of nodule with HGD and ALA-enhanced fluorescence imaging of identical nodule. (Courtesy of Norman Nishioka, MD, Boston, Mass.) *Also shown on page 372.*

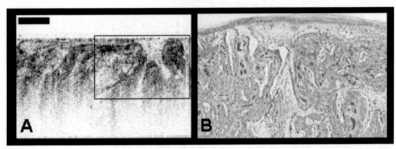

Figure 18-4. (A) OCT image of esophageal adenocarcinoma. Scale bar 500 μm. (B) Corresponding histopathology (H&E, orig. mag x 40). (Courtesy of Brett Bouma, PhD and Gary Tearney, MD, PhD, Boston, Mass.) *Also shown on page 377.*

chapter **14**

Interventional Radiology

Karen T. Brown, MD; Anne Covey, MD;
and Lynn A. Brody, MD

INTRODUCTION

The role of interventional radiology in the care of patients with malignant disease continues to grow. Procedures may involve diagnosis, treatment or palliation. The trend toward minimally invasive medicine is well served by percutaneous image guided interventions (IGI). New advances in IGI, including robotics, navigation, and virtual reality, make the field ever more exciting and offer new choices in less invasive cancer treatment.

What follows is a compendium of common procedures performed by interventional radiologists that might serve to help the gastrointestinal oncology physician better care for his or her patients.

GASTROINTESTINAL PROCEDURES

GASTROSTOMY/GASTROJEJUNOSTOMY

Patients with a functional GI tract who are unable to obtain adequate nutrition by mouth are ideal candidates for enteral feeding via gastrostomy or transgastric jejunostomy. Percutaneous gastrostomy catheters may also be used for decompression in patients with chronic bowel obstruction. Decompression gastrostomy is most commonly performed for patients with advanced ovarian cancer. Symptoms of nausea and abdominal distension can be alleviated, and in some cases patients are able to resume oral intake. Although there is no nutritional benefit, since the drainage gastrostomy empties the stomach, most patients derive a lifestyle benefit from this.

Gastrostomy and gastrojejunostomy catheters can be placed endoscopically or surgically.[1,2] Percutaneous image guided placement is safe and effective, and most useful in cases where endoscopy in unsafe, impractical, or impossible, such as with head and neck or esophageal cancers. In patients with ascites, endoscopic illumination may be quite difficult. Percutaneous gastrostomy placement may be safely performed in these patients by using gastropexy to fix the stomach to the anterior abdominal wall. This is accomplished via metallic "T-fasteners" introduced through the percutaneous access needle. Finally, percutaneous gastrostomy or gastrojejunostomy catheter placement generally requires less sedation than endoscopic catheter placement, and may be more appropriate in cases where sedation is an issue.

Percutaneous gastrostomy catheter placement is performed using fluoroscopic guidance, though ultrasound guided gastrostomy placement has been described.[3] Some interventional radiologists administer barium (either orally or via a nasogastric tube) the night prior to the procedure, so that the colon is filled with barium at the time of the procedure to minimize the risk of puncturing the colon. All relevant abdominal imaging should be reviewed prior to the procedure.

Several catheters in different sizes (10 to 28 French), and with different locking mechanisms (pigtail, mushroom, inflatable balloon) are available. Larger catheters (24 to 28 French) are preferred for decompression, especially in obstructed patients who want to eat. Catheters may be placed using either "push" or "pull-through" techniques. Both methods involve primary percutaneous puncture of the stomach after insufflation with air, commonly using an 18-gauge needle. Gastropexy may be performed based on the clinical situation or operator preference. With the "push" technique, the puncture tract is serially dilated and the gastrostomy tube is advanced into the stomach through the abdominal wall, then held in position by an inflatable balloon or locking loop on the catheter. This technique is also employed in placing transgastric jejunostomy catheters. In this case, after accessing the stomach, a directional catheter is advanced to the jejunum under fluoroscopic guidance, using water soluble contrast to opacify the bowel.

In the "pull-through" technique, the percutaneous access needle is exchanged for a directional catheter, which is advanced retrograde under fluoroscopic guidance from the stomach to the mouth. A snare is then advanced through the catheter exiting the mouth. The snare is used to pull the gastrostomy catheter to the stomach and out through the anterior abdominal wall, similar to PEG placement. This technique is increasingly popular as it allows for large catheters (up to 28 French) to be placed primarily. The complication rates are low and the long-term patency of these large catheters is high.

Complications include site infection, peritonitis, tube malfunction, and dislodgement. When gastropexy is performed, or after a tract has been established (2 to 4 weeks), catheter replacement may be performed without imaging guidance. Contraindications to gastrostomy include previous gastrectomy, gastric varices, and uncorrectable coagulopathy.

GASTROINTESTINAL STENTS

Stents may be delivered per oral into the esophagus, or per rectum into the colon to palliate patients with malignant obstruction and to treat malignant fistulae (Figure 14-1). These stents are most often self-expanding metallic stents covered with silicone or PTFE to prevent tumor ingrowth in malignant obstruction and to seal fistulae or perforations. Left sided colonic stents have been used to reestablish luminal patency and palliate bowel obstruction (as occurs in 10% to 30% cases of colorectal cancer). Colonic stenting has also been proposed as a preoperative adjunct in patients with obstruction as a bridge to definitive one-stage laparoscopic resection, avoiding the increased mortality of emergent surgery[4] and the need to create, and then close, a colostomy. Following esophageal stent placement for malignant obstruction, most patients are able to resume a near normal diet.[5] When used to seal fistulae, esophageal stents offer an immediate

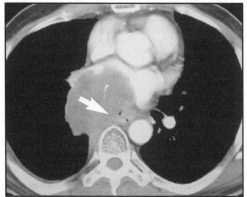

Figure 14-1A. Esophageal stent. CT shows subcarinal mass compressing the esophagus with small air bubbles outside the lumen of the esophagus (arrow).

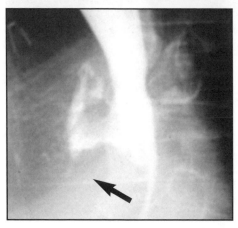

Figure 14-1B. Prestent esophagram shows narrowing of distal esophagus and ulceration into the mass (arrow).

success of 73% to 100%, with a 20% to 39% recurrence rate, most often due to new fistula formation or stent migration.[6]

TREATMENT OF BILIARY DISEASE

PERCUTANEOUS BILIARY PROCEDURES

Interventional radiologists play an important role in the diagnosis and treatment of biliary obstruction. Biliary obstruction may be due to either extrinsic compression of the bile ducts or an obstructing focus within the duct. Benign causes include stone disease and strictures. This chapter will focus on biliary obstruction in the oncology patient population.

Bile duct obstruction is commonly seen in primary biliary cancers, including cholangiocarcinoma and gallbladder cancer.[7] Primary hepatocellular carcinoma, as well as metastases from common tumors such as colorectal carcinoma, may also cause bile duct obstruction. This occurs in one of two ways—either the tumor grows into the biliary

Figure 14-1C. Following stent placement, the esophagus is patent with rapid emptying into the stomach and the ulcer is no longer seen.

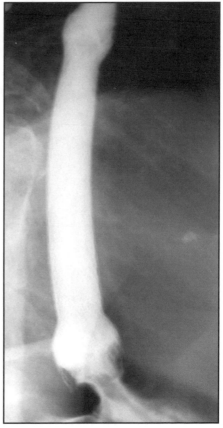

tree, and the polypoid intraductal tumor causes biliary obstruction, or mass effect from the parenchymal tumor causes extrinsic compression of the bile duct. Pancreatic and ampullary or duodenal carcinomas frequently cause low bile duct obstruction. Metastatic disease to the bile duct epithelium may occur; most often from melanoma or from solid tumors of the GI tract. Biliary obstruction may also be caused by masses causing extrinsic compression of the extrahepatic biliary tree, as in cases of periportal lymphadenopathy from metastatic disease or lymphoma.

Biliary obstruction may be classified based on the level of the occlusion, as either "high", "mid," or "low." Low obstruction typically refers to obstruction occurring at the ampulla or distal common bile duct. High obstruction is caused by lesions at or above the common hepatic duct. Mid bile duct obstruction is everything in between. Obstruction at or above the confluence of the right and left hepatic ducts may result in isolation of part or parts of the biliary tree. For example, a tumor at the hilus may cause obstruction of both the left and right hepatic ducts. The right hepatic duct is typically shorter than the left and, not uncommonly, the obstruction may extend from the confluence to isolate the right anterior and posterior ducts from each other, as well as from the left duct. With larger central tumors, isolation may progress to the subsegmental level. This has tremendous implications for developing drainage strategies. One must realize that a stent or catheter will only decompress the system in which it is placed, and other ducts with which that system connects. Isolated ducts will not be effectively drained. For example, in the case of a central mass causing isolation of the right anterior, right posterior, and left hepatic ducts, a drainage catheter or stent placed via one of those systems will drain only that system, while the other two systems will remain undrained. In these cases, multiple catheters or stents may be necessary for effective palliation. In some cases, adequate drainage cannot be achieved. The situation is further complicated by issues related to contamination and cholangitis.

We refer to isolation as: 1) *complete*—the isolated ducts are never opacified cholangiographically; 2) *effective*—the isolated ducts are opacified, but the contrast that fills them does not drain; or 3)*impending*—the opacified ducts can be drained at the current time, but there is central narrowing that is likely to progress. Particularly in cases of effective isolation, it is almost certain that the incompletely drained ducts will become contaminated, and may cause cholangitis and even sepsis. Not infrequently, multiple drainage catheters or stents are necessary to individually drain each isolated system. At times, this may not be practical or possible, and optimal drainage cannot be achieved.

The level of obstruction commonly dictates management directed toward palliation. Management is also influenced by expected survival and lifestyle issues. Since proper identification of the level of obstruction is so important, it is essential to have good cross-sectional imaging prior to any intervention. Similarly, since the risks involved in percutaneous or endoscopic access to the biliary tree are not trivial, noninvasive imaging tools should be used for diagnostic purposes. Direct cholangiography should be used for diagnostic purposes only under unusual circumstances.

Since biliary drainage procedures are, for the most part, palliative in nature, the goal(s) of intervention should be well delineated at the start. Commonly accepted indications for drainage include hyperbilirubinemia precluding chemotherapy, pruritis, and cholangitis. Preoperative drainage may be requested at the discretion of the hepatobiliary surgeon. Diminished appetite and malaise may also improve after biliary drainage, and these symptoms should be taken into consideration when deciding whether or not to proceed with drainage. We do not consider asymptomatic ductal dilatation, hyperbilirubinemia alone, or even jaundice a suitable reason to intervene in most cases. One must remember that an asymptomatic patient cannot be made to feel better, but they can be made to feel worse. Particularly as the level of obstruction gets higher, the likelihood of complete drainage decreases, the number of drainage catheters increases, and the complexity of management grows.

Mid- and low bile duct obstruction are generally easier to palliate than disease at or above the confluence, as a single stent or drain can successfully decompress the entire biliary tree. Obstruction at this level is accessible to the gastroenterologist, and should first be approached endoscopically, unless surgically altered anatomy, gastric outlet obstruction, or a duodenal mass impair access to the ampulla. Endoscopic treatment obviates the need for percutaneous puncture or exteriorized catheters. Tools for relieving low bile duct obstruction available to the endoscopist include plastic and metallic stents, as well as nasobiliary drainage catheters for very short-term use. Endoscopically placed metallic stents are self-expanding with typical diameters of 8 to 12 mm. Covered and bare stents are available. Patency of covered stents may be longer, but care must be taken not to occlude the cystic duct (or any side duct), as cholecystitis has been reported in this situation.[8] Most metallic stents are not removable, and their presence may complicate or even preclude surgery. Therefore, prior to placement, care should be taken to assure that the patient has a diagnosis of malignancy and is not a surgical candidate. The average patency of metallic stents is 7 months. Metallic stents are particularly well-suited to patients whose survival is not likely to exceed the patency of the stent. In patients who do not possess the aforementioned characteristics, plastic stents may sometimes be placed. Plastic stents are typically smaller in diameter than metallic stents, and average patency is considerably shorter, on the order of 3 months. These stents are removable, and can be changed either as needed, or at regularly scheduled intervals.

Patients with high bile duct obstruction or those with low or midobstruction who cannot be accessed or successfully treated endoscopically, should be treated percutaneously. Percutaneous biliary drainage is done primarily under fluoroscopic guidance. Relevant cross-sectional imaging is reviewed to guide selection of the access site/duct. The imaging is reviewed to assess for patency of the portal vein(s), atrophy, tumor volume, ascites, and previously placed stents or catheters. The indication for drainage is carefully considered. It is important to discuss with the referring clinician, as well as the patient, what the likelihood is that the goal of drainage will be met. This is typically dependent upon the amount of functional liver that can be drained, the level of obstruction and the indication for drainage. For example, drainage of only a small amount of functional liver, occasionally just a few ducts, is all that is necessary to ameliorate pruritis, whereas achieving a normal bilirubin typically requires drainage of at least 30% of the liver. In patients with compromised hepatic function, and high bile duct obstruction with isolation, this may not be possible.

Access may be into the right or left liver. The right ducts are typically accessed via a lower intercostal approach, generally between the mid and anterior axillary line. The left ducts are accessed from the epigastric region, though rarely a left intercostal approach may be employed depending on the individual anatomy. At the discretion of the operator, ultrasound may be used to guide the puncture of a duct. Often it is easier to see the left ducts sonographically. A 21- or 22-gauge needle is used for initial access, and a limited cholangiogram is then performed. The needle is converted to a larger introducer, through which standard sized angiographic catheters and steerable guidewires can be placed. The catheters and guidewires are used to negotiate across the occlusion and gain access to the small bowel. The angiographic catheter can then be exchanged for a biliary drainage catheter. These catheters range in size from 8 to 12 French, and have multiple sideholes beginning in the distal loop of the catheter and extending proximally to a point above the level of obstruction. The catheters are available in various lengths and with various numbers of sideholes for applicability to a wide range of anatomy and level of obstruction. These types of catheters are referred to as internal/external catheters, meaning that the bile can drain either internally (into the small bowel) or externally (into a drainage bag). The catheters can function like internal stents if they are closed to external drainage. Some patients cannot tolerate closing their catheters to external drainage, and there may then be management issues related to losing large volumes of fluid and electrolytes.

At times, it is not possible to cross the obstruction when the patient is initially drained. In these cases, and in other select circumstances, an "external" drainage catheter is placed. These catheters must remain open to external drainage (Figures 14-2A and B). Repeated attempts to convert an external catheter to an internal-external catheter are warranted, and these are often successful after decompression of the bile ducts above the level of obstruction (Figure 14-2C).

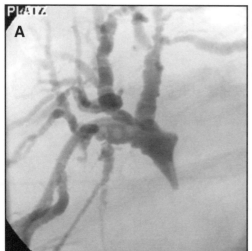

Figure 14-2. Biliary drainage catheters. (A, B) Cholangiogram through an external drainage catheter placed at the hepatic hilus in a patient with bile duct occlusion.

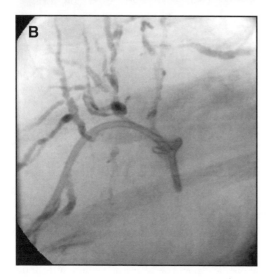

   Irrespective of the catheter type, catheter care is the same. We recommend flushing the catheters twice daily with 10 cc of saline. The catheters are flushed internally but are not aspirated. This helps clear debris from the side holes of the catheter. If the catheter is attached to an external drainage system, the external tubing and drainage bags are changed weekly. The drainage catheters themselves require routine exchange every 10 to 12 weeks. The catheters are also changed as needed if proper function ceases. This is often manifest by leakage of bile around the catheter, difficulty flushing the catheter, and symptoms of cholangitis. Prior to the initial drainage, and for every future procedure, prophylactic antibiotics are recommended.

Figure 14-2C. Internal/external drainage catheter in a different patient with ampullary carcinoma. As opposed to the external catheters which provide external drainage only, internal/external catheters allow for preservation of bilioenteric circulation and provide added stability based on the length of the catheter within the duct.

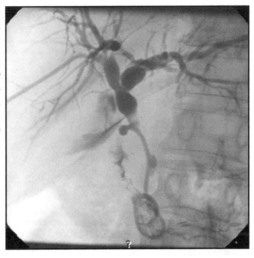

Complications related to percutaneous drainage include bleeding and sepsis. Most sepsis occurs in patients presenting with cholangitis, in the setting of bile contaminated from previous procedures. Most early hemobilia is related to venous bleeding, and will frequent resolve with time, or exchanging the catheter for one of slightly larger diameter. Delayed hemobilia, or that resulting in significant blood loss, is more likely related to arterial injury, and will necessitate arterial embolization in most cases.

Most patients dislike exteriorized catheters, for both physical and psychological reasons. When possible, every attempt is made to convert the catheters to internal stents. The same criteria for placement of endoscopic stents apply here: the patient should have a diagnosis of cancer (or recurrent cancer in the appropriate circumstance) in whom surgical resection for cure is not possible. Additionally, either the goal of drainage should have been met, or there are no possible additional procedures that may be necessary (eg, drainage of other parts of the biliary tree). Clearly, the patient must also have a patent and functional small bowel. Occasionally, plastic stents will have been placed endoscopically, but could not be exchanged, or failed due to tumor overgrowth. These stents must also be addressed, as their presence precludes placement of metallic stents (the plastic stent would be trapped). These stents may be pushed into the small bowel and eliminated in the feces (Figure 14-3), or may be removed percutaneously using a snare. If the stent cannot be removed percutaneously, endoscopic removal is necessary. Most percutaneous stents currently in use are self-expanding metallic stents. Plastic stents may be placed but are rarely indicated.

As noted previously, self-expanding metallic stents are recommended for most patients with malignant biliary obstruction who are not surgical candidates. Placement of metallic stents improves quality of life, owing to the absence of external tubes and their associated maintenance and risks, which include skin infection, bile leakage, and catheter obstruction or dislodgment. Even patients with longer life expectancies should be considered for metal stent placement, as several months of catheter-free existence is often preferable, even though there exists the possibility of having to undergo repeat drainage if the stent fails.

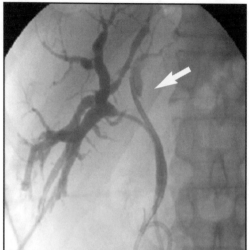

Figure 14-3A. Removal of endoscopic plastic stent. Right sided percutaneous biliary drainage was performed to maximize biliary drainage in a patient with hilar cholangiocarcinoma and an indwelling left sided endoscopic stent (arrow) in anticipation of stent placement.

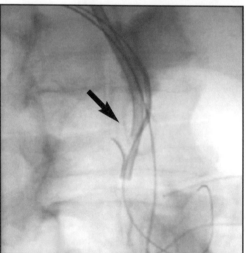

Figure 14-3B. Removal of endoscopic plastic stent. The distal flange of the stent was catheterized with a balloon catheter (arrow).

Metallic stents are deployed through the same tract established for biliary drainage using small (6 to 9 French) delivery systems. Most stents are self-expanding, though balloon expandable stents are used on rare occasions. Self-expanding stents have intrinsic radial force and, once released from the delivery device, eventually expand to their stated diameter. Most percutaneously placed stents are 8 to 10 mm in diameter, but stents from 4 to 12 mm may be placed. With a larger lumen and intrinsic radial force, these stents have a longer primary patency than plastic stents, with a median patency of 7 months. Self-expanding metallic stents are very flexible and remain patent despite relatively acute angulation. This is a useful feature when the tumor involves the confluence

Figure 14-3C. Removal of endoscopic stent. The stent was displaced into the duodenum using a balloon catheter.

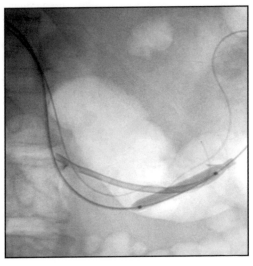

of hepatic ducts (Figure 14-4). In the case of high bile duct obstruction, multiple stents may be placed simultaneously. Multiple ducts may be stented using both "Y" and "T" configurations.

In addition to establishing biliary drainage, percutaneous access to the bile ducts provides a means for additional diagnostic and therapeutic procedures including biopsy of bile duct masses,[9,10] stone retrieval, percutaneous choledochoscopy, and placement of catheters for novel treatments such as local radiation (brachytherapy) or photodynamic therapy.

When the cause of bile duct occlusion is uncertain, bile duct biopsy can be performed through the tract created for biliary drainage. Because the specimens obtained are from the mucosa and superficial portion of the fibromuscular layer of the duct,[10] this is most effective for mucosal and intraductal lesions, including cholangiocarcinoma and intraductal metastases, and is less effective in diagnosing extraductal lesions, such as pancreatic cancer or liver or nodal metastases causing extrinsic compression. After cholangiography is performed, a forceps, brush, or atherectomy device is advanced to the obstruction and a specimen is obtained. Reported sensitivities of forceps biopsy range from 30% to 100% for malignancy, but in most studies a high false negative rate effectively makes a "negative" biopsy nondiagnostic in most cases.

Biliary stone disease is surprisingly common in cancer patients, due to concurrent gallstone disease or biliary stasis, particularly related to narrowing at a bilioenteric anastomosis. Small stones may pass from the gallbladder through the cystic duct into the common bile duct. When large, these are apparent preoperatively and can be removed endoscopically. Smaller stones, however, can be missed during surgery and identified by cholangiography in patients with persistent symptoms or hyperbilirubinemia. After maturation of a T-tube or biliary drainage tract, these stones can be safely treated in the majority of cases using either a basket or snare to remove them percutaneously, a balloon to push them through the papilla into the small bowel, or a laser lithotripsy device to disintegrate them.[10] When associated with papillary stenosis or anastomotic strictures,

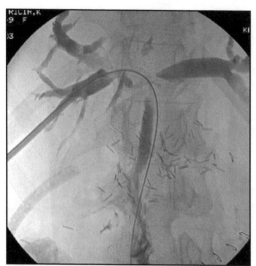

Figure 14-4A. Biliary stent. Isolated left and right ducts in a patient s/p choledochojejunostomy.

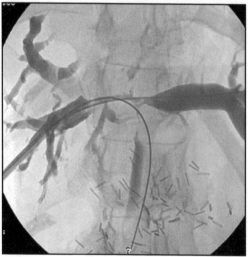

Figure 14-4B. Biliary stent. The left sided ducts were catheterized from the right sided puncture.

balloon sphincterotomy is performed to allow stone fragments to pass. In contradistinction to endoscopic sphincterotomy, where there is a high incidence of sepsis and pancreatitis, such complications following balloon sphincterotomy are uncommon.[11]

Percutaneous choledochoscopy is a technique in which a fiberoptic scope similar to a bronchoscope is advanced percutaneously along the course of a biliary drainage catheter and used to visualize bile ducts, intraluminal masses, and stones in detail. Currently, the most common applications are intrahepatic stone retrieval and intraductal biopsy. Choledochoscopy is performed after the maturation of a percutaneous tract following biliary drainage, which usually takes 2 to 4 weeks. When used in concert with

Figure 14-4C. Two Wallstents were placed to drain bile internally, from the left hepatic duct to the right hepatic duct (arrows) and from the right hepatic duct into the common bile duct (curved arrow), in this patient with cholangiocarcinoma.

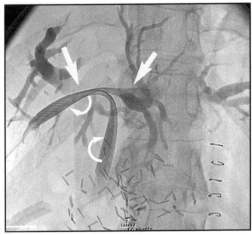

fluoroscopic cholangiography, the choledochoscope can easily be manipulated into the duct of interest. Once a stone is visualized, a basket, snare, or balloon catheter can be advanced through the instrument channel and used to remove the stone percutaneously or to push the stone into the small bowel (Figure 14-5).

PERCUTANEOUS CHOLECYSTOSTOMY

Percutaneous cholecystostomy (PC) is indicated in patients with acute calculus or acalculous cholecystitis who are unable to undergo urgent cholecystectomy due to comorbid disease or debilitated condition. Because of the low procedure-related morbidity, in addition to its therapeutic role, PC is commonly used as a diagnostic tool in patients with unexplained sepsis.[12]

PC is performed using ultrasound or CT guidance. A transhepatic approach is generally preferred to minimize the risk of bile peritonitis and leakage during catheter placement and exchange procedures. PC allows for rapid decompression of the diseased gallbladder as well as access for cholecystography and potential further intervention. Overdistension of the gallbladder at the time of placement is avoided because bile in diseased gallbladders is often infected, and overdistention may worsen sepsis in these already compromised patients.[12]

After resolution of the acute episode, cholecystography can be very helpful in determining the presence and level of obstruction. In cases of acalculous cholecystitis, patency of the cystic duct is known to be restored when normal bile begins draining from the catheter. Once the patient's clinical condition improves, the catheter is capped and left in place until the tract matures, at which point it can be removed. In other instances, PC catheters are left in place until the time of definitive treatment, which is usually cholecystectomy. Occasionally, percutaneous stone removal through the PC can be performed as a definitive procedure in high-risk patients with calculus cholecystitis. Although recurrent stone disease will cause biliary symptoms within 5 years in 20 to 50% of cases, this less invasive treatment may be preferable in patients with limited life expectancy.

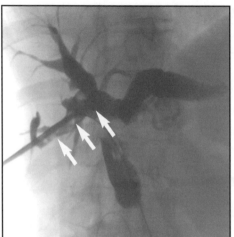

Figure 14-5A. Cholangiography in a patient with Asian cholangiohepatitis demonstrates multiple intrahepatic duct stones (arrows).

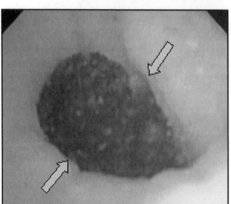

Figure 14-5B. Choledochoscopy. An obstructing stone is identified in the right bile duct. *For a full-color version, see page CA-VII of the Color Atlas.*

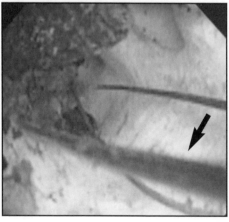

Figure 14-5C. Choledochoscopy. A basket was advanced through the instrument channel and used to remove the stone. *For a full-color version, see page CA-VII of the Color Atlas.*

PC may also provide biliary drainage in some patients with mid or low bile duct occlusion. The gallbladder is quite capacious, and in some cases it can enlarge to completely decompress the intrahepatic bile ducts, making percutaneous biliary drainage quite difficult. In the presence of low bile duct occlusion and a distended gallbladder, PC is technically simple and provides drainage of all bile segments. Alternatively, the gallbladder may be accessed with a needle and cholecystography performed to delineate the intrahepatic bile ducts, thus facilitating percutaneous transhepatic biliary drainage.

Complications of PC include bleeding, sepsis, bile peritonitis, gallbladder perforation, and catheter dislodgement. Removal of a PC prior to the formation of a mature tract can also cause bile peritonitis. Tract maturation usually occurs within 4 weeks even in debilitated patients, but may take longer in patients on immunosuppressive drugs.

PERCUTANEOUS TREATMENT OF HEPATIC NEOPLASMS

EMBOLOTHERAPY

The liver receives oxygenated blood from both the hepatic artery and the portal vein. While the portal vein supplies the majority of the blood supply to the hepatic parenchyma, the hepatic artery is the predominant source of blood for most hepatic tumors, even those that are not "hypervascular." This allows a variety of agents designed to induce in-situ cell death to be delivered to hepatic neoplasms via the hepatic artery. Embolic agents may be delivered alone (bland embolization), or in combination with chemotherapeutic agents (chemoembolization). In combination with embolization, the delivery of chemotherapeutic agents via the hepatic artery has been theorized to result in both prolonged contact and higher concentrations of drug within the tumor, with few or no systemic effects.[13,14] This is an attractive theory for treating chemotherapy sensitive tumors. As an alternative to chemoembolization, chemotherapeutic agents may be administered via hepatic artery infusion pumps to achieve high "first pass" extraction by the liver as another means of achieving higher concentrations of drug within the tumor(s) with diminished systemic effects.[15] In the United States, these pumps are most often placed surgically, but they can be placed percutaneously.

Even in cases of tumors which are thought to be insensitive to chemotherapy, such as hepatocellular carcinoma (HCC), increased concentration and dwell time of a drug might result in response to an agent used for chemoembolization that is not effective when administered systemically. Some early studies demonstrated higher concentration of doxorubicin within chemoembolized tumors, though these involved very few patients.[14] More recent biodistribution studies do suggest that the combination of doxorubicin, ethiodized oil, and an embolic agent results in the highest concentration of doxorubicin in a treated tumor, compared to infusing doxorubicin alone or in combination with ethiodized oil.[13] *In vivo* and *in vitro* laboratory studies also suggest that ischemia promotes cellular uptake of a radio-labeled doxorubicin analogue, most likely secondary to reduced active transport of the analogue out of the cell.[16]

Hypervascular tumors are known to be sensitive to ischemia; in fact early treatment of such tumors involved hepatic artery ligation alone. There are practitioners who concentrate on maximizing the ischemic effect of embolization, rather than adding chemotherapy to the embolic material. Bland embolization is used to treat hypervascular tumors such as HCC and metastatic neuroendocrine tumors.[17,18] Other tumors shown to be hypervascular by contrast enhanced cross sectional imaging, or angio-

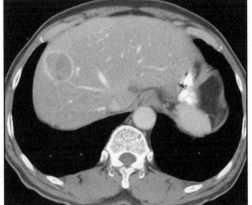

Figure 14-6A. Embolization of solitary HCC. Pre-embolization CT demonstrates an enhancing mass in the right liver.

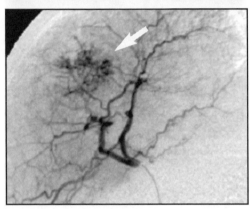

Figure 14-6B. Embolization of solitary HCC. Hepatic angiogram shows corresponding hypervascular mass (arrow) which was embolized.

graphically, can also be treated by bland embolization. In order to maximize the ischemia-induced tumor necrosis, very small particles of embolic material, typically either polyvinyl alcohol particles (PVA) or tris-acryl spheres (Embospheres [Biosphere Medical, Rockland, Mass]) are injected into the vessels supplying the tumor as selectively as possible to effect terminal vessel blockade and cell death. At our institution, embolization will often be initiated with particles as small as 40 or 50 µm in diameter. Larger particles (though rarely larger than 300 µm) may be employed depending on tumor characteristics, including the presence of shunting or the inability to achieve stasis of the vessel(s) supplying the tumor(s) using very small particles alone (Figure 14-6 and 14-7).

A recent randomized, controlled study from Spain failed to demonstrate any significant difference in survival between patients with HCC treated with chemoembolization or bland embolization, using gelfoam as the embolic material in both groups. The study did demonstrate that chemoembolization provided a significant survival benefit compared to conservative treatment.[19] To date, there has been no study demonstrating superiority of chemoembolization over particle embolization alone for prolonging survival in patients with HCC or for palliation (most commonly for control of hormonal symp-

Figure 14-6C. Embolization of solitary HCC. One day after embolization, noncontrast CT shows retention of contrast laden microspheres in the tumor.

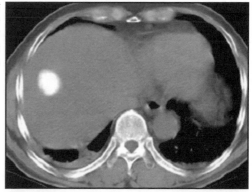

Figure 14-6D. Following resection 6 weeks later, no viable tumor was present, and hepatic vessels containing microspheres were identified in the background of necrosis. *For a full-color version, see page CA-VIII of the Color Atlas.*

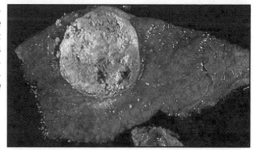

Figure 14-6E. Another look at resection 6 weeks later, no viable tumor was present, and hepatic vessels containing microspheres were identified in the background of necrosis. *For a full-color version, see page CA-IX of the Color Atlas.*

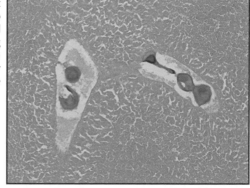

toms or, occasionally, for pain related to tumor bulk). Further, there are no conclusive data regarding the optimal mix and type of chemotherapeutic agent(s), embolic material(s), and contrast used for chemoembolization. It is our belief that for the treatment of hypervascular tumors, bland embolization is simpler, less expensive, and obviates potential side effects related to chemotherapeutic agents. One might expect that in treating hypovascular tumors, chemoembolization would be more efficacious. We do not treat hypovascular tumors with any form of embolization, as patients at our institution who

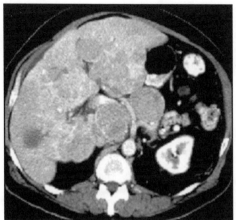

Figure 14-7A. Embolization of neuroendocrine liver metastasis. Pre-embolization CT demonstrates innumerable right and left hemi-liver metastases.

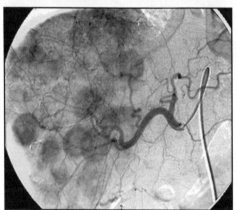

Figure 14-7B. Embolization of neuroendocrine liver metastasis. Hepatic angiogram shows multiple discrete hypervascular masses.

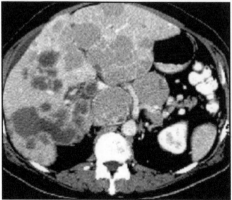

Figure 14-7C. Embolization of neuroendocrine liver metastasis. Follow-up CT after right hepatic artery embolization demonstrates multiple necrotic foci corresponding to prior tumor deposits compared to the untreated left metastases, which are solid.

might be treated this way at other medical centers typically receive intra-arterial chemotherapy via surgically placed pumps.

Embolization is performed from a femoral approach; almost always from the right femoral artery. Patients receive prophylactic antibiotics, typically a first generation cephalosporin or equivalent. In patients likely to have bile colonized with bacteria, such as those who have undergone previous pancreaticoduodenectomy or other type of surgery producing a bilioenteric anastomosis, or even those with biliary stents, coverage (and longer treatment) with tazobactam/piperacillin (Zosyn [Wyeth, Madison, NJ]) is recommended because of the higher incidence of infection and abscess formation in these patients.[20] Patients also receive antinausea prophylaxis. The procedure is performed with conscious sedation.

Recent, good quality, contrast enhanced imaging is crucial prior to the embolization. This maximizes the ability to correlate angiographic findings with cross sectional findings, and provides a basis for follow up and assessment of results. After arterial anatomy is delineated, a catheter (or microcatheter as needed) is advanced as distally as necessary and/or possible. The need for super-selective catheterization will vary depending on the type, number and distribution of tumors. For focal HCC or other tumors treated to prolong survival, super-selective catheterization is preferred. For multifocal HCC or neuroendocrine metastases, typically either the right or left hemiliver is treated initially, with the patient returning after a few weeks for treatment of the other hemiliver in the case of HCC, or as symptoms dictate in the case of neuroendocrine metastases.

Postembolization syndrome (PES) consists of pain, fever, and nausea. Most patients will experience PES to at least some extent. PES is self-limited, generally lasting between 1 and 3 days. Patients also typically demonstrate leukocytosis and elevation of liver function tests. Complications from embolization may be related to arterial access, such as bleeding, vessel injury, femoral pseudoaneurysm formation, etc, or to the embolization itself. Rarely do treated tumors become infected. Patients at greatest risk for liver abscess are those likely to have bile colonized with bacteria, as discussed above. Cholecystitis may also occur, though in our experience this is surprisingly infrequent, even when the cystic artery has been embolized. Images obtained soon after the embolization may raise the question of infection or abscess formation, as tumors typically contain gas, and the gallbladder wall is often thickened, even when the cystic artery appeared to have been preserved on the angiographic images. These imaging findings should be ignored in the absence of compelling clinical evidence to the contrary.

PERCUTANEOUS TUMOR ABLATION

Although surgical resection is the treatment of choice for HCC, many tumors are either too advanced when diagnosed, or occur in a background of cirrhosis that might be severe enough to preclude surgical resection. In addition, surgical resection is expensive. In areas where hepatitis B and C are endemic, the incidence of disease is quite high. If the percentage of resectable patients is increased by screening, the costs of surgical resection could severely strain the health care system. Combining these facts with the understanding that while the 5-year survival following resection is around 50%, the disease-free 5-year survival is only around 20%, it is easy to think of HCC as a chronic disease and attempt to find some method of treatment other than surgical resection. Embolotherapy is the mainstay in patients with high volume disease. For patients with 1 to 3 small lesions (generally <5 cm), percutaneous ablative therapies have been devised.

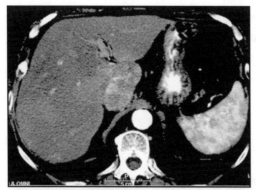

Figure 14-8A. Tumor ablation. HCC recurrence in the caudate following cryoablation.

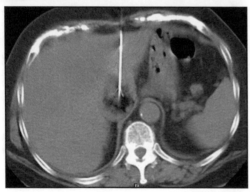

Figure 14-8B. Tumor ablation. Ethanol injection into the tumor shows good coverage of ETOH within the lesion but not in the surrounding liver.

Some of these ablative treatments may be applied to other hepatic neoplasms or, in the case of thermal ablation, even be used outside of the liver.

CHEMICAL ABLATION

Ethanol has been the most commonly used agent for the chemical ablation of HCC. Absolute ethanol results in coagulative necrosis; causing cell dehydration and denaturation as well as small vessel occlusion, presumably due to endothelial cell damage. Percutaneous ethanol injection (PEI) gained popularity in 1995 when Livraghi and his group published a study of 746 patients with HCC treated with PEI who demonstrated survival results similar to those who underwent surgical resection.[21] Small HCC tumors are well suited to treatment with PEI, as the typical HCC is a "soft" tumor occurring in the background of a "hard" (cirrhotic) liver. This, combined with the fact that small HCC tumors are often encapsulated, facilitates injection and promotes uniform distribution and containment of the alcohol within the lesion. While recent studies have shown that radiofrequency ablation (RFA) is more effective and requires fewer treatments than PEI, PEI may still be preferred for treatment of HCC tumors that might not be safely or effectively treated with RFA based on tumor location[22] (Figure 14-8).

Figure 14-8C. Tumor ablation. Solitary hepatic recurrence of colon cancer in a patient s/p right hepatectomy.

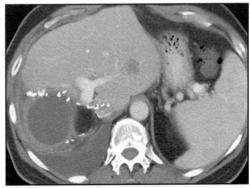

Figure 14-8D. Tumor ablation. Radiofrequency probe centered in lesion.

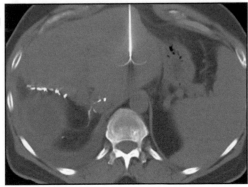

PEI is indicated for the treatment of patients with 1 to 3 HCC tumors, each of which is less than 5 cm in diameter. The treatment of larger tumors may be precluded by potential alcohol toxicity. The volume of alcohol to be injected is calculated using the formula $4/3\pi(r + 0.5)^3$, where r is the radius of the tumor in centimeters. PEI is performed using a 22-gauge needle, with either CT or ultrasound guidance. The alcohol is well seen on CT imaging, appearing as black as air. Alcohol can only be used in soft tumors such as HCC; because most metastases are quite hard, it is not possible to inject them with any significant amount of ethanol. Typically, in this situation alcohol will leak back along the course of the needle, rather than infusing into the tumor.

PERCUTANEOUS ACETIC ACID TREATMENT

Acetic acid also effects coagulative necrosis, causing protein denaturation and destruction of interstitial collagen. The ability to break down collagen allows for better infiltration of tumor septae and tumor penetration. Using acetic acid, tumor necrosis can be achieved with much smaller volumes (30%) and fewer sessions compared with PEI.[23] Large volume injections can cause renal toxicity and metabolic acidosis. Hemoglobinuria may be seen with volumes greater than 10 cc.

THERMAL ABLATION

Tissue can be killed using either heat or cold. Percutaneous cryotherapy has recently become possible, though probes are still larger than those used for injection of chemical ablative materials or even radiofrequency ablation (RFA). More than one tumor can be treated at a time, though multiple probes are often needed for each tumor. Experience is still limited. Treatment of tumors in liver, lung, and kidney has been performed.[24,25] Cryotherapy is reportedly less painful than RFA.

Radiofrequency ablation uses heat to induce coagulative necrosis of the target tissue. Cell death occurs instantly at temperatures greater than 60°C. Necrosis can be achieved at lower temperatures if the temperature is maintained for longer times. At temperatures between 100 and 110°C vaporization, carbonization and charring may occur. RFA involves inserting a probe with an insulated shaft and noninsulated tip into a tumor using imaging guidance. During RFA, the patient is turned into a part of the electrical circuit. After grounding pads are applied to the patient, the probe is attached to a generator, which produces AC current in the radiofrequency range (300 to 500 kHz). This causes ionic agitation at the probe tip, which, in turn, causes frictional heating. Tissue immediately adjacent to the electrode heats by resistive heating, whereas deeper tissues heat by conduction. As the necrotic "sphere" (the lesions themselves are rarely perfectly spherical) grows, the tissue desiccates and impedance rises (see Figure 14-8).

Probes range in size from 15- to 17-gauge. Coaxial and flexible systems have been developed to combat some of the logistical issues associated with imaging guided RFA, which typically involve trying to fit the patient in the CT gantry with the probe in place. MRI compatible probes have also been developed.

RFA is limited in two major ways: by the size of the treated area produced by a given probe and by "heat sinks." Manufacturers have used many methods in order to increase the size of the treated area in one "burn." Since lesion size is proportional to power, the generators have become more powerful over the last few years. Some probes are internally cooled by circulating saline, many probes are configured in arrays of multiple tines, the size and diameter of which have continued to increase, and some employ pulsed power. Various methods of infusing saline into the tumor during the ablation are also being investigated.[26] Currently, the largest diameter of cell death that can be created using a single burn cycle with one probe is 7 cm. Larger lesions can be created by heating overlapping spheres of tissue.

"Heat sinks" refer to vessels of large enough size that the flowing blood "takes away" enough heat to preclude reaching a high enough temperature adjacent to the vessel to achieve cell death. In order to combat this problem, some have employed occlusion balloons to block regional blood flow during RFA. The use of a Pringle maneuver, in which the hepatic vascular inflow is temporarily occluded by placement of a vascular clamp across the porta hepatic, during laparoscopic RFA has been shown to increase the size of ablation in a pig model.[27]

Another problem associated with adjacent structures involves not the efficacy but the safety of RFA. In certain circumstances the location of a tumor relative to the bowel, heart, bile duct, adrenal gland, or renal pelvis might preclude safely ablating the tumor. In these cases, it might be possible to create a "safe window" by injecting saline to move the tissue to be spared out of the way. Alternatively, a surgical rather than percutaneous approach might be safer in such cases.

Results of RFA have been promising, especially in treating HCC tumors 3 cm in diameter or less.[15] While the greatest experience with RFA has been in treating liver tumors, it has also been used to treat tumors in the lung, adrenal gland, kidney, soft tissues, and bone.

COMBINATION THERAPY

Any of the minimally invasive treatment methods described above can be used conjunctively with one another.[28,29] The two methods we routinely use together are embolotherapy with percutaneous ethanol injection, or embolotherapy and RFA. The biggest problem with any ablative treatment is local recurrence. It follows that the use of two different treatment methods may reduce the recurrence rate. In the case of embolotherapy and PEI, we found that when PEI was performed after embolotherapy it was possible to inject higher volumes of ethanol into the target tumor, and there appeared to be better coverage than when PEI was used alone. Embolizing the arterial blood supply to a hypervascular tumor might be expected to shorten treatment time for RFA by reducing the "heat sink" and allowing for immediate direct deposition of heat into the target tissue. It might also enhance the effects of RFA, resulting in a larger area of tissue destruction, as is seen with balloon occlusion of the artery at the time of RFA or with the Pringle maneuver. RFA has also been combined with PEI in a rat model, resulting in an increase in the extent of coagulation necrosis.[30]

INTRA-ARTERIAL DELIVERY OF A RADIOPHARMACEUTICAL

Administering local radiation therapy by injecting radiolabeled embolic agent is another method that can be used to treat virtually any type of liver tumor.[90]Yttrium labeled microspheres are beta emitting microspheres that measure 20 to 30 μm in diameter and can be administered intra-arterially. Patients must be evaluated for shunting to the lungs before each treatment and cannot be treated if their total pulmonary dose will result in a cumulative dose exceeding 30 Gy. These spheres have a low toxicity profile, with the most common side effects being self-limited nausea and fatigue. Liver function studies are transiently elevated, as with embolization, and GI symptoms may occur if there is inadvertent deposition of particles into the gastric or gastroduodenal arteries. The response rate is around 20% with mean duration of response of 127 weeks, and median time to progression of 44 weeks. Outpatient treatment is feasible, because beta radiation does not require medical confinement.

ASCITES

Most ascites is due to liver disease, and medical management is the mainstay of therapy for this group of patients. In cases of medically refractory ascites or in ascites of other etiologies, in particular malignant ascites (representing approximately 10% of cases), other treatment options must be considered. There are many procedures aimed at controlling ascites now in the armamentarium of the Interventional Radiologist, and more are no doubt forthcoming.[31,32]

Repeated large volume paracentesis (LVP) is the most common means of managing refractory ascites. Safe drainage of up to 4 to 6 L per session seems relatively uncontroversial. Reports of draining more than 20 L at one time exist. The biggest problem with LVP is the need for patients to return repeatedly for the procedure. Concerns also exist regarding the loss of protein from the ascitic fluid.

Control of ascites using percutaneously placed exteriorized catheters has been reported by several authors.[33-35] Catheters have been used for both benign and malignant etiologies, though more reports describe their use in malignant disease. Nontunneled catheters are easily placed, but have been reported to be associated with a high rate of infection and catheter related sepsis. Tunneled catheters have been advocated by several authors, and appear to provide effective relief for most patients. It is currently unclear whether or not the Pleur-x (Denver Biomedical, Golden, Colo) offers a substantial advantage over nonvalved cuffed catheters such as the Tenckhoff catheter. Potential complications include infection, which is thought to be less common than with nontunneled catheters, occlusion, dislodgment, and loss of protein, as with repeated LVP. The catheters are likely to be successfully managed by the patients and their families, though they do carry the psycho-social issues and physical constraints associated with other types of exteriorized catheters. There are small series describing the use of subcutaneous peritoneal ports, which could ameliorate some of those issues. However, one study noted a 33% infection rate. Additionally, a trained health care worker is typically needed to access the port.

The role of percutaneous peritoneovenous shunting remains unclear. Potential benefits of shunting include the lack of repeated trips to a health care provider, lack of an exteriorized device, and the continued reintroduction of the ascites volume and proteins into the circulation. Reports on the success and complications associated with the procedure are quite varied. Recently, a few reports have been published describing percutaneous placement of Denver peritoneovenous shunts (Denver Biomedical) by interventional radiologists.[36] However, most reports come from the surgical literature. Reported complications include shunt malfunction from occlusion and disseminated intravascular coagulation (DIC). The occurrence of the latter appears to be reduced by completely draining the ascites at the time of shunt placement. Theoretical concern of decreasing survival by disseminating tumor cells in cases of malignant ascites has not been reported in the literature.

Placement of a transjugular intrahepatic portosystemic shunt (TIPS) can control ascites in patients with portal hypertension. TIPS are contraindicated in patients with encephalopathy or heart failure, and are not well tolerated in cases of poorly compensated cirrhosis. TIPS plus medical therapy has been shown to be superior to medical management of ascites alone. Compared with LVP, TIPS has been shown to lower the rate of ascites recurrence and the risk of developing hepatorenal syndrome, but with an increased incidence of encephalopathy. Many studies show no survival benefit to TIPS compared with other therapies, though other studies have suggested improved survival in certain populations. TIPS may take several weeks to result in resolution of ascites, and may not be effective in all cases.

ABSCESS DRAINAGE

Image-guided percutaneous drainage techniques have had tremendous impact on the management of fluid collections within the abdomen and pelvis, most of which are postoperative. Reoperation is obviated in most cases. Postoperative collections may result from leaks (bowel contents, bile, urine, or pancreatic fluid), lymphatic obstruction or injury (lymphocele), or the presence of residual blood or ascites. Drainage is most often performed for suspected infection, typically in the setting of fever and leukocytosis. Drainage may also be performed to relieve symptoms from mass effect, control a leak (sometimes in conjunction with diversion of the source of the leaking fluid), or for characterization of the fluid.

CT imaging, preferably with both oral and intravenous contrast, is our preferred modality for diagnosing a postoperative fluid collection. It affords excellent visualization of the fluid, and is often able to provide characterization of the fluid as well. CT scanning may demonstrate urine or bowel leaks, and is also accurate in characterizing blood. Enhancement of the wall of a collection may support clinical concerns for infection and, in the case of multiple collections, can be helpful in deciding which collection to drain. CT also allows planning of the drainage, and will demonstrate rare cases where a collection cannot be safely accessed percutaneously, as in deep collections surrounded by bowel, vessels, and/or bone.

Drainage may be performed using CT, ultrasound, or fluoroscopic guidance, depending on the nature and location of the collection, as well as operator preference. As with most interventional procedures, abscess drainage is performed using conscious sedation. Depending on the nature of the fluid, locking loop catheters ranging from 8 to 12 French are placed primarily. Gram stain and culture is performed routinely. Specimens may be sent for measurement of amylase, creatinine, bilirubin, or triglycerides, depending on the clinical situation. In managing urinomas after cystectomy or partial nephrectomy, typically associated with a leak from the ureter, collecting system, ileal conduit or neobladder, diverting nephrostomies are almost always necessary. Biliary diversion may be necessary in cases of bile leak, but generally only in the setting of obstruction.

While most catheters are placed percutaneously, a transrectal, transvaginal, or perineal approach may also be used. Management of the catheters is similar irrespective of the source or the approach. The catheters are flushed twice daily to help ensure patency. If postprocedure imaging shows incomplete drainage, fibrinolytic therapy is initiated. This may be performed using tissue plasminogen activator (tPA) or urokinase. While initial reports described benefits of lytic therapy in managing empyema, this has become a very popular tool in the management of abdominal and pelvic fluid collections as well, often speeding resolution of the collection and obviating additional procedures to reposition a catheter or place multiple catheters.[37,38]

When the output of the drain is essentially equal to the volume of daily flush, investigation is performed to determine whether the collection has resolved, or whether low output is due to catheter malfunction. This may involve CT scanning or studying the cavity fluoroscopically by injecting contrast material into the drainage catheter. A contrast study performed after the cavity has resolved, or at least decreased significantly in size, may demonstrate the source of a leak. Even with a known leak from bowel, bile duct, or urinary system, a fistula may be impossible to demonstrate if the collection of fluid/cavity is large. It is difficult to force contrast along the fistula, since it is easier to fill the capacious space. As the space decreases, as well as the inflammatory changes in the wall of the cavity, it is usually possible to demonstrate the fistula. Most leaks will close if the cavity outside the perforation closes, unless there is obstruction of the system from which the fluid is leaking, distal to the leak. Generally, when the cavity is completely resolved, the drain can be removed.

In addition to managing postoperative fluid collections, interventional radiological techniques may be applied to diverticular or appendiceal abscesses, as a preoperative procedure.

PERCUTANEOUS BIOPSY

Percutaneous imaging-guided needle biopsy may be used to diagnose primary or metastatic cancers and occasionally benign neoplasms. In the case of organ dysfunction, needle biopsy may provide tissue (liver or kidney) for histologic evaluation. Imaging guided aspiration may also be used to sample an abscess or infected tumor in order to provide an organism to guide antibiotic treatment. A specific diagnosis should be made in 80% to 95% of biopsies. Complications may occur but are generally self-limited or easily treated. Needle tract seeding has been reported but is quite rare. It is important to remember that there is no such thing as a "negative" biopsy. If malignancy is not documented then a specific benign diagnosis should be made. If nonspecific findings such as normal site tissue, fibrous tissue, or inflammatory, reactive, or atypical cells are present in the biopsy specimen, then a repeat biopsy or close follow-up are warranted. In certain cases, incisional or even excisional biopsy may be warranted.

Percutaneous biopsy needles range in size from 14- to 25-gauge, and may be of either coring or noncoring design. Larger needles (20- to 14-gauge) needles are typically used to perform core biopsies, where pieces of tissue are obtained for pathologic evaluation. Smaller needles (25- to 20-gauge) are commonly used to obtain specimens for cytological evaluation, or for acquisition of material for culture or chemical analysis. At our institution, the majority of tumor biopsies are performed using 22-gauge needles to provide material for cytology. Core biopsies are generally performed to facilitate a specific diagnosis in suspected sarcomas, hepatocellular carcinoma and lymphomas. In biopsies performed for patients with known or suspected non-Hodgkin's lymphoma, material is also obtained for flow cytometry. Key to maximizing the likelihood of obtaining diagnostic material is onsite evaluation of each specimen by a skilled cytotechnologist or cytopathologist. If the initial specimen is not felt to provide diagnostic material, additional tissue can be obtained immediately. It is important for the interventional radiologist to be aware of special handling instructions or tissue preparations that may be unique to his or her institution.

Good quality imaging is essential for demonstrating the lesion and planning the biopsy. It is optimal to have a study demonstrating the target lesion using the modality that will be used to guide the procedure. For example, if a mass is only demonstrable by MRI, performing the biopsy with CT or ultrasound guidance will be challenging, at best. This is less relevant with larger lesions, where the likelihood that a mass will not be demonstrated by multiple modalities is lower, or the mass can be biopsied based on landmarks alone. Percutaneous biopsy can be performed using CT, ultrasound, fluoroscopic, or MRI guidance, depending on available resources, operator preference and experience and the nature of target. The biopsy should be planned to minimize both potential complications and the need for the patient to cooperate with complicated positioning or breathing instructions.

While the basic principles of percutaneous needle biopsy apply irrespective of the target tissue, there are a few considerations that are location specific.

LUNG/MEDIASTINAL BIOPSY

Lung biopsies can be performed under CT or fluoroscopic guidance. In our experience, lung biopsies are easier and faster under fluoroscopic guidance, as the real-time modality allows for adjustment of the needle with breathing. This is more important with smaller lesions. Mediastinal biopsies generally require CT guidance.

Complications related to lung and mediastinal biopsy involve hemorrhage and pneumothorax. True hemorrhagic complications are rare in biopsy of parenchymal lung masses performed in noncoagulopathic patients. Serious bleeding complications may occur in coagulopathic patients. Hemoptysis is not uncommon, occurring in up to 30% of cases. This is almost uniformly self-limited, and advising the patient properly will avoid them being frightened. True bleeding complications may occur during or after mediastinal biopsy, and may result in hemothorax or hemopericardium. Hemorrhagic pericardial tamponade is quite rare, but is life threatening. While hypoxemia can occur with either pneumothorax or pericardial tamponade, tamponade can be suspected by the concomitant development of hypotension with narrowed pulse pressure, as well as diminished amplitude of the ECG complex. Immediate CT scanning provides diagnostic confirmation, and allows guidance for placement of a small drainage catheter into the pericardial space, which in our experience of three cases, has provided effective treatment.

Pneumothorax occurs in 25% to 30% of patients undergoing percutaneous lung biopsy. Treatment is required in approximately 5% of cases overall.[39] The risk of pneumothorax is increased with deeper lesions and increased number of pleural surfaces traversed, but is surprisingly unrelated to the size of the needle. Treatment is more often necessary in patients with underlying COPD. No treatment is required for stable pneumothorax in an asymptomatic patient. Once the pneumothorax has been shown to be stable over at least 2 hours, an asymptomatic patient can be discharged. Patients who are symptomatic, or with an enlarging pneumothorax are treated with small caliber (typically 8 French) thoracostomy catheters, typically placed in the second anterior intercostal space. Once the lung is re-expanded and the absence of an air leak can be documented, the catheter is removed. Occasionally, an air leak will persist beyond a few hours, and admission to the hospital is then required. Rarely, a reliable patient can be sent home with a Heimlich valve (a one way valve which allows air out but not in) and can be managed as an outpatient.

ADRENAL BIOPSY

Adrenal adenomas are common benign tumors, occurring in as many as 10% of patients. The adrenal gland is also a fairly common site of metastatic disease. While MRI can often reliably distinguish an adenoma from a metastasis,[40] needle biopsy is sometimes required for definitive diagnosis. It is often necessary for the needle to traverse aerated lung when performing percutaneous adrenal biopsy and pneumothorax is the most common complication of this procedure. Adrenal biopsy is typically performed using CT guidance.

LIVER BIOPSY

Many benign tumors such as FNH, adenoma, or hemangioma can be reliably diagnosed by high quality cross-sectional imaging. Biopsy of these lesions is rarely conclusive, though the absence of malignant tissue may further support imaging findings that may be suggestive, but not diagnostic, of a benign entity. Metastatic disease can generally be documented using a cytologic specimen obtained from a fine needle biopsy.[41] Special studies can often be performed to determine the primary tumor type when needed. A core biopsy is sometimes necessary to diagnose hepatocellular carcinoma, as well-differentiated tumors can be difficult to distinguish from normal liver based on cytology alone. In patients with a liver mass in the background of cirrhosis or viral hepatitis, an alpha-fetoprotein level >500 ng/mL is considered diagnostic for HCC. Biopsy of hepatic masses is most commonly performed using CT or ultrasound guidance, largely depending upon operator preference.

PANCREAS BIOPSY

Most patients with pancreatic cancer still present with unresectable disease. Needle biopsy may be requested for tissue diagnosis so that treatment can be initiated. Pancreatic cancer often incites a scirrhous reaction and there is often abundant fibrous tissue associated with the tumor; it is often more fruitful to biopsy peripancreatic lymph nodes or liver metastasis, when present. Biopsy of the pancreas may be safely performed from an anterior approach through the stomach or liver, or from a posterior approach through the inferior vena cava when necessary. CT guidance is most common, but ultrasound guided biopsy may also be performed. Pancreatitis may occur rarely after needle biopsy.

RETROPERITONEAL AND PELVIC BIOPSY

Most retroperitoneal and pelvic biopsies are performed to diagnose the etiology of lymphadenopathy. Core or fine needle biopsy is performed depending on the indication/clinical suspicion. As with other sites of metastatic disease, FNA is generally sufficient to document metastases, while core material may be necessary to diagnose lymphomas or sarcomas. In women with pelvic masses that may be adnexal, the diagnosis of ovarian cancer should be excluded prior to biopsy. Percutaneous biopsy can result in peritoneal contamination, and might relegate the patient to intraperitoneal chemotherapy which would otherwise not have been indicated. That said, the ovary may be the site of metastatic disease and adnexal biopsy may be indicated in certain patients.

BIOPSY FOR "ORGAN DYSFUNCTION"

Most liver biopsies done to evaluate for hepatic dysfunction are performed by our gastroenterology colleagues without imaging guidance. Occasionally, due to anatomic considerations such as obesity, known hepatic cysts, or hemangiomas, core biopsy is performed using ultrasound or CT guidance. In coagulopathic patients, transjugular liver biopsy obviates the need to puncture the hepatic capsule. In this procedure, a special needle is advanced from the jugular vein (generally the right internal jugular) into one of the hepatic veins, preferably the right. The needle is then advanced through the wall of the vein into the hepatic parenchyma and the biopsy is performed. Any bleeding should be contained within the liver or back along the needle track into the hepatic vein.

Biopsy of the kidney in cases of nephropathy is typically done with either ultrasound or CT guidance. At some institutions this is done by our nephrology colleagues, while at others it lies within the province of Interventional Radiology.

CENTRAL VENOUS ACCESS

Good central venous access is essential in the treatment of patients with cancer and the role of the interventional radiologist has increased dramatically in this area. With the use of ultrasound and fluoroscopy, intravenous contrast, and specialized catheters and guidewires, interventional radiologists can place central venous catheters more safely and reliably than physicians relying on landmarks alone.[42] Access requirements vary from patient to patient, and as a result, many different types of catheters are available. These are characterized by catheter size, type (implantable vs external), number of lumens, and potential dwell time.

Central venous access should be considered when long term treatment is anticipated, or when treatment with desiccant chemotherapy or total parenteral nutrition is indicated. Complications of central venous access include pneumothorax, infection, catheter malposition, venous stenosis, and pericatheter thrombosis. Internal jugular access for catheter placement and proper catheter tip positioning minimize the risk of symptomatic venous thrombosis, and with ultrasound guidance, the risk of pneumothorax is essentially eliminated. Subclavian access is associated with a higher risk of pneumothorax, development of venous stenosis, and pericatheter thrombosis causing symptomatic upper extremity edema. The preferred site of access, therefore, is the internal jugular vein because of the low risk of complications. Access via the right internal jugular vein is preferred over the left, because of a shorter and straighter intravascular course to the right atrium.

In patients who have had multiple prior catheters, conventional access sites may be occluded. Interventional radiology techniques are especially valuable in such cases, as central venous access can often be achieved by recanalizing an occluded vein or using collateral veins. Occasionally, alternative access sites must be employed. Catheters may be placed from a translumbar approach into the inferior vena cava, from a trans-hepatic approach into one of the hepatics vein, or via a transfemoral approach.

Implantable ports are ideal for long-term intermittent use, as is often the case for patients receiving chemotherapy. When not accessed, they are completely contained under the skin; as such, these catheters have a low risk of infection and no lifestyle restrictions (once the incision has healed patients can shower, swim, play golf, etc). As with all central venous access, the preferred access site is the right internal jugular vein, and the catheter is tunneled under the skin of the anterior chest wall to the port reservoir placed in a subcutaneous pocket. Because ports require an incision and the creation of a "pocket" in the chest wall, as well as a needle stick for access, coagulopathy or anticoagulation is a relative contraindication. Ports may remain in place indefinitely, often for several years, and need to be flushed only every 4 to 6 weeks. Chest wall ports can be placed safely, even in patients who have undergone ipsilateral axillary lymph node dissections from breast cancer or melanoma surgery.[43] Ports may also be placed in the arm, via the brachial or basilic vein. However, the risk of central venous stenosis or occlusion is higher than with jugular access for chest port placement.

Exteriorized tunneled catheters are also commonly used, including Broviac/Hickman catheters, leukapheresis, and dialysis catheters. Most catheters are available with one, two or three lumens, and come in many sizes. Larger catheters (13.5 French to 15.5 French) are commonly used for dialysis or leukapheresis, where higher flow rates are required. As with ports, these catheters are generally placed in the internal jugular vein and tunneled to the anterior chest wall. Because the catheters are exteriorized, it is not necessary to puncture the skin to use them. However, they are more lifestyle limiting and require more care. Additionally, these catheters are not ideal for noncompliant patients, small children, or patients with small children, as they may be removed inadvertently with traction.

Peripherally inserted central catheters (PICCs) are placed in an upper extremity vein, often at bedside by a nurse or IV team, and measured so that the tip ends centrally. They are nontunneled catheters, and may be used for short to intermediate term therapy. Because they are placed in an arm vein and have a long intravascular course, complications include symptomatic venous thrombosis. They are, however, very easy for patients to take care of at home and very acceptable cosmetically.

SVC STENTS

Malignant occlusion of the superior vena cava is a potential consequence of thoracic malignancies, most commonly lung cancer. Obstruction may be due to direct tumor involvement, extrinsic compression by tumor, or lymphadenopathy. Benign cases of superior vena cava occlusion in cancer patients occur as well, most commonly due to malpositioned venous access devices.

Often radiographic occlusion is seen in patients with no clinical symptoms, due to abundant thoracic collateral channels predominantly draining into the azygous system or inferior vena cava. In such cases, no treatment is indicated. In some patients, however, superior vena cava obstruction is associated with the superior vena cava syndrome, consisting of upper extremity, head and neck swelling, headache, mental status changes, and dyspnea.

In symptomatic patients with radiosensitive tumors, radiation has been the treatment of choice. While this is often successful, it requires daily therapy for several weeks and improvement occurs slowly over days to weeks. Recanalization of the superior vena cava with balloon angioplasty or metallic stenting, on the other hand, offers rapid and often dramatic relief of symptoms, typically within 24 hours. Although some success has been reported with angioplasty alone, the recurrence or failure rate after percutaneous transluminal angioplasty, particularly in patients with malignant obstruction, is quite high because of the elastic recoil that takes place secondary to the compressing tumor or fibrosis. Stent placement is the most durable method of reestablishing blood flow.

Contrast-enhanced chest CT is critical for procedure planning to define the level and length of obstruction. CT may also suggest the presence of acute thrombus, which may require thrombolysis prior to stenting. When venous access is also required (as is often the case in patients with cancer), an approach via the subclavian or internal jugular vein is preferred, and a venous access device is placed through the stent at the end of the procedure. Alternatively, a transfemoral approach may be used. Once venography is performed, the occlusion is crossed with a catheter and guidewire. If acute thrombus is present, pharmacologic thrombolysis (tPA, urokinase) is indicated prior to balloon dilation or stent placement to minimize the risk of procedure-related pulmonary embolism and stent occlusion by thrombus.

It is our practice to place unilateral stents from the brachiocephalic vein of the punctured side to the high right atrium. This is supported by a recent study by Dinkel, in which 84 patients with SVC syndrome underwent either unilateral or bilateral stenting (ie, double barreled stents into the SVC from both brachiocephalic veins) for malignant SVC syndrome. They found no difference in technical success or clinical response, but a trend toward longer primary patency in the unilaterally stented group.[44]

Pre-stent angioplasty may be performed and an appropriate diameter self-expanding stent is then deployed across the occlusion. Technical success approaches 100%, and symptomatic relief is seen in 80% to 99%. Peri- and postprocedure anticoagulation is controversial and ranges from baby aspirin to full, lifetime anticoagulation with warfarin.[45]

Recurrent symptoms following successful stent placement suggest stent occlusion and should be evaluated with contrast chest CT. Common causes include tumor overgrowth, neointimal hyperplasia and, rarely, stent migration. Recurrent obstruction may be treated with thrombolysis, balloon angioplasty, or repeat stenting. Complications related to SVC stent placement include hemorrhagic pericardial tamponade and pulmonary embolus, either of which can result in death.

INFERIOR VENA CAVA FILTERS

The association between venous thrombosis and malignancy has been known for more than a century. When venous thrombosis involves the deep system of the lower extremities anywhere from the IVC to the popliteal vein, the risk of pulmonary embolism is markedly increased.[46] The need to treat calf vein DVT in cancer patients remains controversial.

In the United States, 550,000 cases of pulmonary embolism are diagnosed annually, nearly one-third of which are fatal. The incidence of pulmonary embolism in cancer patients is three times that in the general population. First-line treatment for DVT or PE is systemic anticoagulation. Indications for IVC filter placement include contraindication to anticoagulation (hemorrhagic stroke, GI bleed or other recent hemorrhage, brain metastases), inability to achieve adequate anticoagulation, propagating thrombus or recurrent pulmonary thromboemboli despite therapeutic anticoagulation, and planned surgery. Free-floating IVC thrombus seen on CT or ultrasound is also a relative indication, as these thrombi have a high likelihood of embolizing. In such patients, mechanical filtration of the venous return from the pelvis and lower extremities is required to prevent pulmonary emboli.

Several IVC filters are commercially available, including the Greenfield (Boston Scientific, Natick, Mass) stainless steel and titanium filters, Vena-Tech (LG Med, France), Simon Nitinol (Nitinol Med Tech, Woburn, Mass), Bird's Nest (Cook Inc, Bloomington, Ind), and Trap-Ease (Cordis Corp, Miami Lakes, Fla). Recently, two optionally retrievable filters, the Recovery (Bard, Tempe, Az) and the Gunther Tulip (Cook Inc) were approved for use in the United States.[47]

Filters can be deployed from a femoral or jugular approach. A jugular approach is preferred in the majority of patients for several reasons. The vast majority (>90%) of pulmonary emboli arise from lower extremity thrombi, and catheterization of the femoral vein not only risks dislodging a clot that is already present, but risks causing a clot as well; local thrombus develops after manual compression of the femoral vein in 2% to 35%.[46] Also, after internal jugular puncture, patients recover more comfortably with their head elevated, in contrast to the flat position required after femoral approach. Finally, if a venous access device is needed, it may be placed concurrently, using the same puncture site.

Venography is first performed to evaluate IVC and renal vein anatomy, measure the diameter of the IVC, determine the location of the renal veins, and evaluate for the presence of possible IVC thrombus. IVC anomalies occur uncommonly and include duplication (persistence of a left IVC draining into the left renal vein), interruption of the IVC, and left-sided IVC. Renal vein anomalies such as a circumaortic or retroaortic left renal vein are more common, and may influence the type of filter placed as well as the positioning of the filter. In patients with extensive retroperitoneal tumor, the IVC may be occluded or too narrow for filter placement. In these patients, this effective interruption of the IVC approximates a filter (serving as an "auto-filter") and filter placement is not indicated. Ideally, filters are placed immediately below the most caudal renal vein, but they may be placed in a suprarenal portion of the IVC if the thrombus extends more centrally. Most filters are designed to be placed in vessels of 20 to 28 mm, and in the unusual case of a "mega-IVC," a Bird's Nest filter can be placed safely in IVCs up to 40 mm. Each filter has advantages and disadvantages, and selection of a specific filter often depends on the experience of the radiologist.

Complications of filter placement include nontarget placement, recurrent pulmonary embolism, IVC occlusion, migration, contrast reactions, and access complications. The frequency of complications reported in the literature is difficult to interpret, as ranges of 3% to 69% for filter migration, 2% to 28% access site thrombosis and 6% to 30% IVC occlusion are reported.[46] For more realistic numbers, a study of 1765 filters placed in 1731 patients over 26 years at the Massachusetts General Hospital was reported in 2000.[48] In this large cohort, symptomatic IVC thrombosis occurred in 2.7%, recurrent PE in 5.6% (fatal in 3.7%).

Recently, an optionally retrievable IVC filter was approved for use in the United States. The term "optionally retrievable" refers to the fact that this filter may be removed up to 161 days after placement, but also may function as a permanent filter if the contraindication to anticoagulation unexpectedly persists. This filter can provide short-term mechanical filtration for patients at high-risk for pulmonary embolism and prevent the long-term complications associated with permanent filter placement. Indications include preoperative prophylaxis in high-risk patients who have no long-term contraindication to anticoagulation, protection during lower extremity or IVC thrombolysis, DVT in pregnancy, and trauma. An additional advantage is the ability to retrieve and reposition malpositioned filters after deployment. Currently, the Recovery is the only FDA-approved retrievable filter, though others are awaiting approval.

GENITOURINARY PROCEDURES

Obstruction of the urinary tract is not uncommon in cancer patients, and may be caused by primary GU neoplasms, other pelvic masses, lymphadenopathy or other metastases, or ureteral strictures or fibrosis. Stone disease may also occur in this patient population. Relief of obstruction may be indicated for renal insufficiency or frank renal failure, pyonephrosis, or pain control. Asymptomatic obstruction may also be treated to preserve or maximize renal function. Percutaneous urinary drainage may also be required to provide urinary diversion, in cases of fistulae or leaks.

Good quality preprocedure imaging is essential to identify the cause and level of the obstruction and get a look at the bladder, as well as defining relevant anatomic details. It helps determine the treatment options available, as well as whether the patient is best approached percutaneously or cystoscopically. Generally, patients with essentially normal bladders, who are able to fill and empty their bladder, should undergo attempted retrograde ureteral stent placement as a primary treatment approach. This obviates the need for percutaneous catheters, with their attendant physical and psychological issues. A percutaneous approach to urinary drainage should be undertaken in cases of unsuccessful cystoscopic, retrograde stent placement, when the bladder is filled with or compressed by tumor, or to provide urinary diversion. Urinary diversion is generally provided by a percutaneous nephrostomy catheter. For cases in which permanent diversion is desired, nephrostomy placement may be combined with embolization of the ureter. Ureteral occlusion may be accomplished by placement of coils, gelatin sponge pledgets, or detachable latex balloons using the percutaneous nephrostomy site for access.[49,50]

There are four main tools employed by interventional radiologists who perform percutaneous urinary drainage procedures. These are: nephrostomy, nephroureterostomy, transloop retrograde nephrostomy, and ureteral stent. Initial percutaneous access is performed using fluoroscopic and/or sonographic guidance. A nephrostomy catheter enters the patient via the flank and terminates in the renal pelvis. Most catheters have a locking-loop that forms a pigtail, and serves as a retention device. A nephroureterostomy catheter is essentially a nephrostomy catheter with an "attached" ureteral stent, so that the catheter enters the kidney, has a loop within the renal pelvis, then extends to the bladder where it terminates in another pigtail. This catheter can drain both the kidney and the bladder when allowed to drain externally. These catheters can be capped and can act as an internal stent, allowing urine from the collecting system to drain into the bladder. This can allow a trial of internal stent use. If the patient tolerates a capped nephroureterostomy catheter, the catheter can then be converted to an internal stent. Occasionally, patients who cannot tolerate an internal stent may be able to cap their nephroureterostomy intermittently. Patients who undergo conversion of a percutaneous catheter to an internal ureteral stent are typically referred to a urologist for future cystoscopic stent exchanges. Stents can be changed by the Interventional Radiologist from a transurethral approach using fluoroscopic guidance. This is reasonably easy in women, but may be difficult in men.

Ureterointestinal anastomotic strictures occur in 4% to 8% of patients who have undergone cystectomy and creation of a neobladder or ileal conduit. In these patients, open ureteral implantation has traditionally been the treatment of choice. Balloon dilation (cutting/angiographic), however, now offers a minimally invasive treatment option and is successful in approximately 50% of cases, obviating the need for long-term catheter drainage.[51,52] Another option for patients with an ileal conduit is to use antegrade access to the kidney to allow for crossing the obstruction into the conduit, and then retrograde placement of a nephrostomy tube. The end of this catheter then protrudes from the patient's stoma and is placed in the stoma bag. Therefore, the lumen of the catheter does not become obstructed from mucus produced by the conduit, and the catheter can easily be changed from below. If nephroureterostomy catheters are placed in these patients the catheters should not be capped, as the intestinal mucosa of the conduits or neobladders, secretes mucus that will occlude the distal portion of the catheter. These patients are not candidates for internal stent placement for the same reason. In patients with ileal conduits, a nephroureterostomy catheter can easily be converted to a retrograde nephrostomy, as discussed previously. This option is preferred by patients because there is no additional external appliance to maintain (Figure 14-9).

Exteriorized urinary drainage catheters typically require routine exchange at roughly three month intervals. Antibiotic coverage for these procedures is essential. Like all exteriorized catheters, nephrostomy and nephroureterostomy catheters will be colonized within a few days, and thus transient bacteremia may result from even routine exchange. If a catheter occludes, patients may develop urosepsis. Because these catheters become colonized, when they are properly functioning there is no need to treat positive cultures from the catheter in the absence of clinical signs or symptoms.

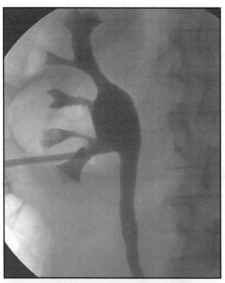

Figure 14-9A. Urinary drainage catheters. Nephrostomy placed for urinary diversion in a patient with a postoperative urinoma (not shown).

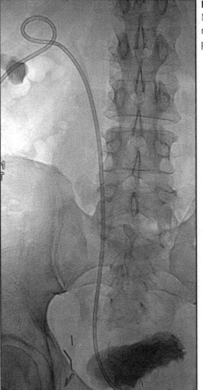

Figure 14-9B. Urinary drainage catheters. Nephroureteral catheter in a patient with retroperitoneal fibrosis associated with pancreatic cancer.

Figure 14-9C. Urinary drainage catheters. Retrograde nephrostomy catheter in a patient with ureteroenteric anastamotic stricture after cystectomy for bladder cancer. The locking loop of the catheter is positioned in the kidney and the catheter drains into the urostomy bag.

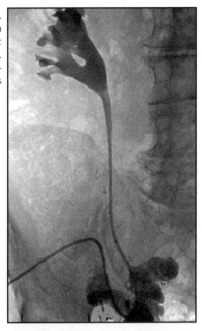

Figure 14-9D. Urinary drainage catheters. Ureteral stent in a patient with malignant ureteral obstruction from ovarian carcinoma.

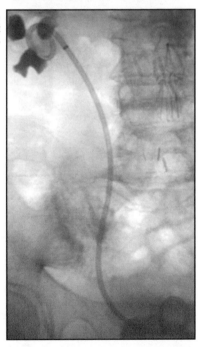

INTERVENTIONS IN THE CHEST

PLEURAL EFFUSIONS

Malignant pleural effusions are common in patients with cancer, most frequently in breast carcinoma, lung carcinoma, and lymphoma. These effusions are exudative in nature, and result from weeping of fluid from pleural metastases or lymphatic obstruction by tumor. The accumulation of fluid in the pleural space may be associated with dyspnea, cough or chest pain.

Malignant effusions in patients with lymphoma or small cell lung cancer may improve significantly or even resolve with systemic therapy, but the majority of symptomatic patients with malignant pleural effusions will require some form of drainage for relief. Treatment options include repeated thoracentesis, tube thoracostomy, VATS and pleurodesis.

Thoracentesis may be performed on an outpatient basis or at bedside, but because malignant effusions recur in the vast majority, it does not represent a definitive treatment option.

Several different chest tubes, made of polyurethane or silicone, are available for drainage of pleural effusions, ranging in size from 8 to 36 French. Surgical chest tubes, placed at the bedside or in the operating room, are usually 24 to 36 French catheters. When placed at bedside, chest tube placement is a "blind" procedure relying on landmarks to access the effusion. Therefore, this technique is limited to patients with moderate to large free-flowing effusions, and poor catheter position is a common occurrence. These catheters tend to be rather uncomfortable, as well.

Although surgical teaching is that a large catheter is required for successful drainage, recent data suggests that smaller caliber catheters are equally effective. Large caliber tubes are certainly associated with more pain and limitation of mobility. The small bore (8 to 15.5 French) catheters placed by interventional radiologists (and some surgeons) generally have multiple side holes, flexible pigtail locking-loops, and are able to change position within an effusion as it resolves. Several studies have demonstrated no significant difference between large and small bore catheters in the successful management of malignant pleural effusions.[53,54]

Placement of chest tubes using CT, ultrasound, or fluoroscopic imaging has the additional advantage of making it possible to place the catheter into a desirable location to maximize drainage. In other words, using guidance, catheters can be placed "where the fluid is" rather than at an external anatomic landmark. This is most important in patients with small or loculated effusions.

Using imaging guidance, an appropriate puncture site is marked. The pleural space is accessed with an 18- to 21-gauge needle and fluid is aspirated. A guidewire is advanced into the pleural space, and this guidewire may be used to disrupt septations in multiloculated effusions. The tract is then dilated, and a catheter is advanced over the wire into a dependant portion of the pleural space. One to 1.5 L may be aspirated immediately, after which the catheter is attached to a closed system water-seal device. Gravity drainage is usually sufficient, but suction may improve drainage in a minority of patients.

A chest radiograph is obtained immediately following drainage to provide a new baseline and to evaluate for lung re-expansion. In chronic effusions, the lung may not be compliant and an ex-vacuo air collection may be seen in the pleural space after drainage of pleural fluid. This usually resolves over days to weeks, but may persist in some cases.

Daily outputs are measured and are critical in the tube management decision making process. Low catheter output (<25 cc/day) indicates either tube malfunction or resolution, and a chest radiograph can usually differentiate between the two. If the catheter is malpositioned or malfunctioning, it may be exchanged over a guidewire. If the effusion has resolved, as happens in a significant minority of patients with malignant pleural effusions, the catheter may be removed without further intervention.

The majority of patients with malignant pleural effusions, however, will not have a durable, long-term response to thoracentesis or catheter placement alone. In this group of patients, mechanical or chemical pleurodesis may be performed. Mechanical pleurodesis and/or chemical pleurodesis are performed during video-assisted thorascopy, while chemical pleurodesis can be performed at bedside via a chest tube. While surgical pleurodesis offers a slightly higher success rate and shorter hospital stay, it is more expensive, more invasive, and associated with higher morbidity.[55,56]

Chemical pleurodesis is achieved by instilling a sclerosing agent (asbestos-free talc, bleomycin, doxycycline) into the pleural space to incite an inflammatory reaction that ultimately causes the visceral pleura to adhere to the parietal pleura, thereby eliminating the potential space in which fluid can accumulate. The choice of agents is operator dependent, and each has pros and cons. Talc is inexpensive and readily available, but has been associated with acute respiratory distress syndrome. Talc also forms a thick slurry and can occlude smaller bore (8 to 10 French) catheters. Bleomycin is slightly less effective and quite expensive. Doxycycline is relatively effective, inexpensive, and available, and has, therefore, been our agent of choice.

In order for pleurodesis to be successful, the pleural space should be completely drained with good apposition of the visceral and parietal pleura. Injecting a sclerosant into an incompletely drained effusion can turn a simple effusion into a multiloculated effusion, often necessitating further intervention. Once adequate drainage is documented by imaging, 1% lidocaine is injected into the pleural space and intravenous analgesics administered prior to pleurodesis. The sclerosant (5 gm of talc in 100 cc NS, 500 mg doxycycline in 100 cc NS, 60 IU Bleomycin in 100 cc D5W) is injected into the pleural space, the catheter is clamped, and the patient is instructed to change position every 15 minutes for 2 hours to distribute the agent in the pleural space. The tube is then reopened and removed when drainage is less than 100 cc/day.

Chemical pleurodesis is effective in 61% to 90% patients, but often requires prolonged hospitalization of 5 to 12 days to adequately drain the pleural space;[56] in a patient population with a median life expectancy of 6 to 12 months and a 30-day mortality of 29% to 50%,[57] this may not be acceptable.

An alternate approach is to treat malignant pleural effusions with a long-term tunneled chest catheter (Pleur-x, Denver Biomedical). This is a 15.5 French silastic catheter with an airtight valve in the hub, allowing the catheter to remain in place indefinitely and be accessed for intermittent drainage using a vacuum bottle. These catheters may be placed on an outpatient basis with appropriate teaching, and intermittent drainage may be performed by the patient at home. Mechanical pleurodesis is spontaneously achieved by almost 50% of patients at 30 days.[58]

To improve drainage of complex pleural collections, intrapleural fibrinolytic agents, including tPA and urokinase, may be instilled into the pleural space. These agents promote enzymatic debridement of fibrinous septae in the pleural space and when injected through a chest tube can reestablish catheter patency and improve drainage of complex, multiloculated effusions and even empyema.[57,59]

BRONCHIAL STENTS

Patients with occlusion of the central airways by intrinsic tumor or extrinsic compression present with dyspnea, obstructive pneumonia, and often have the sensation of impending suffocation.[60] When not amenable to resection, intraluminal malignant lesions can be effectively palliated bronchoscopically with laser ablation, electrocautery, brachytherapy, or photodynamic therapy. Placement of plastic or metallic stents is a useful adjuvant to reestablish and maintain airway patency in these cases, and it is the treatment of choice for endobronchial obstruction due to extrinsic compression.[61-63] In fact, 78% to 98% of patients stented can be expected to have immediate relief of respiratory symptoms related to central airway obstruction.[62]

As in the biliary tract, plastic stents have the advantage of being removable and replaceable, but require rigid bronchoscopy for placement and are subject to occlusion by inspisated mucus or granulation tissue. Self-expanding metallic stents provide a larger lumen and may be placed via flexible bronchoscopy, but they are permanent.

Successful stent deployment requires a coordinated effort by a multidisciplinary team. CT with 3-dimensional reconstruction is useful in determining the length and level of obstruction, as well as the anatomy of the airway. Flexible or rigid bronchoscopy is then performed (usually by a surgeon or pulmonologist) to confirm the imaging findings and provide access to the lesion. The scope is then removed over a guidewire in the side port and an angiographic catheter advanced central to the obstructing lesion. A self-expanding metallic stent is then advanced over the guidewire and deployed to cover the obstructed portion of the airway. Lastly, the bronchoscope is readvanced over the guidewire to confirm adequate coverage by the stent prior to completion of the procedure.

Long-term follow-up data is limited because the life expectancy of these patients is measured in weeks. Wood et al published Washington University's series of 53 patients stented for malignant disease, in whom 85% had adequate palliation with a mean follow-up of 4 months, with 28% requiring additional bronchoscopic procedures to reestablish stent patency.[63] A study from Norway, in which 14 patients were treated with endobronchial stents for malignant obstruction, had a median survival of 11 weeks, with a range of 0.5 to 34 weeks.[60]

EMERGING THERAPIES AND FUTURE DIRECTIONS

The field of interventional radiology has undergone several metamorphoses since its inception almost 30 years ago, when Charles Dotter performed the first percutaneous dilation of a superficial femoral stenosis in a patient who had refused amputation. Minimally invasive image guided techniques have replaced many open surgical procedures and provide new options for patients with previously untreatable diseases.

Progress continues and many new and exciting techniques are emerging. Gene therapy is a promising new tool based on the transfer of genetic material to a target cell population. Preclinical and clinical studies in the treatment of liver metastases in which viral vectors containing either a "suicide gene" or corrective copies of a defective gene are injected directly into the hepatic artery or portal vein to reverse the malignant phenotype and induce apoptosis or growth arrest of tumor cells are being investigated. The role of interventional radiology is not only to provide access for local delivery, but in the development of maximally effective delivery systems.

Chemotherapy containing liposomes, including new "stealth" liposomes that evade destruction by the immune system are currently in clinical trials for the treatment of melanoma, breast carcinoma, ovarian carcinoma, and AIDS-related Kaposi's sarcoma. Currently delivered systemically, catheter-directed delivery has the potential to maximize pharmacokinetics and minimize systemic toxicity.

In addition to novel treatment strategies, future trends in interventional radiology promise to include more effective and efficient ways to perform current procedures. Robots with arms and wrists have allowed complex open surgical procedures, including coronary artery bypass grafting surgery (CABG) and hepatic resection, to be performed through tiny incisions and have facilitated surgical procedures on newborns and fetuses. The development of robotics has promised to revolutionize the field of surgery in replacing open surgical procedures with minimally invasive ones and developing entirely new procedures to treat disease. In the arena of interventional radiology, where essentially all procedures are "minimally invasive," robotics can be used to improve accuracy of needle placement when performing a biopsy, radiofrequency ablation, or targeted access to an organ or vessel.

A precursor to robotics includes an electromagnetic targeting system based on the Global Positioning System, which is commercially available for both CT and ultrasound. Using a sensor on a needle in a weak magnetic field, the exact position and orientation of a needle with respect to the target is displayed on a monitor in multiple planes, facilitating and optimizing needle placement.

REFERENCES

1. Preshaw RM. A percutaneous method for inserting a feeding gastrostomy tube. *Surg Gyn Obstet.* 1981;152:659-660.

2. Gauderer MW, Ponsky JL, Izant RJ. Gastrostomy without laparotomy: a percutaneous endoscopic technique. *J Ped Surg.* 1989;15:872-875.

3. Hoffer EK. US guided percutaneous gastrostomy: a portable technique. *JVIR.* 1996;7(3):431-434

4. Morino M, Bertello A, Garbarini A, et al. Malignant colonic obstruction managed by endoscopic stent decompression followed by laparoscopic resections. *Surg Endosc.* 2002;16:1483-1487.

5. Lee SH. The role of oesophageal stenting in the non-surgical management of oesophageal strictures. *BJR.* 2001;74:891-900.

6. Abadal JM, Echenagusia A, Simo G, Camunez F. Treatment of malignant esophagorespiratory fistulas with covered stents. *Abd Imag.* 2001;26:565-569.

7. Khan SA, Davidson BR, Goldin R, et al. Guidelines for the diagnosis and treatment of cholangiocarcinoma: consensus document. *Gut.* 2002;51(S6):V1-19.

8. Isayama H, Komatsu Y, Sasahira N, et al. A prospective randomised study of covered versus uncovered diamond stents for the management of distal malignant biliary obstruction. *Gut.* 2004;53:729-734

9. Savader SJ, Prescott CA, Lund GB, Osterman FA. Intraductal biliary biopsy: comparison of three techniques. *J Vasc Intervent Radiol.* 1996;7:743.

10. Jung GS, Huh JD, Lee SU. Bile duct: analysis of percutaneous transluminal forceps biopsy in 130 patients suspected of having malignant biliary obstruction. In: Blumgart LH, Fong Y eds. *Surgery of the liver and biliary tract.* New York, New York: Saunders; 2002.

11. Baum S, Pentecost MA, eds. *Angiography*. New York, NY: Little Brown and Company; 1997:485-490.

12. Byrne MF, Suhocki P, Mitchell RM, et al. Percutaneous cholecystostomy in patients with acute cholecystitis: experience of 45 patients at a US referral center. *J Am Coll Surg*. 2003;197:206-211.

13. Raoul JL, Heresbach D, Bretagne JF, et al. Chemoembolization of hepatocellular carcinomas. A study of the biodistribution and pharmacokinetics of doxorubicin. *Cancer*. 1992;70(3):585-590.

14. Nakamura H, Hashimoto T, Oi H, Sawada S. Transcatheter Oily Chemoembolization of hepatocellular carcinoma. *Radiology*. 1989;170:783-786.

15. Kemeny M. Hepatic artery infusion of chemotherapy as a treatment for hepatic metastases from colorectal cancer. *Cancer*. 2002;8 Suppl 1:S82-8

16. Kruskal JB, Hlatky L, Hahnfeldt P, et al. In vivo and in vitro analysis of the effectiveness of doxorubicin combined with temporary arterial occlusion in liver tumors. *JVIR*. 1993;4:741-747.

17. Brown KT, Nevins AB, Getrajdman GI, et al. Particle embolization for hepatocellular carcinoma. *JVIR*. 1998;9:822-828.

18. Brown KT, Koh BY, Brody LA, et al. Particle embolization of hepatic metastases for control of pain and hormonal symptoms. *JVIR*. 1999;10:397-403.

19. Llovet JM, Real MI, Montana X, et al. Arterial embolisation or chemoembolization versus symptomatic treatment in patients with unresectable hepatocellular carcinoma: a randomized controlled trial. *Lancet*. 2002;359:1734-39.

20. Geschwind JF, Shaifali K, Ramsey DE, et al. Influence of a new prophylactic antibiotic therapy on the incidence of liver abscesses after chemoembolization treatment of liver tumors. *JVIR*. 2002;13:1163-6

21. Livraghi T, Giorgio A, Marin G, et al. Hepatocellular carcinoma and cirrhosis in 746 patients: long-term results of percutaneous ethanol injection. *Radiology*. 1995;197:101-108.

22. Livraghi T, Goldberg SN, Lazzaroni S, et al. Small hepatocellular carcinoma: treatment with radio-frequency ablation versus ethanol injection. *Radiology*. 1999;210:655-661.

23. Ohishi K, Nomura F, Ito S, Fujiwara K. Can small hepatocellular carcinoma be cured by percutaneous acetic acid injection therapy? *Hepatology*. 1996;23:994-1002.

24. Goldberg SN, Dupuy DE. Image-guided radiofrequency tumor ablation: challenges and opportunities—Part I. *JVIR*. 2001;12:1021-1032.

25. Dupuy DE, Goldberg SN. Image-guided radiofrequency tumor ablation: challenges and opportunities—Part II. *JVIR*. 2001;12:1135-1148.

26. Giorgio A, Tarantino L, de Stefano G, et al. Percutaneous sonographically guided saline-enhanced radiofrequency ablation of hepatocellular carcinoma. *AJR*. 2002;181:479-484.

27. Scoutt DJ, Fleming JB, Watumull LM, et al. The effect of hepatic inflow occlusion on laparoscopic radiofrequency ablation using simulated tumors. *Surg Endosc*. 2002; 16(9):1286-91

28. Kitamoto M, Imagawa M, Yamada H, et al. Radiofrequency ablation in the treatment of small hepatocellular carcinomas: Comparison of the radiofrequency effect with and without chemoembolization. *AJR*. 2003;181:997-1003.

29. Tanaka K, Nakamura S, Numata K, et al. The long term efficacy of combined transcatheter arterial embolization and percutaneous ethanol injection in the treatment of patients with large hepatocellular carcinoma and cirrhosis. *Cancer*. 1998;82(1):78-84.

30. Goldberg SN, Kruskal JB, Oliver BS, et al. Percutaneous tumor ablation: increased coagulation by combining radio-frequency ablation and ethanol instillation in a rat breast model. *Radiology.* 2000;217:827-831.

31. Yu AS, Hu K. Management of ascites. *Clin Liver Dis.* 2001;5(2):541-568.

32. Zervos EE, Rosemurgy AS. Management of medically refractory ascites. *Am J Surg.* 2001;181:256-64.

33. Barnett TD, Rubins J. Placement of a permanent tunneled peritoneal drainage catheter for palliation in malignant ascites: A simplified approach. *JVIR.* 2002;13:379-383.

34. O'Neill MJ, Weissleder R, Gervais DA, Hahn PF, Mueller PR. Tunneled peritoneal catheter placement under sonographic and fluoroscopic guidance in the palliative treatment of malignant ascites. *AJR.* 2001:615-618.

35. Richard HM, Coldwell DM, Boyd-Kranis RL, Murthy R, Van Echo DA. Pleurx tunneled catheter in the management of malignant ascites. *JVIR.* 2001;12:373-375.

36. Park JS, Won JY, Park SI, Park SJ, Lee DY. Percutaneous peritoneovenous shunt creation for the treatment of benign and malignant refractory ascites. *JVIR.* 2001; 12:1445-1448.

37. Bakal CW, Sacks D, Burke DR, et al. Quality improvement guidelines for adult percutaneous abscess and fluid drainage. *JVIR.* 2003;12:S223-225.

38. Maher MM, Kealey S, McNamara A, et al. Management of visceral interventional radiology catheters: a troubleshooting guide for interventional radiologists. *Radiographics.* 2002;22:305-322.

39. Westcott JL, Rao N, Colley DP. Transthoracic needle biopsy of small pulmonary nodules. *Radiology.* 1997;202:97.

40. Schwartz LH, Ginsberg MS, Burt BE, et al. MRI as an alternative to CT-guided biopsy of adrenal masses in patients with lung cancer. *Ann Thorac Surg.* 1998;65:193-197.

41. Dodd LG, Mooney EE, Layfield LJ, Nelson RC. Fine-needle aspiration of the liver and pancreas: a cytology primer for radiologists. *Radiology.* 1997;203:1-9.

42. Reeves AR, Shashadri R, Terotola SO. Recent trends in central venous catheter placement: a comparison of interventional radiology with other specialties. *JVIR.* 2001; 12:1211-1214.

43. Gandhi RT, Getrajdman GI, Brown KT, et al. Placement of subcutaneous chest wall ports ipsilateral to axillary lymph node dissection. *JVIR.* 2003;14(8):1063-1065.

44. Dinkel HP, Mettke B, Schmid F et al. Endovascular treatment of malignant superior vena cava syndrome: is bilateral Wallstent placement superior to unilateral placement? *J Endovasc Ther.* 2003;10(4):788-797.

45. Chatziioannou A, Mourikis AD, Dardoufas K, et al. Stent therapy for malignant superior vena cava syndrome: should be first line therapy or simple adjunct to radiotherapy? *Eur J Rad.* 2003;47:247-250.

46. Kinney TB. Update on inferior vena cava filters. *JVIR.* 2003;14:425-440.

47. Kercher K, Sing RF. Overview of current inferior vena cava filters. *Am Surg.* 2003; 69:643-648.

48. Athanasoulis CA, Kaufman JA, Halpern EF, et al. Inferior Vena Caval filters: review of a 26-year-old single-center experience. Radiology. 2003;26(3):54-66.

49. Farrell TA, Wallace M, Hicks ME. Long-term results of transrenal ureteral occlusion with use of Gianturco coils and gelatin sponge pledgets. *JVIR.* 1997;8(3):449-452.

50. Schild HH, Gunther R, Thelen M. Transrenal ureteral occlusion: results and problems. *JVIR.* 1994;5(2):321-325.

51. Yagi S, Goto T, Kawmoto K, et al. Long-term results of percutaneous balloon dilation for ureterointestinal anastomotic strictures. *Int J Urol.* 2002;9(5):241-246

52. Bierkens AF, Oosterhof GO, Meuleman EJ, Debruyne FM. Anterograde percutaneous treatment of ureterointestinal strictures following urinary diversion. *Eur Urol.* 1996; 30(3):363-368.

53. Parulekar W, DiPrimio G, Matzinger F, et al. Use of small-bore vs. large-bore chest tubes for treatment of malignant pleural effusions. *Chest.* 2001;120:19-25.

54. Tattersall DJ, Traill C, Gleeson FV. Chest drains: does size matter? *Clin Rad.* 2000; 55:415-421.

55. Colt HG. Thorascopic management of malignant pleural effusions. *Clin Chest Med.* 1995;16(3):505-513.

56. Patz EF, McAdams P, Erasmus JJ, et al. Sclerotherapy for malignant pleural effusions: a prospective randomized trial of bleomycin vs doxycycline with small-bore catheter drainage. *Chest.* 1998;113:1305-1311.

57. Jerjes-Sanchez C, Ramirez-Rivera A, Elizalde JJ, et al. Intrapleural fibrinolysis with streptokinase as an adjunctive treatment in hemothorax and empyema: a multicenter trial. *Chest.* 1996;109(6):1514-1519.

58. Pollak JS, Burdge CM, Rosenblatt M, et al. Treatment of malignant pleural effusions with tunneled long-term drainage catheters. *JVIR.* 2004;12:201-208

59. Erickson KV, Wost M, Bynoe R, et al. Primary treatment of malignant pleural effusions: video-assisted thoracoscopic surgery poudrage vs tube thoracostomy. *Am Surg.* 2002; 68(11):955-959.

60. Vonk-Noordegraaf A, Postmus PE, Sutedja TG. Tracheobronchial stenting in the terminal care of cancer patients with central airways obstruction. *Chest.* 2001;120:1811-1814.

61. Monnier P, Mudry A, Stanzel F, et al. The use of the covered Wallstent for the palliative treatment of inoperable tracheobronchial cancers: a prospective, multicenter study. *Chest.* 1996;110:1161-1168.

62. Seijo LM, Sterman DH. Interventional pulmonology. *NEJM.* 2001;332(10):740-749.

63. Wood DE, Liu YH, Vallieres E. Airway stenting for malignant and benign tracheobronchial stenosis. *Ann Thorac Surg.* 2003;76:167-174.

chapter 15

Maintenance of Luminal Patency: Dilation, Endoprosthetics, and Thermal Techniques

Patrick R. Pfau, MD

INTRODUCTION

Advanced malignancy may result in obstruction of the gastrointestinal lumen in patients with esophageal, gastric, pancreatobiliary, colorectal, or metastatic cancers resulting in significant patient morbidity and mortality. Traditional methods of relieving or bypassing malignant obstruction through surgery or chemoradiotherapy are often difficult in patients with a poor performance status or those who need immediate relief of obstruction.

A number of successful endoscopic methods have been developed and are used in clinical practice that provide safe and prompt relief to patients with malignant GI obstruction.

ESOPHAGUS

Esophageal cancer remains an infrequent disease in the United States with approximately 12,000 cases diagnosed per year. However, the incidence of adenocarcinoma of the esophagus and gastroesophageal junction is increasing at a rate greater than any other malignancy. Further, cancer of the esophagus remains a deadly disease with a 5-year survival of less than 10%.[1]

Cancer of the esophagus presents often at an advanced stage and local recurrence is a common problem post esophageal resection. Malignant dysphagia is the most common symptom, occurring in 70% of patients with esophageal cancer.[2] Obstruction of the esophagus can also lead to nausea, vomiting, anorexia, aspiration, and malnutrition.

Surgery in esophageal cancer is now primarily limited to patients thought to be potentially resectable for cure. Radiation with or without chemotherapy is still frequently used for palliation of dysphagia but can be complicated by esophagitis, strictures, and more importantly, does not provide immediate relief of dysphagia. These limitations have led to the development of endoscopic modalities to treat the malignant dysphagia associated with cancer of the esophagus.

Figure 15-1. Through-the-scope (TTS) radial balloon esophageal dilator and polyvinyl wire-guided dilator.

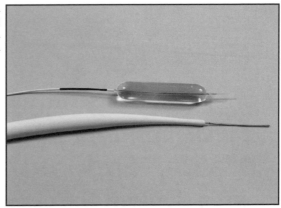

DILATION

Dilation of esophageal strictures has long been used as a temporizing endoscopic therapy for malignant dysphagia. Dilation can provide immediate improvement in swallowing and may be used prior to more definitive therapy such as surgery, radiation, or other endoscopic interventions. However, dilation is not a permanent solution to maintain luminal patency. Further, malignant strictures are complex and often have an unpredictable response to dilation in terms of relief of symptoms and duration of relief of symptoms.[3] Thus, endoscopic dilation of esophageal cancer should be used as a bridge to a more permanent relief of a patient's dysphagia through other methods.

Endoscopic dilation is performed with either polyvinyl wire-guided dilators or through the scope (TTS) balloon dilators (Figure 15-1). A third type of dilator, the Maloney dilator, is passed without endoscopic guidance, should be avoided in malignant strictures due to the complexity of these strictures and potential increased chance for perforation.

Savary dilators are passed over a wire that is placed under direct vision at the time of endoscopy. The endoscope first is negotiated through the tumor and the wire is placed through the working channel of the endoscope. The dilators are then passed over the wire through the tumor, slowly and progressively enlarging the esophageal lumen by using larger diameter dilators. Size of dilators used is primarily an estimation by the endoscopist knowing that dilation of the luminal diameter to 13 to 15 mm is often needed to provide symptomatic relief of a patient's dysphagia. Tight complex strictures and particularly strictures through which the guidewire but not the endoscope can be passed should be performed under fluoroscopy to improve the safety of the procedure.

Radial TTS balloon dilators may be passed under endoscopic visualization through the malignant stricture and then dilated to a predetermined size and force. Theoretical advantages are that the force with which the TTS balloon is applied is in a radial direction without an additional longitudinal force seen in wire-guided dilation.[4] As with wire-guided dilation, more than one dilation session may be needed to stretch the luminal diameter to provide adequate improvement in swallowing.

Dilation is generally safe with complication rates of 2.5 to 10%, comparable to the dilation of benign strictures.[5] Other than as a bridge to more permanent treatment, dilation is useful as an adjunct treatment to other treatment modalities. Dilation is often used along with photodynamic and thermal treatment of strictures. Dilation also may be used after placement of esophageal endoprosthesis within the lumen of the stent either immediately after placement or if dysphagia occurs because of tumor ingrowth, overgrowth, or in patients who have stents placed for external compression of the esophagus. Finally, endoscopic dilation is the treatment of choice with success rates approaching 100% in restoring luminal patency in patients with postesophagectomy strictures and with strictures secondary to scarring from radiation treatment.

THERMAL TECHNIQUES

Thermal techniques, particularly laser therapy, through the endoscope have been used to palliate advanced cancer for over 20 years. BICAP, tumor probes, argon plasma coagulation, and carbon dioxide lasers have been used to treat esophageal carcinoma, but by far the most experience and data are with the neodymium:yttrium aluminum garnet (Nd:Yag) laser.

Laser is a noncontact light treatment that is applied through the working channel of the endoscope and has thermal and photobiochemical effects on the cancerous tissue. The depth and degree of tumor ablation is dependent on power of the laser, duration of exposure, tissue absorption of the light, and the distance of the laser from the tissue.[6]

Practically, treatment is applied with the use of a Nd:YAG probe passed through an endoscope and the laser light is applied with direct endoscopic visualization. Treatment that begins distal to proximal is preferred, even if dilation is needed prior to treatment. However, proximal endoscopic laser treatment can be useful and may be the only endoscopic method possible when the lumen is nearly completely obstructed. Treatment is applied in a circumferential manner, slowly enlarging the esophageal lumen. Total energy is recorded during treatment but endoscopic evidence of a coagulation effect and then vaporization of the tumor tissue is the primary way that determination of adequate treatment is made. The goal of treatment is vaporization of tumor tissue to restore luminal integrity. Repeat treatment 24 to 48 hours after the first treatment is often needed to debride necrotic tumor tissue with the endoscope and possibly apply more therapy.

Success of laser therapy, with resumption of oral intake as the marker of success, is approximately 85% with success rates ranging in the literature from 64% to 100%.[7-10] The tumor length and circumference as well as degree of tumor obstruction affect the ability of Nd:YAG laser to successfully palliate dysphagia secondary to esophageal cancer.[8] Laser therapy is most suited for short tumors, less than 5 cm, exophytic discrete strictures, and proximal lesions that are not suitable for other modes of endoscopic treatment, particularly esophageal stenting. Complication rates range from 1% to 15% with perforation, creation of a tracheo-esophageal fistula, and bleeding being the most common problems associated with laser treatment.[11] The greatest limitation is the need for frequent treatment sessions with dysphagia free intervals lasting only 2 to 4 months. If laser is the sole palliative treatment modality the patient is committed to multiple endoscopies and repeat laser applications.

Argon plasma coagulation (APC) is a relatively new endoscopic thermal technology that causes tissue coagulation and destruction through a noncontact probe that transfers energy via electrically charged argon gas. The largest study examining endoscopic APC treatment of malignant dysphagia had a success rate of 84%, approaching the success found with Nd:YAG laser.[12] However, APC treatment requires even more frequent sessions and is limited in the palliative treatment of esophageal cancer because of limited tissue destruction depth to only 2 to 3 mm.[13] No data exists directly comparing APC to Nd:YAG laser for the palliative treatment of malignant dysphagia.

While laser or APC treatment are both limited as a primary treatment to treating short, discrete strictures or proximal tumors, both have been found to be useful when used as adjuvant therapy, particularly in association with esophageal stents. Laser therapy is effective in treating tumor ingrowth or tumor overgrowth at the proximal or distal aspect of the stent by recanalizing a lumen through the stent. Laser treatment in a stent is safe, extremely easy to perform, and possibly more cost-effective than placing a second esophageal stent within the lumen of the original stent.

PHOTODYNAMIC THERAPY

Photodynamic therapy is another thermal technique used in the palliation of esophageal cancer that couples the use of a photosensitizer with the delivery of light directly to the tumor resulting in selective destruction of tumor cells. In the treatment of advanced esophageal cancer, photosensitizers are usually porphyrin based, the most commonly used being porfimer sodium or Photofrin II (Axcan, Birmington, Ala). Photosensitizers are selectively taken up and concentrated in tumor cells, resulting in a high therapeutic index. Reasons why photosensitizers are retained to a greater degree in tumor cells is complex and not completely understood. Theories include that larger amounts of porphyrins are thought to pass through a tumor's neovasculature, the lymphatics of tumors may poorly drain the sensitizer, and transport of the sensitizer into tumor cells may be greater because photosensitizers bind to low-density lipoproteins which preferentially are carried into the tumor cells.[14]

Activation of the photosensitizer is performed by delivery of light to the area of the tumor. In esophageal cancer this is performed via laser light carried to the tumor by a flexible endoscope and applied with a cigar-shaped cylindrical diffusing fiber that allows light to be transmitted circumferentially within the esophagus. The sensitizer is given intravenously 48 hours before the delivery of the light with the endoscope. Red light with a standardized wavelength and light dosimetry have been developed for advanced esophageal cancer to produce a light penetration of approximately 5 mm resulting in maximal tumoricidal efficacy while minimizing complications.[15]

Delivery of the light to the sensitized tissue causes generation of oxygen radicals and molecular oxygen. The generated oxygen radicals affect cell plasma and organelle membranes particularly in mitochondria resulting in a direct cytotoxic effect. Tumor vasculature endothelium is thought to be affected greater than normal tissue resulting in vasoconstriction, thrombosis, and tumor death as a result of hypoxia.[14] Besides direct tumor cell death and tissue necrosis, PDT is thought to have other antitumor effects including induction of apoptosis, stimulation of the immune system, and an overall increased cytokine based inflammatory response.

The length of the tumor is treated in as many stages as needed at the first treatment session, usually with the use of a 2.5 or 5.0 cm cylindrical fiber passed through the endoscope. The tumor is treated in a distal to proximal step-wise fashion with attempts to ensure the length of the tumor has been exposed to the laser light. Forty-eight hours after the first treatment an upper endoscopy is repeated to debride necrotic tumor and retreat any residual tumor that is seen (Figure 15-2). Timing of retreatment is not standardized and should be based upon the recurrence of symptoms, the physical amount of tumor recurrence, and other treatment options that may be available to the patient.

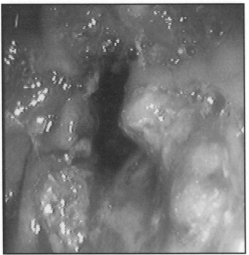

Figure 15-2A. Endoscopic app-earance of an obstructing eso-phageal cancer. *For a full-color version, see page CA-X of the Color Atlas.*

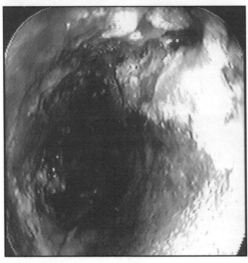

Figure 15-2B. Endoscopic visu-alization of same patient 48 hours after application of photo-dynamic therapy showing ex-tensive tissue necrosis and tumor debris. *For a full-color version, see page CA-X of the Color Atlas.*

Through anecdotal experience it has been shown that multiple treatment sessions over a period of months may be applied safely and effectively.

Multiple nonrandomized retrospective studies have stated success rates for PDT in esophageal cancer to range from 60% to 90% with success usually defined as improve-ment in dysphagia scores.[10,16] Multiple sessions are often required because of return of dysphagia symptoms with duration of each treatment session ranging from 9 to 14 weeks.[17,18] No definitive improvement in survival has been found with the use of PDT. PDT has been found to be successful and safe before and after radiation/chemotherapy and successful in treating tumor overgrowth and ingrowth within esophageal stents.[19]

Figure 15-2C. Post-treatment image demonstrating no endoscopic evidence of tumor with restoration of the esophageal lumen. *For a full-color version, see page CA-XI of the Color Atlas.*

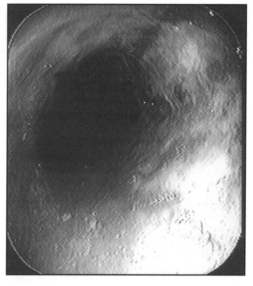

The most frequent toxicity associated with PDT is skin photosensitivity. This is secondary to the propensity for the photosensitizer to collect in the skin and then be activated upon exposure to sunlight. Risk for skin photosensitivity is generally limited to the first 4 weeks post-treatment. Exposure to sunlight usually results in mild erythema and sunburn but second degree burns and blistering burns are frequently reported. Patient education is essential and patients should be instructed to avoid direct sunlight for the first 30 days after each treatment with protective eyewear, headwear, and clothes to be worn when going outside for any extended time period.

Mild procedure related toxicities with PDT include chest pain, nausea, and occasional self-limited fevers secondary to inflammation. Transient increase in dysphagia is common secondary to debris, necrosis, and swelling immediately after therapy. This is easily treated 48 hours after treatment by endoscopic clearance of the necrotic debris.

Major complications include esophageal stricture or fistula with incidence of post-PDT stricture formation ranging from 0% to 21% and fistula formation from 0% to 14%.[14] As more experience has been gained with PDT and uniform light dosimetry is applied these complication rates have become less frequent. Fistula formation can be further lessened through correct staging with endoscopic ultrasound and bronchoscopy if tracheal involvement is suspected. Treatment of post-PDT strictures is easily managed with endoscopic dilation while fistulas require a covered esophageal stent for treatment.

Two randomized studies have compared PDT to Nd:YAG laser for the palliation of advanced esophageal cancer.[20,21] These studies showed better and longer relief of dysphagia with PDT (84 days vs 53 days) as compared to laser. Mild toxicities, particularly photosensitivity, were more common with PDT, but major complications (most notably perforation) occurred more frequently with laser treatment.

Advantages of PDT are ease of use and relatively low serious complication rates. PDT is especially useful for proximal esophageal cervical tumors and gastroesophageal junction tumors where it is sometimes difficult to place an esophageal stent. Further, as opposed to esophageal stents, previous chemoradiotherapy does not increase or affect the complication rate of PDT. PDT is also very efficient for near complete obstruction of the lumen in which case only the small PDT fiber needs to be advanced through or into the tumor.

Major drawbacks of PDT include the need for multiple repeated treatments and cost, with PDT being arguably the most expensive of modalities available for esophageal cancer dysphagia palliation. Finally, the skin photosensitivity and the need to avoid sunlight for 4 to 6 weeks is an important aspect to consider in patients with average survival rates of 6 months or less.

ESOPHAGEAL STENTS

The first endoscopic stenting of malignant dysphagia was performed with plastic endosprosthesis. The originally designed plastic stents were difficult to deploy and extremely rigid leading to an unacceptable high complication rate. Further, the original plastic stents had a limited diameter leading to only minimal improvement in a patient's dysphagia.

Since the early 1990s, self-expanding metal stents (SEMS) have become the primary stents used to palliate inoperable esophageal cancer. Placement of the various types of SEMS is based on the same principles using a combination of endoscopy and fluoroscopy. Endoscopy should always be performed first to measure the length of the tumor, determine the position of the tumor (cervical, midesophagus, or crossing the gastroesophageal junction), and estimate the luminal diameter. Selection of stent length should be at least 2 to 3 cm above and below the proximal and distal aspects of the tumor. Cervical tumors within a few centimeters of the upper esophageal sphincter are thought to be a relative contraindication to stent placement because of the possibility of respiratory compromise and permanent foreign body sensation caused by the proximal aspect of the stent. Recently however, groups have reported acceptable success rates with minimal complications when stenting cervical tumors.[22] Stent diameters range from 16 to 24 mm with a general rule to use smaller diameter stents for midesophageal tumors to prevent perforation and larger diameter stents in GE junction tumors to prevent stent migration.

Esophageal stents come with or without polyurethane coverings to prevent the late complication of tumor ingrowth through the stent. Care should be used in placing covered stents across the GE junction because of increased chance of migration without the bare metal to embed into the esophageal mucosa and submucosa to hold the stent in place.[23] Studies have shown that the newer covered stents, which are of greater central and proximal diameter and have areas of uncovered stent on both ends of the stent, do not have an increased migration rate even when crossing the cardia.[24]

If a malignant stricture is present at the time of endoscopy, it may need to be first dilated to 9 to 11 mm prior to the placement of the stent so that the delivery system that measures from 7 to 11 mm can pass through the stricture. Before removing the endoscope the proximal and distal aspects of the tumor are marked to aid in placement of the stent under fluoroscopy. This can be performed with external markers, internal clips placed onto the esophageal mucosa, or a contrast agent that can be injected into the submucosa just above and below the tumor. A stiff guidewire is then placed through the endoscope across the stricture into the stomach, and the endoscope is subsequently removed leaving the wire in place. The stent is placed under fluoroscopic control, ensuring the stent extends 2 to 3 cm above and below the malignant stricture to allow com-

Figure 15-3A. Gastroesophageal junction tumor prior to placement of esophageal stent. *For a full-color version, see page CA-XI of the Color Atlas.*

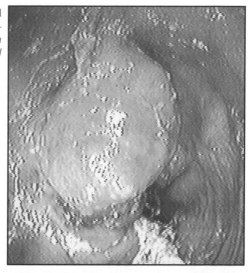

Figure 15-3B. Appearance of stent immediately after deployment shows a recreated lumen. *For a full-color version, see page CA-XII of the Color Atlas.*

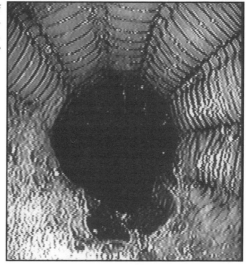

plete covering of the tumor (because of the shortening that occurs in some stents after deployment). Based upon the type of stent used repositioning of the stent can be performed during or just after deployment. The endoscope can be passed back into the esophagus to check the proximal position of the stent (Figure 15-3). SEMS then fully expand to their desired maximal diameter, expanding the esophageal lumen over the next 1 to 2 days. This ensures maximal palliation while lessening the immediate complications that were seen with the rigid plastic stents. On Day 0 or 1, chest x-ray/abdominal films or barium swallow may be performed to verify correct stent location and improvement in luminal diameter (Figure 15-4).

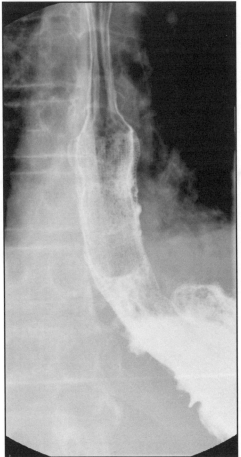

Figure 15-4. Barium swallow of patient on day 1 postesophageal stent shows contrast freely flowing through the esophageal lumen and verifies stent placement in distal esophagus, bridging the gastroesophageal junction.

Available SEMS in the United States include the Wallstent II (Microvasive, Natick, Mass), the Ultraflex stent (Microvasive) and the Gianturco Z-stent (Wilson Cook Medical, Winston-Salem, NC) (Figure 15-5 and 15-6). The majority of stents are covered as this significantly decreases the rate of tumor in-growth through the stent and the need for re-intervention because of recurrent dysphagia. Stents are still available in uncovered versions for tumors crossing the GE junction or tumors causing external compression to potentially lessen the migration rate. Though each patient must be individualized generally the larger stents should be placed across the GE junction to avoid migration and the smaller diameter stents should be placed in tight midesophageal strictures to avoid the possibility of perforation with stent expansion. Finally, because of the significant amount of reflux associated with stents placed across the GE junction a recently developed version of the Z-stent—the Dua antireflux stent—has become available (Figure 15-7). This stent has a valve or windsock on the distal aspect of the stent,

Figure 15-5A. The covered esophageal Wallstent.

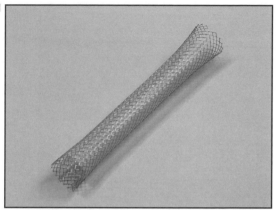

Figure 15-5B. The covered covered esophageal Z-stent. *For a full-color version, see page CA-XII of the Color Atlas.*

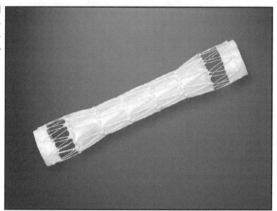

Figure 15-6. Illustration of an esophageal Flamingo stent bridging a distal esophageal tumor. *For a full-color version, see page CA-XIII of the Color Atlas.*

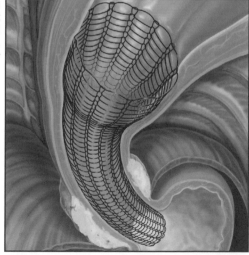

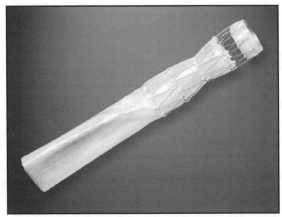

Figure 15-7. Covered Dua stent with distal sleeve to prevent acid reflux into esophagus post-stent deployment. *For a full-color version, see page CA-XIII of the Color Atlas.*

which theoretically reduces the amount of acid reflux across the stent into the esophagus post stent deployment.[25]

A recent study compared the various makes of esophageal stents (Ultraflex stent, Z-stent, and Flamingo Wallstent [available in Europe]) for efficacy and safety in 100 consecutive patients.[26] Each stent type resulted in a significant improvement in dysphagia and similar reintervention rates of 24% to 33%. There was no statistical difference in complication rates between the different stents, but a trend of higher major complications of 1.5 to 2 times was seen with placement of the Z-stent. A smaller comparative study found Ultraflex stents to have lower procedure-related mortality and complication rates when compared to esophageal Wallstents.[27]

A recently developed self-expanding plastic stent (Polyflex [Rusch, Duluth, Ga]) has been shown to have similar success, complication, and re-intervention rates compared to historical numbers reported with SEMS.[28] However, data on self-expanding plastic stents are still very limited with no direct comparison to metal stents.

Multiple series exist which examine patient outcomes using esophageal self-expanding metal stents to treat malignant dysphagia. Examining the larger studies in the literature technical deployment is successful in greater than 95% of cases. Dysphagia scores routinely improve in 75% to 95% of patients, with dysphagia scores improving a mean of 2 in most studies using a 4 or 6 point scale.[9,10,13,29,30] Successful palliation is near immediate in the first 24 to 48 hours poststent insertion.

Chest pain postprocedure occurs in almost 100% of patients secondary to the expansile force of the stent. Major immediate and early complications include perforation, fistula formation, bleeding, and aspiration of gastric contents. On average major complications occur in as many as 10% to 20% of patients after having an esophageal stent placed.[9,10,13] Studies have shown an increased major complication rate in patients who have received prior or are receiving concurrent chemotherapy and/or radiation, particularly an increased perforation rate because of the presumed weakened tissues.[31,32]

Later complications include stent migration and tumor ingrowth and overgrowth. Stent migration has been reported to occur in 0% to 6% of placed SEMS with increased migration rates when the stent is placed across the cardia.[9,10,13,29,30] Migration is likely increased with covered stents, but if larger diameter covered stents are used migration rates of covered stents do not appear to be significantly increased. With uncovered stents tumor ingrowth was common, 8% to 35%, with resultant recurrent dysphagia and need for repeat intervention to maintain luminal patency.[9,10,13] The problem of tumor ingrowth has been for the most part solved with the increasing use of covered stents. With covered stents, tumor overgrowth at the distal or proximal edge of the stent has become the more frequent problem. This may be due to infiltration of the tumor over the edge or through the uncovered aspect of the stent. Benign epithelial hyperplasia, granulation tissue, and tissue fibrosis where the edge of the bare stent contacts the esophageal mucosa can also lead to stent obstruction. Other causes of dysphagia are food impaction within the stent and angulation of the stent as it crosses the GE junction. Re-intervention with dilation, second stent placement, or application of thermal techniques occurs at a mean of 80 days after stent placement, but with proper patient screening and stent selection reintervention is not needed in the majority of patients for more than 120 days.

Survival poststenting has been found to be between 3 and 6 months in the majority of studies with mortality related to the advanced state of the cancer. Thirty day mortality post-stent placement has been reported to be as high as 26%, with up to 3% to 16% mortality directly attributed to the stent placement.[13,33,34]

SEMS has a distinct advantage over other endoscopic modalities in that stents can successfully treat tracheo-esophageal fistulas and obstruction of the esophageal lumen secondary to extrinsic compression from metastatic tumor, mediastinal masses, or lymphadenopathy. Placement of a covered metal stent with the covered aspect of the stent sealing the fistula has become the treatment of choice in patients with esophageal cancer associated with a fistula. Studies are small but success rates in sealing a fistula have been found to be 90% or greater with covered esophageal stents placed under combined endoscopic and fluoroscopic control.[32,34,35] Dysphagia scores decrease post-stent placement in patients with external compression, but not to as great a degree as found when stents are placed to relieve intrinsic malignant blockage of the esophagus. The main complication rate of placing a stent for extrinsic compression is stent migration due to the fact that no luminal tumor is present to better anchor the stent within the esophagus.

Four studies have compared thermal therapy, primarily Nd:YAG laser to esophageal stent therapy in treating malignant dysphagia.[36-39] Two studies show a greater degree of improvement in dysphagia with SEMS while two other studies showed no difference in efficacy between esophageal stents and laser therapy. More complications overall were found in patients treated with laser than stents and the use of laser therapy required more frequent endoscopic reintervention to maintain swallowing. One of four studies did show a survival advantage with laser and a faster decrease in health related quality of life in patients who had SEMS placed. The stent group in this study had a median survival of only 4.7 weeks with a poor improvement in dysphagia post-stent likely secondary to selection of patients with a very poor pretreatment health and performance status.

UPPER GASTROINTESTINAL OBSTRUCTION

Malignant obstruction of the upper GI tract may occur with a variety of tumors found not to be resectable for cure including gastric cancer, duodenal cancer, compression from pancreatobiliary cancer, and (rarely) metastatic disease. The most commonly encountered is duodenal obstruction from pancreatic cancer which occurs in 15% to

30% of cases of nonresectable pancreatic cancer.[40] Malignant upper GI obstruction leads to significant patient morbidity including nausea, vomiting, abdominal pain, esophagitis, and malnutrition. Further, these symptoms interfere with patients' ability to receive and tolerate chemotherapeutic medications.

The traditional treatment of gastric outlet and duodenal obstruction is surgical bypass, most commonly a palliative gastrojejunostomy which has been found to have high success rates of 90% or greater in relieving obstructive symptoms. However, surgical bypass can carry a complication rate as high as 25% to 35% with a perioperative mortality of 2%.[40,41] Patients with worse outcomes include patients with malignant ascites, carcinomatosis, multiple areas of obstruction, and clinically-advanced disease associated with poor performance status.[42]

Because of these reasons less invasive methods to palliate upper intestinal obstruction have been sought. Endoscopic-guided balloon dilation, thermal treatment with Nd:YAG laser, or dithermal snare debulking through the endoscope have been tried in gastric and duodenal obstruction with only moderate and short-term success.[42,43] Thus, dilation and thermal methods have largely been abandoned as a primary treatment because of their very short temporizing benefit requiring multiple interventions. The optimal nonsurgical method to restore gastric and duodenal luminal patency has become the placement of expandable metal stents across the areas of malignant obstruction. The majority of early data on using SEMS in treating gastroduodenal obstruction is found in interventional radiology literature where expandable esophageal stents were placed in the area of gastric or duodenal obstruction under fluoroscopic control. Endoscopic placement of SEMS in the stomach or duodenum was limited because delivery systems were not long enough to place stents through upper endoscopes.

Combined endoscopic and fluoroscopic placement of enteral stents has become possible and more common with the development of the Enteral Wallstent (Microvasive Endoscopy) and delivery system placed through a therapeutic endoscope (Figure 15-8). Advantages of endoscopic/fluoroscopic placement of SEMS over placement with fluoroscopy alone are greater control of the stent device, greater ability to visualize, and subsequently cross tight stenoses, and a distinct mechanical advantage in tumors in the duodenum where passing the stent through an endoscope avoids gastric looping of the delivery system while shortening the entire system—increasing technical ease and success.[44]

Placement of enteral stents follow the same general principles as placing esophageal stents except that the proximal aspect of the tumor and stent can be directly visualized before and during deployment (Figures 15-9 and 15-10). Attempts are first made to traverse the strictured tumor with the endoscope. If the endoscope can traverse through and past the malignant stricture, the distal and proximal aspects of the tumor should be marked with radiopaque dye or endoclips. Stent size should extend 2 to 3 cm past the proximal and distal aspects of the tumor. If the endoscope diameter is too large to traverse a tight stricture, a wire with the use of a biliary catheter is used to cross the stricture under fluoroscopic control. Using the wire as a guide, the catheter is then placed through the stricture and dye is injected through the catheter to obtain radiologic images of the length and features of the stricture. The entire system is then passed over the wire, through the endoscope, and across the stricture. Balloon dilation may be necessary to pass the stent delivery system through the stricture. Proximal and distal aspects of the stent and its deployment can be directly visualized under fluoroscopy with the aid of endoscopic visualization. If the stent does not appear to fully open, a second stent can

Figure 15-8. Enteral Wallstent with associated 255 cm delivery system allowing placement of stent via the endoscope.

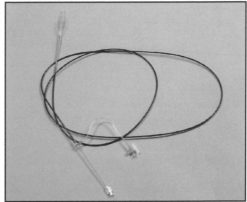

Figure 15-9A. Endoscopic visualization of narrowed duodenal lumen secondary to metastatic cancer. *For a full-color version, see page CA-XIV of the Color Atlas.*

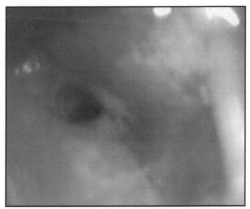

Figure 15-9B. Status postplacement of enteral stent restoring the duodenal lumen. At the superior aspect of the lumen a biliary Wallstent can be seen emanating from the papilla that was previously placed for bile duct obstruction secondary to the cancer. *For a full-color version, see page CA-XIV of the Color Atlas.*

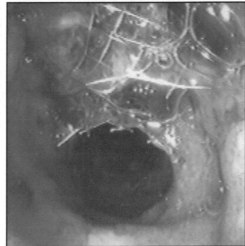

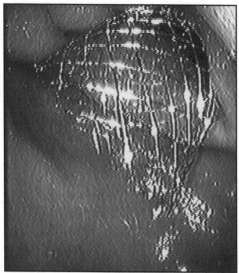

Figure 15-10. Enteral Wallstent seen extending proximally through the pylorus into the stomach. Stent was placed through pylorus into duodenum for malignant gastric outlet obstruction. *For a full-color version, see page CA-XV of the Color Atlas.*

be deployed with overlapping of the two stents, again ensuring there is stent proximal and distal to the tumor.

Data on outcome of SEMS placed by endoscopy in patients with malignant gastro-duodenal obstruction is limited by the fact that studies in the literature are retrospective and small (less than 50 patients).[40,43-50] Technical placement of the stents is almost always successful with success rates of 90% to 100%. Larger studies report improvement in symptoms and improvement in diet in approximately 80% of patients. Almost all patients are able to tolerate some oral intake after stent placement, but not necessarily a full solid diet. Studies in which weight and Karnofsky score have been measured have found a slight increase in both after placement of an enteral stent for malignant upper tract obstruction.

Immediate complications are primarily bleeding and perforation. Reported rates of immediate complications are less than 5%,[40,43-50] but are likely under-reported in the literature and slightly higher in practice. Late complications include tumor overgrowth and ingrowth. This may lead to the need for endoscopic reintervention in approximately 15% to 25% of patients with enteral stents. Reintervention usually consists of a second stent placed across the tumor or restoration of the lumen with thermal methods such as APC or Nd:YAG laser. The other main late complication is stent migration. SEMS migration may be asymptomatic or lead to bleeding or perforation as the edges/ends of the stent contact normal mucosa. Obstruction because of altered angulation of the stent in the lumen may occur as the already expanded stent migrates distally in the small intestine. Stent migration occurs in <5% of cases and is a less frequent problem than the migration seen with esophageal metallic stenting.

Two studies have compared surgical bypass with enteral stent placement for gastric or duodenal obstruction.[45,51] One study showed similar survival in both groups of 90 days. Patients who had enteral stents placed had less inpatient hospital days and lower overall hospital charges than the surgical group. The second comparative study found a lower 30-day mortality rate with stents as opposed to surgery (0% vs 18%). Limitation of these studies must be noted as both studies were retrospective and had very small amount of patients. Likely no accurate prospective study will be performed comparing surgical versus endoscopic palliation of upper GI obstruction as surgery remains the first treatment of choice in a patient group with a high performance status and relatively extended expected survival. Enteral stenting is performed more frequently in patients who tend to be more ill, more symptomatic, have a shorter expected survival, and who would not tolerate surgery.

Finally, survival postenteral stenting is short, with median survival ranging from 7 to 20 weeks in most studies.[40,43,45-47,49] As with methods to maintain esophageal lumen patency, enteral stenting is a palliative modality in patients with advanced gastric or pancreato-biliary malignancies who cannot undergo surgery for cure or palliation. No data have shown that enteral stenting has a definitive impact on survival.

COLORECTAL OBSTRUCTION

Colon cancer may present with complete or near complete luminal obstruction in up to 30% of patients.[52] Patients who present with obstruction often have advanced disease and are usually found to have Dukes stage C or D disease at the time of surgery.[53] Metastatic disease, peritoneal carcinomatosis, and extrinsic compression from genitourinary tumors may also cause malignant large bowel obstruction.[54] Patients with malignant obstruction of the colon will frequently present malnourished, dehydrated, and severely ill.

The traditional therapy of malignant large bowel obstruction, like that of upper GI obstruction, is surgery. The three-stage surgery for obstructing colon cancer —decompressing colostomy, a second operation for resection of the tumor, and a third to reconnect the large intestine—has largely been discontinued because of the number of procedures, time needed for treatment, and high associated morbidity and mortality. Presently, a two-step surgery may be performed: a Hartmann's procedure, initially performed for decompression and resection, followed by a second surgery to restore bowel continuity. Finally, a one-step procedure can be performed with primary resection and anastomosis on an unprepped bowel, if extensive perioperative cleansing of the bowel can be done. However, overall morbidity is 40% in cases when surgery is performed on an unprepped obstructing colon cancer.[55] Mortality ranges from 5% to 32% for surgical procedures for these patients.[55,56] Appropriate patient selection is important with worse outcome associated with patients who have advanced disease, poor performance status, and associated diffuse disease such as ascites or carcinomatosis.[42]

Due to the morbidity and mortality associated with the surgical treatment of acute malignant large bowel obstruction less invasive modalities have been developed to deal with the obstruction and restore luminal patency. The two main methods used are laser therapy through the colonoscope or the placement of colonic stents via the endoscope with fluoroscopic guidance or with fluoroscopy alone. Nonsurgical treatment, particularly stent placement, has become more frequent in both palliative treatment of colorectal obstruction and as a temporizing resolution of the obstruction so the patient may be subsequently prepped for a one-step surgery.

Laser therapy, usually Nd:YAG has been used to recanalize the colonic lumen in a method similar to how laser is used to palliate nonresectable esophageal cancer. A laser probe is passed through the working channel of a colonoscope. Thermal energy provided under direct endoscopic visualization is used to partially ablate the tumor in a circumferential manner, creating a workable colon lumen so that the obstruction can be relieved.

Success rates of treating obstruction in colon cancer with laser are 75% to 90% with relief of obstructive symptoms and the ability to pass stool.[54] Repetitive sessions are almost always needed because of recurrent symptoms. Complication rates range from 2% to 15% with the most common complications being bleeding or perforation, both of which can require urgent surgery. Limitations of laser for obstructive colon cancer are the need for multiple sessions, often in frail patients; limited success with larger and longer tumors; and finally, laser therapy is more technically difficult and less successful in tumors proximal to the sigmoid colon.

SEMS are increasingly being used to acutely decompress the colon in patients with either obstructing colon cancer or metastatic and extrinsic tumors causing large bowel obstruction. Technique for deployment is similar to deployment in the upper digestive tract and like upper tract tumors colonic stents were originally primarily placed by interventional radiologists because of the lack of a colonic stent that could be placed through the colonoscope. Data concerning the placement of colonic stents are found in both the radiology and gastroenterology literature and whether colonic stents are placed by radiologists or gastroenterologists is institution based. Three colonic stents are available in the United States. The Enteral Wallstent is the same stent used for stent placement in the upper GI tract and is the only colonic stent that has a delivery system that that can pass through the working channel of a colonoscope. The colonic Z-stent (Wilson-Cook Medical) and the Bard (Tempe, Ariz) colonic stent do not pass through the colonoscope, but are placed under fluoroscopy sometimes with a colonoscope alongside the stent and its delivery system to provide some endoscopic visualization. Placement of the enteral Wallstent through the colonoscope has the advantage of direct visualization of the tumor and the stent at deployment. TTS stents improve the mechanical advantage during placement and allow placement of colon stents in the more proximal colon. Placement of colonic stents without endoscopic guidance is limited to the very distal colon because of the inability of the delivery system with fluoroscopy alone to maneuver through the sigmoid colon.

Outcome data in the endoscopic and radiology literature derives mostly from retrospective series of 80 patients or less. Technical success in placing colonic metal stents can be achieved in greater than 90% of patients. Clinical success, defined as relief of obstruction in palliative cases or as a temporizing measure prior to surgery, approaches 90%.[44,50,54,57]

The largest prospective study examining colonic stents to treat obstruction as a bridge to surgery found that 85% of patients could undergo a primary anastomosis without the need for a colostomy after stent placement. Only 41% of patients could be treated successfully with one operation if surgery was performed without prior colonic stenting.[58] Further, complications and in-patient stay were less when colonic obstruction was first treated with a SEMS. A review of all publications concerning colonic stents published in the literature from 1990 to 2000 revealed an 85% technical success rate and 95% of stent patients able to undergo a one-stage operation.[57] Clinical success rates with relief of the obstruction for patients treated for palliation were in the range of 85% to 95%.[57] Stent patency at 3 and 6 months has been found in greater than 90% of patients[59] and many reports exist of palliation secondary to colon stent lasting greater than 1 year after the placement of the stent.

Placing stents in the colon can be more challenging than in the upper GI tract because of the angulation and tortuosity of the colon. Though the through the scope Enteral Wallstent allows placement of a colonic stent in the proximal colon, the majority of data still exists on stents placed in the distal colon. Whether success and complication rates are equal for stents placed in the proximal colon is unknown. Perforation occurs in 0% to 7% of cases either at the time of deployment due to stent expansion or later secondary to stent migration.[57] Predilation of a malignant colon stricture may increase the rate of perforation and should be avoided. Migration occurs in 3% to 22% of colon stents placed.[57] Migration of a stent may be asymptomatic, result in perforation, or result in recurrent obstruction because the tumor is no longer stented or because the stent itself causes physical obstruction at an acute angulation of the colon. Bleeding secondary to stent insertion occurs in 0% to 5% of cases and reobstruction of the lumen by tumor occurs in 0% to 15% of patients.[57] Tumor ingrowth or overgrowth may be managed with repeat stenting or with endoscopic guided laser treatment. Complications unique to colon stents placed distally in the rectum are tenesmus and incontinence.

Since there has been a noted increased risk of perforation with dilation prior to the placement of a colon stent, a number of researchers have found success in treating malignant colon obstruction with a combination of Nd:YAG laser and SEMS.[60,61] In these studies Nd:YAG laser photoablation was used to initially restore a completely obstructed or near completely obstructed lumen. This allowed passage of a guidewire and then stent delivery system through the previously blocked lumen. Success rates of laser plus stenting have equaled the success of laser or SEMS alone without any increase in complication rate.

Conclusion

Endoscopic palliation can provide a less invasive and highly successful means to treat GI obstruction secondary to advanced malignant disease. The use of various endoscopic thermal treatment methods and enteral stenting has expanded from clinical tertiary research centers to general clinical practice. Future challenges are to design and perform prospective trials that compare the various endoscopic methods to palliate esophageal cancer and to better compare endoscopic to surgical palliation for upper and lower tract cancer. This will enable the practicing clinician the ability to choose the safest, most efficacious, and even most cost-efficient method to restore GI luminal patency, and provide symptomatic palliation for their individual patient.

References

1. Wong R, Malthaner R. Esophageal cancer: a systematic review. *Curr Probl Cancer.* 2000; 24:297-373.
2. Brierley JD, Oza AM. Radiation and chemotherapy in the management of malignant esophageal strictures. *Gastrointest Endosc Clin N Am.* 1998;8 451-453.
3. Esophageal dilation: guidelines for clinical application. *Gastrointest Endosc.* 1991;37: 122-124, 1991.
4. Grahm DY, Smith JL. Balloon dilation of benign and malignant esophageal strictures. *Gastrointest Endosc.* 1985;31:171-174.
5. Ko G, Song, H, Hong H, et al. Malignant esophagogastric junction obstruction: Efficacy of balloon dilation combined with chemotherapy and/or radiation therapy. *Cardiovasc Intervent Radiol.* 2003;26:141-145.

6. Mayoral W, Fleischer DE. Laser therapy for malignant esophageal strictures. *Techniques in Gastrointestinal Endoscopy.* 1999;1:82-85.

7. Naveau S, Chiesa A, Poynard T, et al. Endoscopic Nd: YAG laser as palliative treatment for esophageal and cardia cancer: parameters affecting long-term outcome. *Dig Dis Sci.* 1990;35:294-301.

8. Low DE, Pagliero KM. Prospective randomized clinical trial comparing brachytherapy and laser photoablation for palliation of esophageal cancer *J Thorac Cardiac Surg.* 1992; 104:173-178.

9. Weigel TL, Frumiento C, Gaumnitz E. Endolumimal palliation for dysphagia secondary to esophageal carcinoma. *Surg Clin N Am.* 2002;82:747-761.

10. Adler DG, Baron TH. Endoscopic palliation of malignant dysphagia. *Mayo Clin Proc.* 2001;76:731-738.

11. Gossner L, Ell C. Malignant strictures. Thermal treatment. *Gastrointest Endosc Clin N Am.* 1998;8:443-454.

12. Heindorff H, Wojdemann M, Bisgaard T, et al. Endoscopic palliation of inoperable cancer of the oesophagus or cardia by argon electrocoagulation. *Scand J Gastroenterol.* 1998; 33:21-23.

13. Leiper L, Morris AI. Treatment of oesophago-gastric tumours. *Endoscopy.* 2002;34: 139-145.

14. Pfau P, Hsi A, Kochman ML. Photodynamic therapy for esophageal carcinoma. *Techniques in Gastrointestinal Endoscopy.* 1999;1:86-90.

15. Lightdale C. Role of photodynamic therapy in the management of advanced esophageal cancer. *Gastrointest Endosc Clin N Am.* 2000;10:397-408.

16. Luketich JD, Christie NA, Buenaventura PO, et al. Endoscopic photodynamic therapy for obstructing esophageal cancer; 77 cases over a 2-year period. *Surg Endosc.* 2000;14: 653-657.

17. Thomas RJ, Abbott M, Bhathal PS, et al. High-dose photoirradiation of esophageal cancer. *Ann Surg.* 1987;206:193-199.

18. Schweitzer VG, Bologna S, Batra SK. Photodynamic therapy for treatment of esophageal cancer: a preliminary report. *Laryngoscope.* 1993;103:699-703.

19. Scheider DM, Siemens M, Cirocco M, et al. Photodynamic therapy for the treatment of tumor ingrowth in expandable esophageal stents. *Endoscopy.* 1997;29:271-274.

20. Lightdale CJ, Heier SK, Marcon SE, et al. Photodynamic therapy with porfimer sodium versus thermal ablation with Nd:YAG laser for palliation of esophageal cancer: a multicenter randomized trial. *Gastrointest Endosc.* 1995;42:507-512.

21. Heier SK, Rothman SK, Heier LM, et al. Photodynamic therapy for obstructing esophageal cancer: light dosimetry and randomized comparison with Nd:YAG laser therapy. *Gastroenterology.* 1995;109:63-73.

22. Profili S, Meloni GB, Feo CF, et al. Self-expandable metal stents in the management of cervical oesophageal and/or hypopharyngeal strictures. *Clinical Radiology.* 2002;57: 1028-1033.

23. Siersema PD, Marcon N, Vakil N. Metal stents for tumors of the distal esophagus and gastric cardia. *Endoscopy.* 2003;35:79-85.

24. Vakil N, Morris AI, Marcon N, et al. A prospective, randomized, controlled trial of covered expandable metal stents in the palliation of malignant esophageal obstruction at the gastroesophageal junction. *Am J Gastroenterol.* 2001;96:1791-1796.

25. Dua KS. Antireflux stents in tumors of the cardia. *Amer J Med.* 2001;111:190S-196S

26. Siersema PD, Hop WCJ, van Blankenstein M, et al. A comparison of 3 types of covered metal stents for the palliation of patients with dysphagia caused by esophagogastric carcinoma: a prospective, randomized study. *Gastrointest Endosc.* 2001;54:145-153.

27. Schmassmann A, Meyenberger C, Knuchel J, et al. Self-expanding metal stents in malignant esophageal obstruction: a comparison between two stent types. *Am J Gastroenterol.* 1997;92:400-406.

28. Dormann AJ, Eisendrath P, Wigginghaus B, et al. Palliation of esophageal carcinoma with a new self-expanding plastic stent. *Endoscopy.* 2003;35:207-211.

29. Segalin A, Bonavina L, Carazzone, et al. Improving results of esophageal stenting: a study on 160 consecutive unselected patients. *Endoscopy.* 1997;29:701-709.

30. Cwikiel W, Tranberg KG, Cwikiel M, et al. Malignant dysphagia: palliation with esophageal stents—long-term results with 100 patients. *Radiology.* 1998;207:513-518.

31. Kinsman KJ, DeGregorio BT, Katon RM, et al. Prior radiation and chemotherapy increase the risk of life-threatening complications after insertion of metallic stents for esophagogastric malignancy. *Gastrointest Endosc.* 1996;43:196-203.

32. Siersema PD, Schrauwen SL, vanBlankenstein M, et al. Self-expanding metal stents for complicated and recurrent esophagogastric cancer. *Gastrointest Endosc.* 2001;54:579-585.

33. Wang MQ, Sze DY, Wang ZP, et al. Delayed complications after esophageal stent placement for treatment of malignant esophageal obstructions and esophagorespiratory fistulas. *J Vasc Interv Radiol.* 2001;12:465-474.

34. Bartelsman JF, Bruno MJ, Jensema, et al. Palliation of patients with esophagogastric neoplasms by insertion of a covered expandable modified Gianturco-Z endoprosthesis: experiences in 153 patients. *Gastrointest Endosc.* 2000;51:134-138.

35. May A, Ell C. Palliative treatment of malignant esophagorespiratory fistulas with Gianturco-Z stents. *Am J Gastroenterol.* 1998;93:532-535.

36. Dallal HJ, Smith GD, Greive DC, et al. A randomized trial of thermal ablative therapy versus expandable metal stents in the palliative treatment of patients with esophageal carcinoma. *Gastrointest Endosc.* 2001;54:549-557.

37. Konigsrainer A, Riedmann B, de Vries A, et al. Expanded metal stents versus laser combined with radiotherapy for palliation of unresectable esophageal cancer: a prospective randomized trial. *Hepatogastroenterology.* 2000;47:724-727.

38. Gevers AM, Macken E, Hiele M, et al. A comparison of laser therapy, plastic stents, and expandable metal stents for palliation of malignant dysphagia in patients without a fistula. *Gastrointest Endosc.* 1998;48:383-388.

39. Adam A, Ellul J, Watkinson AF, et al. Palliation of inoperable esophageal carcinoma : a prospective randomized trial of laser therapy and stent placement. *Radiology.* 1997;202:344-348.

40. Schiefke I, Zabel-Langhennig A, Wiedmann M, et al. Self-expandable metal stents for malignant duodenal obstruction caused by biliary tract cancer. *Gastrointest Endosc.* 2003;58:213-219.

41. Weaver DW, Wieneck RG, Buwman DL, et al. Gastrojejunostomy: is it helpful for patients with pancreatic cancer? *Surgery.* 1987; 102: 608-613.

42. Krouse RS, McCahill LE, Easson AM, et al. When the sun can set on an unoperated bowel obstruction: Management of malignant bowel obstruction. *J Am Coll Surg.* 2002; 195:117-127.

43. Adler DG, Baron TH. Endoscopic palliation of malignant gastric outlet obstruction using self-expanding metal stents: experience in 36 patients. *Am J Gastroenterol.* 2002; 97:72-78.

44. Baron TH, Harewood GC. Enteral self-expandable stents. *Gastrointest Endosc.* 2003;58:421-433.

45. Yim HB, Jacobson BC, Saltzman JR, et al. Clinical outcome of the use of enteral stents for palliation of patients with malignant upper GI obstruction. *Gastrointest Endosc.* 2001;53:329-332.

46. Kim JH, Yoo BM, Lee KJ, et al. Self-expanding coil stent with a long delivery system for palliation of unresectable malignant gastric outlet obstruction: a prospective study. *Endoscopy.* 2001;33:838-842.

47. Maetani I, Tada T, Shimura J, et al. Technical modifications and strategies for stenting gastric outlet strictures using esophageal endoprostheses. *Endoscopy.* 2002;34:402-406.

48. Shand AG, Grieve DC, Brush J, et al. Expandable metal stents for palliation of malignant pyloric and duodenal obstruction. *Br J Surg.* 2002;89:349-350.

49. Singer SB, Asch M. Metallic stents in the treatment of duodenal obstruction: technical issues and results. *Canadian Assoc of Radiol J.* 2000;51:121-129.

50. Mauro MA, Koehler RE, Baron TH. Advances in gastrointestinal intervention: The treatment of gastroduodenal and colorectal obstructions with metallic stents. *Radiology.* 2000;215:659-669.

51. Wong YT, Brams DM, Munson L, et al. Gastric outlet obstruction secondary to pancreatic cancer: surgical vs endoscopic palliation. *Surg Endosc.* 2002;16:310-312

52. Dean GT, Krukowski ZH, Irwin ST. Malignant obstruction of the left colon. *Br J Surg.* 1994;81:1270-1276.

53. Gandrup P. Lund L, Balslev I. Surgical treatment of acute malignant large bowel obstruction. *Eur J Surg.* 1992;158:427-430.

54. Adler DG, Baron TH. Endoscopic palliation of colorectal cancer. *Hematol Oncol Clin N Am.* 2002;16:1015-1029.

55. Makela J, Kiviniemi H, Laitinen S, et al. Surgical management of intestinal obstruction after treatment for cancer. *Eur J Surg.* 1991;157:73-77.

56. Feuer DJ, Broadley KE, Shepherd JH, et al. Systemic review of surgery in malignant bowel obstruction in advanced gynecological and gastrointestinal cancer. *Gynecol Oncol.* 1999;75:313-322.

57. Khot UP, Lang AW, Murali K, et al. Systematic review of the efficacy and safety of colorectal stents *Br J Surg.* 2002;89:1096-1102.

58. Martinez-Santos C, Lobato RF, Fradejas JM, et al. Self-expandable stent before elective surgery vs. emergency surgery for the treatment of malignant colorectal obstructions: comparison of primary anastomosis and morbidity rates. *Dis Colon Rectum.* 2002;45: 401-406.

59. Camunez F, Echenagusia A, Simo G, et al. Malignant colorectal obstruction treated by means of self-expanding metallic stents: effectiveness before surgery and in palliation. Radiology 2000;216:492-497.

60. Tack J, Gevers A, Rutgeerts P. Self-expandable metallic stents in the palliation of rectosigmoid carcinoma: a follow-up study. *Gastrointest Endosc.* 1998;267:271.

61. Spinelli P, Mancini A. Use of self-expanding metal stents for palliation of rectosigmoid cancer. *Gastrointest Endosc.* 2001;203-206.

chapter 16

Gastrointestinal Cancer: Diagnosis and Management of Nutritional Issues

James S. Scolapio, MD and Alan L. Buchman, MD, MSPH

DIETARY AND NUTRITIONAL FACTORS

The evidence connecting food to gastrointestinal cancers is derived from epidemiological studies, case-control studies, and prospective observational studies. However, in many of these studies, it is difficult to determine the independent effects of specific nutrients given the many potential environmental contributors.[1,2]

Esophageal cancer has been linked to low intake of vitamin C, zinc, and selenium, and a protective effect from eating fruits and vegetables has been reported in more than one study. Meat and fish consumption has shown inconsistent associations with esophageal cancer. Despite these positive observations, randomized controlled studies from China have failed to show reduced esophageal cancer mortality in patients treated with multivitamin supplements.[3] As with other malignancies, obesity also appears to be a risk factor.

It has been shown that foods high in salt or have been preserved with salt (eg, pickled, smoked foods) are associated with an increased risk of gastric cancer. Migration studies from Japan have suggested a strong environmental component to gastric cancer.[4] Preserved foods contain nitrates, which form N-nitroso compounds, including nitrosamines, which may increase the risk of gastric cancer. There is consistent data that fruit and vegetable consumption decreases the risk of gastric cancer. Also green tea has been shown to be protective against gastric cancer in a number of studies.[5]

Pancreatic cancer has been linked to excess caloric intake and obesity. The intake of fruits and vegetables may be protective.[2] It has been widely believed that components of the diet, including calcium,[6-8] folate,[9] and selenium[10,11] may be protective against the risk of colon cancer. However, diets with large components of fruits and vegetables,[12,13] and fiber,[14-16] as well as vitamin A, C,[17] and E[17,18] supplements do not appear to offer any protective effect. Dietary fat appears to increase the risk of colon cancer in some studies,[19,20] but not in others in which the development of adenomas was used as a surrogate marker for cancer risk.[14,21,22] Many case control studies have shown a link with high animal (saturated) fat and increased total calorie intake and colon cancer,[20,23,24] although processed meats may be a higher risk.[25] Several epidemiologic studies have suggested a relationship between increased body mass index (BMI) and development of colon cancer.[26,27] This association appears to be stronger for men than for women.[28,29] Central obesity appears more closely linked to colon cancer risk than more peripheral fat deposition. Insulin resistance with subsequent hyperinsulinemia may play a role.[30] It cannot be assumed the proof of association is proof of cause and effect. Establishment of actual cause and effect for particular dietary factors in a prospective fashion is difficult and expensive. In addition, the use of adenoma development as a surrogate marker for risk for development of more advanced carcinogenesis may be problematic.

The American Cancer Society recommends the following dietary guidelines for cancer prevention: 1) Choose most foods from plant sources, 2) Eat more than 5 servings of fruits and vegetables each day, 3) Limit intake of high fat foods, particularly from animal sources, 4) Achieve and maintain a healthy weight, and 5) Limit consumption of alcoholic beverages.[31]

NUTRITIONAL ASSESSMENT

The nutritional management of a patient with gastrointestinal cancer first begins with appropriate nutritional assessment. Multiple factors contribute to malnutrition in cancer patients. Anorexia from tumor cytokines, intestinal obstruction, taste changes, chemotherapy and radiation side effects, and depression are examples. Intestinal malabsorption also contributes to malnutrition in patients with certain types of gastrointestinal cancers. Extensive mucosal infiltrative disease, bacterial overgrowth, and surgical resection all contribute to malabsorption and subsequent weight loss. Increased energy expenditure has also been reported in patients with cancer.[32] Nutrient deficiencies may result in altered cellular immunity with increased risk of infection and delayed wound healing following surgery. Therefore it is important to identify those patients that are at potential risk of malnutrition. Management goals should then include correction of nutritional deficits when possible. There is no gold standard or one laboratory test for measuring the malnutrition of a patient. All current assessment methods may be affected by the underlying illness and not necessary reflect the nutritional reserve of the patient. For example, serum albumin and prealbumin concentrations can be reduced without a history of weight loss or other micronutrient deficiency as hepatic protein synthesis shifts to that of acute phase reactants. Likewise, extracellular fluid shifts can result in low serum albumin and prealbumin concentrations without a clinical history to suggest weight loss or malnutrition. Delayed cutaneous hypersensitivity is an unreliable marker of malnutrition since cancer and medications used to treat cancer can affect results.

A complete history and physical examination is probably the best tool to access the gross nutritional status of an individual patient (Table 16-1). Patients that have lost significant weight (defined as greater than 10%) and have had reduced oral caloric intake over a 2- to 24-week period are at risk of both macronutrient and micronutrient deficiencies. It is known from clinical studies that cancer patients that have lost greater than 10% of their usual weight and have a reduced appetite have shorter median survival and lower chemotherapy response.[33] The important findings on physical examination, besides an accurate weight, include loss of subcutaneous fat, muscle wasting, dependent edema, and ascites. Subjective global assessment (SGA) is a clinical method for the evaluation of nutritional status, and includes historical, symptomatic and physical parameters of patients.[34] The findings from a history and physical examination are subjectively

Table 16-1

NUTRITIONAL ASSESSMENT

History and Physical Examination

History	Unusual dietary habits, medication/vitamin or mineral supplements, change in hair color or texture, poor night vision, dysguesia, dysphagia/odynophagia, abdominal pain/distention, diarrhea, bone pain, muscle pain/cramps/twitching, numbness/parathesias, fatigue, diminished mental activity, weakness
Physical examination	Hair loss/texture, keratomalacia, cheilosis, glossitis, red tongue, parotid enlargement, dentition, skin rash/petechia/bruising, muscle wasting, hepatomegaly, edema, peripheral neuropathy

Anthropometrics

Ideal body weight (IBW)	Males: 48 kg +2.3kg for each in >60
	Females: 45 kg +2.7kg for each in >60
	Calculate % IBW: >5% weight loss in 1 month, >7.5% in 2 months or >10% in 6 months are significant
	Preferred body weight for obese (Hamwi Formula) = (ABW-IBW)(0.25) + IBW *(used clinically; not validated)*
	Adjusted Body Weight for Amputation:
	• Entire Arm (-6.5%)
	• Upper Arm (-3.5%)
	• Hand (-0.8%)
	• Forearm with Hand (-3.1%)
	• Forearm without Hand (-2.5%)
	• Entire Leg (-18.6%)
	• Foot (-1.8%)
Muscle function	Handgrip strength, peak insp pressure
Midarm circumference	Assess skeletal mass
Triceps skin fold	Assess fat stores
Thickness	Operator-dependent variability, unreliable to assess short-term responses

Laboratory Measurements

Nitrogen balance	N intake = grams protein/6.25
	Balance = N intake - (24 urine urea nitrogen [UUN] + 4)
	(requires sufficient calories as well as protein)
Indirect calorimetry	
Visceral proteins	Albumin, pre-albumin, transferrin, retinol-binding protein *(affected by many non-nutritional conditions)*
Immune function	Total lymphocyte count
	Delayed hypersensitivity skin tests *(affected by many non-nutritional conditions)*

weighted to rank patients as well nourished (A), moderately malnourished (B), or severely malnourished (C). (Table 16-2) SGA has 80% reproducible results among multiple observers.[34]

GENERAL DIETARY MEASURES

The most important advice for most cancer patients is to consume a diet liberal in protein, with sufficient calories to maintain weight. Oral intake of 25 to 35 kcal/kg/day and 1.0 to 1.5 g/kg/day of protein will meet the requirements of most non-wasted cancer patients. For those patients that have lost more than 5% of their usual weight, the addition of 500 kcal/day (above the 25 to 35 kcal/day) will help to promote weight gain. Protein should be maximized at a least 1.5 g/ kg/day in those patients with signs of muscle wasting. In patients with advanced cancer, the addition of added calories and protein may not improve lean muscle mass given the inflammatory process (ie, cytokines, associated with cancer itself).

All patients should meet with a registered dietician to determine actual calories consumed. The dietician can also be helpful recommending specific foods and supplements of high caloric density. The addition of flavoring to the food may help improve food intake. Liquid oral supplements such as Ensure (Abbott Laboratories, Abbott Park, Ill), Boost (Novartis, Fremont, Mich), and Carnation Instant Breakfast (Nestlé, Glendale, Calif) may provide the additional calories that a patient requires. The addition of an appetite stimulant may be helpful for patients unable to consume sufficient oral calories.

PHARMACOLOGICAL TREATMENT

Cachexia is a common and major complication of cancer. The severe loss of weight and appetite can produce both physical and emotional disabilities. Cancer cells promote the secretion of host-derived cytokines. Some of these cytokines can result in significant lean tissue loss and depressed appetite. Those that have been studied more recently include tumor necrosis factor alpha, interleukin-6 and proteolysis inducing factor.[35] Medications including pentoxifylline, hydrazine sulfate, melatonin, thalidomide, ibuprofen, and, more recently, infliximab have been used in an attempt to inhibit cytokine-mediated cachexia. These treatments should still be regarded as experimental.

Appetite stimulants including dronabinol, corticosteroids and megestrol acetate (Megace, Bristol-Myers Squibb, New York, NY) may be useful in some patients.[36,37] The administration of megestrol acetate (400 to 800 mg/day) may increase appetite, weight gain (primary fat mass), and quality of life. However, improved morbidity and mortality have not been demonstrated with this treatment.[37] Megestrol acetate comes in an oral suspension that can be given once per day. It may cause adrenal suppression and exacerbate pre-existing diabetes. Thromboembolic events have also been reported in cancer patients treated with 800 mg/day of megestrol acetate. The safest and most efficacious dose is still somewhat controversial and therefore if used, it should be titrated to the lowest effective dose.

Cannabinoids and their derivative dronabinol may stimulate appetite and result in weight gain in cancer patients.[36] Dronabinol is approved by the FDA for treatment of nausea and vomiting associated with chemotherapy. The dose used is 2.5 mg orally three times daily, taken 1 hour after meals. Further controlled trails are needed to identify the optimal dose and patient population that may derive the most benefit.

Table 16-2

SUBJECTIVE GLOBAL ASSESSMENT OF NUTRITIONAL STATUS

I. History

A. Weight change

Overall loss in past 6 months = # _____ kg

Change in past 2 weeks: _____ Increase

_____ No change

_____ Decrease

B. Dietary intake change (relative to normal):

_____ No change

_____ Change: duration = #___ weeks

Type: _____ Suboptimal solid diet_____ Full liquid diet

_____ Hypocaloric liquids _____ Starvation

C. Gastrointestinal symptoms that persisted >2 weeks:

____ None ____ Anorexia ____ Nausea ____ Vomiting ____ Diarrhea

D. Functional Capacity:

_____ No dysfunction (eg, full capacity)

_____ Dysfunction: duration = #_____ Weeks

_____ Working suboptimally

_____ Ambulatory

_____ Bedridden

E. Disease and its relation to nutritional requirements:

Primary diagnosis (specify) _____

Metabolic demand (stress) ____ None ____ Low ____ Moderate ____ High

II. Physical

(for each trait specify 0=normal, 1+=mild, 2+=moderate, 3+=severe)

#_____ Loss of subcutaneous fat (triceps, chest)

#_____ Muscle wasting (quadriceps, deltoids, temporals)

#_____ Ankle edema, sacral edema

#_____ Ascites

#_____ Tongue or skin lesions suggesting nutrient deficiency

III. SGA Rating (select one)

_____ A = Well nourished (minimal or no restriction of food intake or absorption, minimal change in function, weight stable or increasing)

_____ B = Moderatedly malnourished (food restriction, some function changes, little or no change in body mass)

_____ C = Severely malnourished (definite decreased intake, function, and body mass)

Adapted from Detsky AS, McLaughlin JR, Baker JP, et al. What is subjective global assessment of nutritional status? *J Parenter Enteral Nutr.* 1987;11(1):8-13.

Corticosteroids appear to stimulate appetite by the euphoria they produce. Appetite stimulation effects appear to be short lived, and complications from long-term use of corticosteroids are well established. Dexamethasone should only be provided (0.75 mg QID) to terminal cancer patients if increased appetite and quality of life are the short-term goals (eg, weeks).

Cyproheptadine hydrochloride is an antihistamine that presumably increases weight by serotonin antagonism. It has been used primarily in Europe to promote weight gain in cancer patients. A randomized placebo controlled study would suggest lack of benefit of weight gain with this medication.[38]

PERIOPERATIVE NUTRITIONAL SUPPORT

Nutritional support refers to the use of either intravenous (TPN) or enteral tube feeding (TEN) and is usually administered to hospitalized patients. Nutritional support of the hospitalized patient should be instituted promptly when it has been determined from daily calorie counts that a patient is not taking sufficient oral intake of food for seven days or more days. After approximately 7 to 10 days of nil per os (npo), negative nitrogen balance occurs; this increases the risk of infection and interferes with wound healing. Nutritional support may also be considered an adjunctive therapy in malnourished patients in whom sufficient oral intake to promote nutritional repletion is not immediately achievable. Perioperative nutrition refers to the use of nutritional support pre- and postsurgery.

In cancer patients requiring surgery, one needs to ask if there is a benefit to delaying surgery for repletion of nutrition. The available literature would suggest that cancer patients that are severely malnourished (defined as >10% weight loss of usual weight) benefit from 7 to 10 days of preoperative TPN.[39] Although improved mortality has not been reported, a 10% improvement in postoperative complications (eg, reduced postoperative infections) has been reported compared to placebo. Administration of TPN to non-malnourished cancer patients (<10% weight loss) resulted in increased complications from the TPN itself.[40] Therefore, indiscriminate use of preoperative TPN should be avoided. There are no studies that evaluate the benefit of TEN prior to surgery in malnourished cancer patients. The results might be similar and perhaps even better than TPN. The practicality of providing TPN for 7 to 10 days before surgery is difficult. It is difficult to justify hospitalizing a patient for 10 days prior to surgery to administer TPN. Most insurance companies will not approve TPN coverage at home for this indication. Perhaps administering TEN at home via a nasal gastric feeding tube for 7 to 10 days would be more appropriate. However, each clinician must decide if delaying surgery for 10 days prior to surgery is worthwhile, given only a modest 10% decrease in postoperative complications at best, and no benefit on mortality (from short-term nutritional support). Given that lean body mass can be increased only by 1 to 3 pounds/week, short-term TPN will not provide much benefit for the profoundly malnourished patient.

Postoperatively, those cancer patients that are severely malnourished prior to surgery (eg, >10% weight loss) or have an anticipated 7 or more days of inadequate caloric intake following surgery appear to benefit from postoperative TEN given within 48 hours of surgery.[39] Results with TEN appear better than with TPN.[41] It is our opinion in high nutrition risk patients (eg, >10% weight loss, extensive upper abdominal surgical resection) that a jejunal feeding tube should be placed at the time of surgery. The feeding tube can generally be removed as an outpatient during convalescence, once normal oral intake has resumed.

NUTRITION SUPPORT OF SPECIFIC CANCERS

Malnutrition is very common in patients with cancer of the esophagus, primarily because of severe dysphagia. Average weight loss is often some 10 kg at presentation. Surgery is the primary treatment of choice, with radiation and chemotherapy given preoperatively. Side effects of the chemotherapy and radiation can result in further weight loss. Surgical treatment usually involves total or distal esophagectomy requiring bilateral vagotomy, proximal gastrectomy, and anastomosis of the retained portion of the esophagus to the remaining stomach. Postoperative regurgitation of food and bloating are common complications following surgery that can result in further weight loss and debilitation. Esophageal strictures can occur postoperatively and may require repeated dilatation for adequate food passage. Esophageal stent placement may be palliative and improve food and liquid passage for those patients that are not surgical candidates and in whom severe dysphagia results from esophageal luminal cancer growth. Liquid nutritional supplements and small frequent meals may help the postoperative patient who is experiencing dumping and bloating. In those patients that have lost significant (>10%) preoperative weight, placing a jejunal feeding tube at the time of surgery is suggested. Iron and B_{12} deficiency may result postoperatively depending on the amount of stomach removed and should therefore be replaced accordingly.

Patients with gastric cancer frequently present with early satiety, postprandial abdominal pain, and weight loss. Surgical resection usually requires a total gastrectomy with an esophagojejunal anastomosis. Significant weight loss; dumping syndrome; fat maldigestion; and iron, calcium, and B_{12} deficiency can all occur in the postoperative setting.[42] To help with the dumping syndrome small frequent meals (6 to 8 meals/day) should be encouraged and protein should be maximized in the diet. Pectin may be added to the diet to slow gastric emptying and minimize the postprandial fall in blood glucose.[43] Steatorrhea occurs because of secondary pancreatic insufficiency and may be treated with pancreatic enzyme supplementation. Deficiencies of vitamins and minerals can be prevented and treated with adequate oral administration of iron with ascorbic acid and monthly injections of B_{12}. In patients that continue to lose weight despite dietary adjustments, nocturnal jejunal feeding is usually beneficial to prevent further weight loss and maintain hydration.

Pancreatic cancer can result in significant weight loss by the time of diagnosis. If patients were surgical candidates, the same data regarding perioperative nutrition (Section V) would apply to this group of patients. Pancreatic exocrine and endocrine insufficiency can also occur in these patients and exogenous pancreatic enzyme replacement and insulin should be given as clinically indicated. Nocturnal jejunal feeding can supplement the oral intake and provide needed calories and hydration in those patients unable to consume adequate oral calories.

Patients with colorectal cancer usually present with little or no weight loss. Treatment involves resection of the bowel containing the cancer. If postoperative chemotherapy (5-FU) is required is it usually tolerated without significant side effect. If large resections of the right colon are required and the ileocecal valve is compromised, postprandial diarrhea may result. Although cholestyramine may improve bile salt-induced diarrhea, it can also further deplete the bile salt pool if greater than 100 cm of the terminal ileum has been resected and result in fat-soluble vitamin deficiencies. If more than 60 cm of the terminal ileum is resected, B_{12} deficiency may result and replacement is necessary.

Some cancers, including colorectal cancer, are treated with radiation therapy. Although direct tumor treatment with the radiation is the goal, scatter radiation damage can occur. This is especially a nutrition concern when the small intestine is damaged. Radiation enteritis can be classified as acute and chronic. By definition, acute is defined as that occurring within the first 6 weeks of therapy. Acute injury to the small bowel is usually self-limited and presents clinically with nausea and diarrhea. Acute injury does not necessarily predict those patients that will go on to develop chronic radiation injury. Chronic small bowel injury from radiation is marked by inflammation and fibrosis of the small intestine. Fibrosis can result in intestinal obstruction and episodic bleeding. Partial small bowel obstruction can result in bacterial overgrowth and diarrhea. Treatment with broad-spectrum antibiotics may be helpful in decreasing diarrhea if bacterial overgrowth is the cause. Recurrent bowel obstructions can also result in inadequate oral intake over time resulting in significant weight loss. The primary goal should be to surgically correct the obstruction. Often surgeons are reluctant to operate given the extensive damage of the bowel from the radiation, which is often not appreciated until the time of surgery. Selection of an experienced surgeon in the area of radiation injury is critical in the care of these patients. If patients are not surgical candidates, and they are unable to take sufficient fluids and nutrients orally, then placement of a gastric or jejunal feeding tube may be helpful. Often placement of a dual gastric-jejunal tube for gastric venting and jejunal feeding is helpful. There is insufficient data to recommend any specialized elemental formulas or glutamine for these patients. If patients cannot tolerate enteral feeding TPN may be required and can be used successfully provided patients are monitored closely.[44,45] In addition, glutamine has not generally been found to be useful in the treatment of mucositis.[46]

PARENTERAL NUTRITION

Once nutritional support is deemed necessary, which route (parenteral vs enteral) should be used? Indications for parenteral feeding usually include small bowel obstruction, which may develop in cancer patients because of tumor growth; severe diarrhea and malabsorption during active disease and treatment; gastrointestinal hemorrhage; treatment for enterocutaneous or enteroenteric fistulae; and as supportive care in patients that are severely malnourished (SGA "C"). TPN is not generally indicated in patients that have a nonobstructive gastrointestinal tract or when the duration of nutritional support is expected to be less than seven days.

It is thought that the gut atrophies in the absence of enteral nutrition. While this may be the case in animal studies, the data in humans fail to support this concept.[47] It is commonly thought that in the absence of enteral nutrition, bacteria will translocate across the intestinal epithelium, to the mesenteric lymph nodes, and into the systemic circulation—resulting in sepsis and multiorgan failure. Although this has been reported in the rat model, it rarely occurs in humans.[48] When bacterial translocation does occur in humans, it is usually in the setting of small bowel obstruction and unrelated to the route of feeding, and is usually clinically inconsequential.[48]

When is TPN appropriate for the patient with gastrointestinal cancer? TPN may be indicated in patients with severe stomatitis from chemotherapy and/or radiation, patients with intestinal obstruction either related to tumor or radiation therapy, and severe malabsorption and/or diarrhea caused by radiation enteritis. Home TPN may also be considered in such patients. However, Medicare guidelines specify that a permanently inoperative internal body organ (the intestine) be present. Permanence is defined as at least 3 months. Therefore, Medicare and some insurance carriers will not pay for home TPN in the patient when use will be less than 3 months either because of improvement in gastrointestinal function or death. There is no evidence TPN improves outcome of chemotherapy or radiation-related treatment or patient survival with active cancer. TPN is not appropriate in the patient that is expected to succumb within 3 months or less. Patients who are cured of their malignancy, but left with short bowel syndrome or severe radiation enteritis (about 5% of patients) may be candidates for lifetime TPN.[45]

CHOOSING THE ROUTE FOR PARENTERAL NUTRITION DELIVERY

Once it has been determined parenteral nutrition is indicated for a particular patient, a route for delivery must be selected. Parenteral nutrition can be delivered via a peripheral or a central vein. Peripheral PN is generally used when short-term nutritional support is required (eg, <7 to 10 days). The peripheral access can sometimes be used to supply total nutritional needs (25 to 30 kcal/day), especially if a lipid emulsion is used. Lipid emulsions are isotonic. Because of the hypertonicity of the dextrose, thrombophlebitis is a significant risk when concentrations above 10% are used. The amino acid concentration in the TPN solution should also be ≤3.5% to ensure the solution has ~900mOsm. Heparin (1000 units/L) and hydrocortisone (10 mg/L) will reduce the risk of thrombophlebitis. Central parenteral nutrition (CPN), more typically referred to as TPN, is infused into a large central vein. Large veins such as the superior vena cava (SVC) or the inferior vena cava (IVC) can tolerate a greater solution osmolarity (up to 1800 mOsm, typically 35% dextrose and 5% amino acids). It is important that the catheter tip reside in either the SVC or IVC. Should the tip be located in a smaller vessel, catheter thrombosis could result when the hypertonic TPN solution is infused. Catheter location within the right atrium may increase the risk of cardiac arrhythmia. A catheter useful for TPN may include a percutaneously inserted central catheter (PICC) that is typically inserted via the brachial (although occasionally the antecubital) vein, and advance to the SVC. The risk of a pneumothorax can be avoided with this method and therefore should be the choice of access in the authors' opinion. A triple, double, or single lumen (preferred) catheter inserted into the subclavian, internal jugular, or femoral vain may also be used, provided the catheter tip is located within the SVC or IVC. For longer-term use, it is typical that a single lumen Hickman, Broviac, Groshong catheter, or a subcutaneous infusion port, be inserted. Regardless of the catheter type, it is critical that a catheter lumen be reserved for the exclusive use of TPN to minimize infection risk.

WRITING THE TOTAL PARENTERAL NUTRITION PRESCRIPTION: HOW MUCH IS NECESSARY?

A number of studies have investigated energy expenditure and nitrogen excretion in patients with cancer. Cancer patients with active disease may require 1.2 to 1.5 x additional calories above resting energy expenditure. Thirty to 40 kcal/kg/day of ideal body weight and 1 to 1.5 g/kg of ideal body weight (IBW) of protein are usually sufficient for most adult cancer patients. Most hospitalized cancer patients only require nutritional support for 2 weeks or less.

IBW can be calculated using the following equations: 48 kg + 2.7 x number of inches over 60 inches in height (males) or 45 kg + 2.3 x number of inches over 60 inches in height (females). Caloric measurement using indirect calorimetry is usually not needed. A minimum of 200 g of dextrose is necessary daily to meet the needs of brain metabolism. The carbohydrate used in TPN solutions is dextrose monohydrate, which contains 3.4 kcal/mL.

Intravenous fat emulsion is typically used to supply 20% to 40% of the daily calories. Only 6% of daily calories are needed as lipid emulsion to prevent essential fatty acid deficiency. Fat emulsions supply either 1.1 or 2.0 kcal/mL, dependent upon whether a 10% or 20% emulsion is selected. Fluid requirements can usually be met by using 1 mL/kcal or a 1.5 to 2.0 L TPN formula. Patients with cardiac or renal insufficiency may require less and patients with significant diarrhea or fistula losses may require more.

Depending upon the specific order form used, one can order TPN either in terms of absolute amounts of macromolecules (eg, dextrose, lipid, and protein) or by indicating a total volume and final concentration of these TPN constituents. Electrolytes, minerals, trace elements, and vitamins can be written for using standard amounts (eg, multi-trace elements and multiple vitamin solutions unless the addition of a specific nutrient is required to correct or prevent a deficiency or withholding of a specific ingredient is necessary in order to avoid potential toxicity). For example, a 70-kg man that requires 25 kcal/kg/day and 1.0 g/kg/day of protein for maintenance might receive the following formula: 2 L of 20% dextrose (400 g, providing 1360 kcal) + 200 mL of 20% lipid emulsion (400 kcal) with 3.5% amino acids (700 g). Again, depending upon the formulation capabilities of the hospital pharmacy, the complete solution can be provided as a 3 (dextrose, lipid, and amino acids)-in-1 emulsion or as a 2 (dextrose, amino acids)-in-1 solution, with the lipid emulsion hung in a piggybacked fashion. Initially, the TPN rate should be relatively slow (eg, 40 mL/hour) and even slower in the malnourished patient (see refeeding syndrome below). The rate can be advanced as rapidly as every 8 hours in a normally nourished individual without diabetes as long as the blood glucose is <160 mg/dl. During continuous central TPN, the blood glucose should be determined every 6 hrs.

MONITORING PARENTERAL NUTRITION

SAFETY

If used inappropriately or not monitored appropriately, TPN will not have any value to the patient and may even become a life-threatening therapy rather than lifesaving. It is generally recommended to consult the services of a multidisciplinary nutritional support team (NST) in the hospital to assist in writing the TPN prescription, monitoring the therapy, and making adjustments as required. However, it is imperative that the responsible physician understands the importance of appropriate monitoring, especially in the absence of a NST.

Patients should be weighed daily, and accurate inputs and outputs should be recorded. Urine output should be >1000 mL/24 hours in order to assure adequate hydration. If weight gain is planned, anything more than 1 to 2 kg/week indicates fluid retention. This may occur in the first week or two of TPN; decreasing the rate of TPN is usually sufficient, although occasionally diuretic therapy becomes necessary.

In general, electrolytes should be monitored daily the first few days of starting TPN and then at least twice weekly. Acid/base disturbances can often be managed by increasing or decreasing acetate or chloride in the solution. Metabolic acidosis may be caused by diarrhea and can usually be corrected by slightly increasing potassium acetate in the solution. Hypochloremic metabolic alkalosis may result from nasogastric suction in the absence of adequate replacement fluid. Elevated BUN may result because of the provision of insufficient fluid, excessive amino acid infusion, or renal insufficiency.

Mild elevations in the hepatic aminotransferases (ALT, AST), as well as the alkaline phosphatase are often observed within 2 to 14 days of initiating TPN and should be determined at baseline and subsequently on a weekly basis.[49] These elevations are generally transient. More persistent elevation in ALT and/or AST may result from hepatic steatosis from overfeeding or choline deficiency.[49,50] Persistently elevated alkaline phosphatase may signify the development of biliary sludge, which will occur in virtually 100% of patients on TPN that are npo. It is unusual to see a rise in serum bilirubin as a direct result of TPN.[51] A rise in bilirubin is a concern, and other causes besides TPN should be evaluated.

The serum triglyceride concentration should be monitored twice weekly during the first week and weekly thereafter for the first 2 weeks in order to ascertain adequate clearance of the lipid emulsion. It should be obtained 4 to 6 hours after infusion of the lipid emulsion has been completed. Although there is no clear evidence of the deleterious effects of a serum triglyceride concentration <1000 mg/dL, it is generally recommended to decrease the infusion rate and/or volume of the lipid emulsion if the triglyceride concentration is greater than 400 to 500 mg/dL; a concentration of >1000 mg/dL may be associated with the development of pancreatitis.[52]

The human body adapts to starvation and weight loss by decreasing resting energy expenditure. When massive amounts of carbohydrate are supplied to a malnourished cancer patient in an overzealous attempt to renourish him or her, refeeding syndrome may result.[53] This potentially life-threatening complication of either TPN or enteral nutritional therapy occurs when carbohydrate intake stimulates pancreatic insulin release, which results in the flow of potassium and magnesium to the intercellular space, which may result in cardiac arrhythmias. In addition, the demand for phosphate to produce ATP from the infused carbohydrate may result in hypophosphatemia with subsequent hemolytic anemia, seizures, rhabdomyolysis, and/or respiratory muscle dysfunction. In rare cases, respiratory failure may ensue. Prevention of refeeding syndrome can be prevented by the slow introduction of carbohydrate, and the use of protein (amino acids) and lipid. Small amounts of supplemental potassium phosphate and magnesium may be helpful. Serum potassium, magnesium, and phosphate concentrations should be determined daily or more frequently if necessary until the goal caloric support and a stable electrolyte pattern in the normal range can be achieved.

Infectious complications are also common in TPN-treated patients. There are 3 types of catheter infections that can occur.[54] The most common is catheter sepsis, whereby the catheter tip becomes a nidus for bacterial adherence. Bacteria may reach the catheter tip because of catheter contamination from the skin or the catheter hub (used when connecting infusion tubing to the catheter or directly injecting medications). The most common organisms are generally skin flora, including coagulase negative *staphylococci, S. aureus, Klebsiella pneumonia,* and *E. coli.* Such infections can often be treated without the requirement for catheter removal using a 2-week course of systemic antibiotic therapy. Also a highly concentrated solution of vancomycin or amikacin (2 mg/mL) in 2 mL of saline can be instilled into the catheter every 12 hours (antibiotic lock technique).[55]

Should fungemia be identified, the catheter must be removed. Regardless of whether the catheter is removed because of fungemia or refractory bacterial sepsis (sepsis syndrome or the inability to relieve the febrile response after 48 to 72 hours of antibiotic therapy), the patient should remain completely afebrile and have negative blood cultures prior to insertion of a new central venous catheter.

Infection may develop surrounding the anchoring cuff of a subcutaneous tunneled catheter. This type of infection is rarely associated with fever or leukocytosis, but is invariably diagnosed by the presence of purulent drainage from the catheter skin exit site. Often tenderness can be elicited over the catheter cuff. Coagulase negative *staphylococci* and *S. aureus* are the most common organisms involved. Approximately 50% of the time, successful treatment of the infection can be achieved with 2 weeks of systemic antibiotic therapy. If treatment of the catheter *in situ* is ineffective, the catheter should be removed and a new catheter may be placed in a different site without delay in the absence of systemic infection. Systemic antibiotics should however be continued for 5 to 7 days following catheter removal.

The subcutaneous catheter tunnel tract may also become infected. Although it is usually difficult to culture an organism, *S. aureus* is most commonly recovered. Because antibiotic penetration of the tunnel is poor, treatment consists of catheter removal in addition to 1 week of appropriate systemic antibiotic therapy. In the absence of systemic evidence of infection, a new catheter can be inserted in a different site without delay. In order to help prevent the risk of infection, it is imperative that those caring for the catheter learn appropriate catheter care technique. Virtually all catheter-related infections relate either to the skin entrance site or the catheter hub. These must be cleaned appropriately before each use with a bactericidal agent such as povidone-iodine or chlorhexidine; ethanol alone is insufficient. In addition, the skin surrounding the catheter should be cleaned appropriately during dressing changes. We recommend the use of small, sterile gauze covering, with a semipermeable dressing placed over the gauze to anchor it to the skin. Semipermeable membranes alone have been associated with increased infection risk in some studies. Dressings should be changed 2 to 3 times weekly—more often if the area becomes wet or dirty.

Catheter occlusion can take the form of either thrombotic or non thrombotic occlusion, and is generally manifested in difficulty with TPN or medication infusion. Routine heparin flushes are a useful preventative measure. However, fibrin can still accumulate and block the catheter tip. TPA 2 mg, infused in a 2 mL volume (in order to completely fill the catheter) if used within the first 24 to 48 hours, is often successful in dissolving the thrombosis.[56] Following instillation of the TPA into the catheter, aspiration should be attempted after 30 minutes. It may be necessary to repeat the procedure. In the inpatient setting, the catheter is often simply removed and replaced. Although in the outpatient setting, especially in the case of the short bowel patient, every attempt should be made to preserve venous access sites.

Nonthrombotic occlusion may result from calcium-phosphate precipitates or lipid accumulation. Either 0.2 to 0.5 mL of 0.1 N hydrochloric acid or sodium hydroxide may be useful in clearing the obstruction, although occasionally the catheter will require removal and replacement. Care should be taken to avoid the addition of too much supplemental calcium and phosphate simultaneously in the TPN solution. Because the solubility of calcium and phosphate in TPN is dependent on a number of factors, knowledgeable pharmacists should always prepare the formula.

EFFICACY

There is no gold standard or specific laboratory test to measure the efficacy of nutrition with either TPN or enteral feeding. Weight gain in the hospital during a 1- to 2-week course of nutritional support is usually the result of fluid and not lean body mass. Serum visceral proteins such as prealbumin can be measured and followed during the course of therapy if desired. The half-life of prealbumin is 2 days, whereas the half-life of albumin at 21 days is too long to be useful in the inpatient setting. It must be recognized that the serum concentrations of all visceral proteins, including prealbumin, may be affected by many non-nutritional factors including intra- and extravascular fluid shifts in the postoperative patient, or may be depressed because of the protein-losing enteropathy seen in cancer or because of decreased synthesis as the liver turns towards increased production of acute phase proteins during active disease. Although serum concentration of visceral proteins may guide nutritional therapy, they should be interpreted with the caveats described above. It must also be recognized that normal visceral protein synthesis cannot occur in the absence of sufficient energy intake because skeletal muscle will be catabolized as a fuel source.

The nitrogen balance can also be determined if one has a laboratory to perform accurate measurements. A 24-hour urine collection is required. Total urine nitrogen (TUN) is measured and subtracted from the nitrogen intake from TPN (or enteral nutrition for that matter). An additional 2 g is subtracted to account for stool, sweat, and other insensible losses. It is assumed some 95% of nitrogen is generally absorbed and that the average amino acid or protein is 16% nitrogen. Therefore, in order to derive the nitrogen intake, the grams of amino acids (or protein in the case of enteral feeding) are divided by 6.25. If the TUN is not readily available, the urine urea nitrogen (UUN) can be measured. If that is the case, 4 g should be added to the measured nitrogen excretion in order to account for insensible losses and urinary nitrogen losses than are not in the form of urea. Similar to visceral proteins, a positive nitrogen balance requires not only greater nitrogen intake than excretion, but also an energy intake at least equal to energy expenditure. Maintaining a patient in positive nitrogen balance has been associated with better outcome and lower mortality.

HOME PARENTERAL NUTRITION

Patients may require home TPN (HPN) because they have developed short bowel syndrome from multiple bowel resections from cancer, usually from radiation strictures; have chronically draining entero-enteric or enterocutaneous fistulae, or have become severely malnourished in the face of cancer.[57] Such therapy requires assessment of the home environment for appropriateness and safety and proper training of either the patient or a responsible adult especially aseptic catheter care. Patients that have a life expectancy of less than 3 months and are not being actively treated with chemotherapy or radiation should not be treated with HPN in the authors' opinion.

Medicare and most insurance companies have specific guidelines for the reimbursement of HPN. Medicare requires documentation in the medical record that the HPN will be required for at least 3 months and that TEN is not feasible (eg, bowel obstruction). The case manager should evaluate each potential HPN patient prior to discharge to home. If the patient is determined to be a reasonable candidate for HPN, it is important that the patient be metabolically stable prior to hospital discharge. It is appropriate to cycle the TPN to a 10- to 12-hour nocturnal infusion prior to discharge. Nocturnal infusion gives the patient more freedom during the day to ambulate. Nocturnal infusion may also help prevent TPN-associated liver disease and encourage eating during the normal day.

During the cycling process, the patient receives his or her prescribed TPN at a gradually increased rate over a progressively shorter period of time. For example, a patient that receives a 3:1 emulsion containing 2 L of 20% dextrose, 3.5% amino acids, and 200 mL of 20% lipid emulsion over 24 hours (91 mL/hour) would have the same total volume infused over 10 hours (220 mL/hour) as a goal. In order to achieve that goal, the infusion time is shortened by 2 to 4 hour increments during each subsequent 24-hour period. For example, the TPN would be infused at 110 mL/hour for 20 hours, followed by a tapering off of over 30 to 60 minutes. A gradual tapering off is required in order to prevent hypoglycemia because endogenous insulin secretion increases significantly. This can be done either by decreasing the infusion rate by 50% for 15 to 30 minutes and then by another 50% for another 15 to 30 minutes before discontinuing the TPN.

Most pumps used in the home environment can be programmed to automatically and gradually decrease the rate to zero over a 30 to 60 minute period. This time period is not included in the overall infusion time calculation. During cycling of the TPN, the blood glucose should be obtained 2 hours after starting the TPN, just before beginning the taper period (to detect hyperglycemia) and 30 min after the TPN has been discontinued (to detect hypoglycemia). The blood glucose should always be obtained from a peripheral vein opposite the side of the infusion in order to minimize the chance of contamination of the sample from residual dextrose, resulting in a falsely elevated concentration, and to avoid contamination of the catheter. If the blood sugar is >180 mg/dl, regular insulin should be administered subcutaneously. The same amount can be added to the TPN solution just prior to beginning the infusion on subsequent nights. Typically, regular insulin is added 1 unit per 10 g of dextrose (eg, 2 L of 20% dextrose would require 20 units/L or 40 units/bag) if necessary. If post-TPN hypoglycemia is encountered, the patient should be instructed to drink some sugar-fortified juice when the TPN is discontinued and the taper period should be lengthened. Once the goal infusion rate has been achieved (patients with cardiac or renal disease may not tolerate an infusion over 10 to 12 hours and may require a slower rate), the TPN does not require ramping up on subsequent nights.

It is strongly recommended that the home TPN patient receive his or her TPN through a reputable home care company that has considerable experience in the care of such patients; many do not, but welcome the care of such a patient because of the financial remuneration. It is also strongly recommended, because of the complexities involved with HPN, that patients requiring this specialized therapy be referred to a center with a physician experienced in the care of such patients. Because the patient at home should be stable, minimal changes in the TPN prescription should be required. If frequent laboratory monitoring and changes in the TPN formulation are necessary, the patient is probably not ready for discharge.

ENTERAL NUTRITION

In the absence of bowel obstruction, distal fistula, or toxic megacolon enteral nutrition is the preferred form of nutritional support for the cancer patient, provided the patient consents to having a nasogastric or percutaneous placed feeding tube. For nasal gastric feeding, small bore, 8 to 10 French feeding tube should be used rather than the larger tube that is typically used for gastric decompression. Complications (discussed below) are generally fewer with such a tube. Because of postoperative gastroparesis, jejunal feeding may be preferred in specific individuals. Tube placement should be verified radiologically prior to feeding because physical examination, namely ausculatory confirmation, is often inaccurate for determining tube position. In general, feeding is begun at a relatively slow rate (typically 40 mL/hour) and advanced every 8 hours until the goal rate is achieved and if gastric residuals are <200 mL prior to each rate increase. However, if a small bore feeding tube is used or if jejunal feeding is undertaken, it may be difficult to aspirate and to determine an accurate gastric residual volume. In these patients, abdominal pain, distention, and tenderness are used to determine enteral feeding tolerance. The presence or absence of bowel sounds may be helpful, but actually indicates nothing more than an air-fluid interface and feeding can often be undertaken in the absence of bowel sounds. In severely malnourished cancer patients, the formula infusion rate should be increased more gradually to avoid refeeding syndrome (see above). In addition, jejunal feeding in the postoperative patient should be started at as little as 10 mL/hour, although this can often be accomplished in the immediate postoperative phase, and advanced as tolerated. Most isotonic formulas contain 1.0 to 1.5 kcal/mL and include the protein content in this calculation.

The protein content varies among formulas. No formula provides sufficient free water to meet the daily fluid requirement. Therefore, it is important that patients with normal or increased fluid requirements receive at least the equivalent of 25% of the formula's volume as free water. For example, an additional 500 mL of free water should be supplied to the patient that receives 2000 mL of formula daily. This can be provided in 2 to 4 divided doses as a bolus. This amount includes water used to flush medications from the tube. Tap water is fine; sterile or distilled water is unnecessary.

To prevent aspiration, the patient's head and shoulders should be elevated to 30 to 45 degrees at all times. The use of blue dye to detect aspiration should no longer be used, since deaths from the blue dye have been reported.[58] Gastric residuals should also be checked every 4 hours and if <200 mL, the aspirated formula should be returned to the tube as a bolus. The tube should be flushed with 30 mL of water after aspiration. Accurate input and outputs should be recorded, and the patient should be weighed at least three times weekly.

Occasionally, the nasogastric feeding tube may become clogged despite proper flushing as described. Often this is related to protein precipitates. Sugar-free decaffeinated soda is often useful for dislodging this type of occlusion. Sometimes meat tenderizer (papain) is necessary. One teaspoon of nonpotato flake papain meat tenderizer can be mixed in the smallest amount of tap water required to dissolve it and instilled in the catheter. The specific pancreatic enzyme preparations Pancrease (Ortho-McNeil, Raritan, NJ) or Viokase (Axscan Scandipharm, Birmingham, Ala) can be mixed with one crushed 324 mg sodium bicarbonate tablet in 5 mL of tap water, and instilled into the feeding tube. It may be necessary to repeat the procedure. Some medications are not compatible with enteral feedings; therefore, compatibility should be determined prior to using the feeding tube for instillation.

Other complications of tube feeding include esophagitis, esophageal, and/or gastric erosions or ulceration, or esophageal stricture or mucosal bridge formation. Esophageal or gastric erosions may be evident within a week, although longer-term use is generally required before clinically significant disease, including gastrointestinal hemorrhage, may occur. In addition, nasal erosions and nasal cartilage sloughing may result from excessive pressure on the nasal alae and cartilage; therefore, nasogastric feeding should be undertaken via the same nares for a maximum of 4 to 6 weeks.

Gastroenterologists may be asked to place a PEG tube prophylacticly in patients with head and neck cancer who will be receiving radiation postoperatively. Although the practice of placing a PEG prophylactically is acceptable, given the length of time following radiation therapy that patients are unable to take oral nutrients (eg, mean 4 months) and improved quality of life, reports of cancer seeding to the cutaneous skin site have been reported using the traditional pull method of insertion.[59] The endoscopic push or radiology-assisted method, in which the feeding tube does not come into contact with the cancer in the oropharyngeal cavity, is recommended by the authors in patients with head and neck cancer.

REFERENCES

1. Hensrud DD, Heimburger DC. Diet, nutrients, and gastrointestinal cancer. *Gastroenterol Clin North Am.* 1998;27(2):325-346.

2. Silverman DT, Swanson CA, Gridley G, et al. Dietary and nutritional factors and pancreatic cancer: a case-control study based on direct interviews. *J Natl Cancer Inst.* 1998;90(22):1710-1719.

3. Li JY, Taylor PR, Li B, et al. Nutrition intervention trials in Linxian, China: multiple vitamin/mineral supplementation, cancer incidence, and disease-specific mortality among adults with esophageal dysplasia. *J Natl Cancer Inst.* 1993;85(18):1492-1498.

4. Haenszel W, Kurihara M. Studies of Japanese migrants. I. Mortality from cancer and other diseases among Japanese in the United States. *J Natl Cancer Inst.* 1968;40(1):43-68.

5. Kono S, Hirohata T. Nutrition and stomach cancer. *Cancer Causes Control.* 1996;7(1):41-55.

6. Baron JA, Beach M, Mandel JS, et al. Calcium supplements for the prevention of colorectal adenomas. Calcium Polyp Prevention Study Group. *N Engl J Med.* 1999; 340(2):101-107.

7. Bonithon-Kopp C, Kronborg O, Giacosa A, Rath U, Faivre J. Calcium and fibre supplementation in prevention of colorectal adenoma recurrence: a randomised intervention trial. European Cancer Prevention Organisation Study Group. *Lancet.* 2000; 356(9238):1300-1306.

8. Wu K, Willett WC, Fuchs CS, Colditz GA, Giovannucci EL. Calcium intake and risk of colon cancer in women and men. *J Natl Cancer Inst.* 2002;94(6):437-446.

9. Su LJ, Arab L. Nutritional status of folate and colon cancer risk: evidence from NHANES I epidemiologic follow-up study. *Ann Epidemiol.* 2001;11(1):65-72.

10. Clark LC, Combs GF, Jr., Turnbull BW, et al. Effects of selenium supplementation for cancer prevention in patients with carcinoma of the skin. A randomized controlled trial. Nutritional Prevention of Cancer Study Group. *JAMA.* 1996;276(24):1957-1963.

11. Ghadirian P, Maisonneuve P, Perret C, et al. A case-control study of toenail selenium and cancer of the breast, colon, and prostate. *Cancer Detect Prev.* 2000;24(4):305-313.

12. Voorrips LE, Goldbohm RA, van Poppel G, et al. Vegetable and fruit consumption and risks of colon and rectal cancer in a prospective cohort study: The Netherlands Cohort Study on Diet and Cancer. *Am J Epidemiol.* 2000;152(11):1081-1092.

13. Michels KB, Edward G, Joshipura KJ, et al. Prospective study of fruit and vegetable consumption and incidence of colon and rectal cancers. *J Natl Cancer Inst.* 2000;92(21): 1740-1752.

14. Schatzkin A, Lanza E, Corle D, et al. Lack of effect of a low-fat, high-fiber diet on the recurrence of colorectal adenomas. Polyp Prevention Trial Study Group. *N Engl J Med.* 2000;342(16):1149-1155.

15. Gaard M, Tretli S, Loken EB. Dietary factors and risk of colon cancer: a prospective study of 50,535 young Norwegian men and women. *Eur J Cancer Prev.* 1996;5(6):445-454.

16. Terry P, Giovannucci E, Michels KB, et al. Fruit, vegetables, dietary fiber, and risk of colorectal cancer. *J Natl Cancer Inst.* 2001;93(7):525-533.

17. Greenberg ER, Baron JA, Tosteson TD, et al. A clinical trial of antioxidant vitamins to prevent colorectal adenoma. Polyp Prevention Study Group. *N Engl J Med.* 1994; 331(3):141-147.

18. The Alpha-Tocopherol BCCPSG. The effect of vitamin E and beta carotene on the incidence of lung cancer and other cancers in male smokers. *N Engl J Med.* 1994; 330(15):1029-1035.

19. Willett WC, Stampfer MJ, Colditz GA, Rosner BA, Speizer FE. Relation of meat, fat, and fiber intake to the risk of colon cancer in a prospective study among women. *N Engl J Med.* 1990;323(24):1664-1672.

20. Goldbohm RA, van den Brandt PA, van't Veer P, et al. A prospective cohort study on the relation between meat consumption and the risk of colon cancer. *Cancer Res.* 1994; 54(3):718-723.

21. MacLennan R, Macrae F, Bain C, et al. Randomized trial of intake of fat, fiber, and beta carotene to prevent colorectal adenomas. The Australian Polyp Prevention Project. *J Natl Cancer Inst.* 1995;87(23):1760-1766.

22. McKeown-Eyssen GE, Bright-See E, Bruce WR, et al. A randomized trial of a low fat high fibre diet in the recurrence of colorectal polyps. Toronto Polyp Prevention Group. *J Clin Epidemiol.* 1994;47(5):525-536.

23. Armstrong B, Doll R. Environmental factors and cancer incidence and mortality in different countries, with special reference to dietary practices. *Int J Cancer.* 1975;15(4):617-631.

24. Giovannucci E, Rimm EB, Stampfer MJ, et al. Intake of fat, meat, and fiber in relation to risk of colon cancer in men. *Cancer Res.* 1994;54(9):2390-2397.

25. Sandhu MS, White IR, McPherson K. Systematic review of the prospective cohort studies on meat consumption and colorectal cancer risk: a meta-analytical approach. *Cancer Epidemiol Biomarkers Prev.* 2001;10(5):439-446.

26. Boutron-Ruault MC, Senesse P, Meance S, Belghiti C, Faivre J. Energy intake, body mass index, physical activity, and the colorectal adenoma-carcinoma sequence. *Nutr Cancer.* 2001;39(1):50-57.

27. Ford ES. Body mass index and colon cancer in a national sample of adult US men and women. *Am J Epidemiol.* 1999;150(4):390-398.

28. Terry P, Giovannucci E, Bergkvist L, Holmberg L, Wolk A. Body weight and colorectal cancer risk in a cohort of Swedish women: relation varies by age and cancer site. *Br J Cancer.* 2001;85(3):346-349.

29. Giovannucci E, Ascherio A, Rimm EB, Colditz GA, Stampfer MJ, Willett WC. Physical activity, obesity, and risk for colon cancer and adenoma in men. *Ann Intern Med.* 1995;122(5):327-334.

30. Giovannucci E. Insulin and colon cancer. *Cancer Causes Control.* 1995;6(2):164-179.

31. The American Cancer Society 1996 Advisory Committee on Diet N, and Cancer Prevention. Guidelines on diet, nutrition, and cancer prevention: reducing the risk of cancer with healthy food choices and physical activity. *CA Cancer J Clin.* 1996;46(6):325-341.

32. Russell DM, Shike M, Marliss EB, et al. Effects of total parenteral nutrition and chemotherapy on the metabolic derangements in small cell lung cancer. *Cancer Res.* 1984;44(4):1706-1711.

33. Dewys WD, Begg C, Lavin PT et al. Prognostic effect of weight loss prior to chemotherapy in cancer patients. Eastern Cooperative Oncology Group. *Am J Med.* 1980;69(4): 491-497.

34. Detsky AS, McLaughlin JR, Baker JP, et al. What is subjective global assessment of nutritional status? *J Parenter Enteral Nutr.* 1987;11(1):8-13.

35. Jatoi A, Jr., Loprinzi CL. Current management of cancer-associated anorexia and weight loss. *Oncology (Huntingt).* 2001;15(4):497-502, 508; discussion 508-510.

36. Herrington AM, Herrington JD, Church CA. Pharmacologic options for the treatment of cachexia. *Nutr Clin Pract.* 1997;12(3):101-113.

37. Loprinzi CL, Ellison NM, Schaid DJ, et al. Controlled trial of megestrol acetate for the treatment of cancer anorexia and cachexia. *J Natl Cancer Inst.* 1990;82(13):1127-1132.

38. Kardinal CG, Loprinzi CL, Schaid DJ, et al. A controlled trial of cyproheptadine in cancer patients with anorexia and/or cachexia. *Cancer.* 1990;65(12):2657-2662.

39. Satyanarayana R, Klein S. Clinical efficacy of perioperative nutrition support. *Curr Opin Clin Nutr Metab Care.* 1998;1(1):51-58.

40. The Veterans Affairs Total Parenteral Nutrition Cooperative Study Group. Perioperative total parenteral nutrition in surgical patients. *N Engl J Med.* 1991;325(8):525-532.

41. Bozzetti F. Nutrition and gastrointestinal cancer. *Curr Opin Clin Nutr Metab Care.* 2001;4(6):541-546.

42. Bae JM, Park JW, Yang HK, Kim JP. Nutritional status of gastric cancer patients after total gastrectomy. *World J Surg.* 1998;22(3):254-260; discussion 260-251.

43. Jenkins DJ, Bloom SR, Albuquerque RH, et al. Pectin and complications after gastric surgery: normalisation of postprandial glucose and endocrine responses. *Gut.* 1980; 21(7):574-579.

44. Jain G, Scolapio J, Wasserman E, Floch MH. Chronic radiation enteritis: a ten-year follow-up. *J Clin Gastroenterol.* 2002;35(3):214-217.

45. Scolapio JS, Ukleja A, Burnes JU, Kelly DG. Outcome of patients with radiation enteritis treated with home parenteral nutrition. *Am J Gastroenterol.* 2002;97(3):662-666.

46. Buchman AL. Glutamine: commercially essential or conditionally essential? A critical appraisal of the human data. *Am J Clin Nutr.* 2001;74(1):25-32.

47. Buchman AL, Moukarzel AA, Bhuta S, et al. Parenteral nutrition is associated with intestinal morphologic and functional changes in humans. *J Parenter Enteral Nutr.* 1995; 19(6):453-460.

48. Sedman PC, MacFie J, Palmer MD, Mitchell CJ, Sagar PM. Preoperative total parenteral nutrition is not associated with mucosal atrophy or bacterial translocation in humans. *Br J Surg.* 1995;82(12):1663-1667.

49. Buchman AL, Ament ME. Liver disease and total parenteral nutrition. In: Zakim D, Boyer TD, eds. *Hepatology: A Textbook of Liver Disease.* 3rd ed. Philadelphia: WB Saunders; 1996:1812-1821.

50. Buchman AL, Ament ME, Sohel M, et al. Choline deficiency causes reversible hepatic abnormalities in patients receiving parenteral nutrition: proof of a human choline requirement: a placebo-controlled trial. *J Parenter Enteral Nutr.* 2001;25(5):260-268.

51. Scolapio JS, Tarrosa VB, Stoner GL, Moreno-Aspitia A, Solberg LA Jr., Atkinson EJ. Audit of nutrition support for hematopoietic stem cell transplantation at a single institution. *Mayo Clin Proc.* 2002;77(7):654-659.

52. Toskes PP. Hyperlipidemic pancreatitis. *Gastroenterol Clin North Am.* 1990;19(4):783-791.

53. Solomon SM, Kirby DF. The refeeding syndrome: a review. *J Parenter Enteral Nutr.* 1990;14(1):90-97.

54. Buchman AL, Moukarzel A, Goodson B, et al. Catheter-related infections associated with home parenteral nutrition and predictive factors for the need for catheter removal in their treatment. *J Parenter Enteral Nutr.* 1994;18(4):297-302.

55. Messing B, Peitra-Cohen S, Debure A, Beliah M, Bernier JJ. Antibiotic-lock technique: a new approach to optimal therapy for catheter-related sepsis in home-parenteral nutrition patients. *J Parenter Enteral Nutr.* 1988;12(2):185-189.

56. Atkinson JB, Bagnall HA, Gomperts E. Investigational use of tissue plasminogen activator (t-PA) for occluded central venous catheters. *J Parenter Enteral Nutr.* 1990;14(3):310-311.

57. Scolapio JS, Fleming CR, Kelly DG, Wick DM, Zinsmeister AR. Survival of home parenteral nutrition-treated patients: 20 years of experience at the Mayo Clinic. *Mayo Clin Proc.* 1999;74(3):217-222.

58. Maloney JP, Ryan TA. Detection of aspiration in enterally fed patients: a requiem for bedside monitors of aspiration. *J Parenter Enteral Nutr.* 2002;26(6 Suppl):S34-41; discussion S41-32.

59. Sinclair JJ, Scolapio JS, Stark ME, Hinder RA. Metastasis of head and neck carcinoma to the site of percutaneous endoscopic gastrostomy: case report and literature review. *J Parenter Enteral Nutr.* 2001;25(5):282-285.

chapter 17

Chemoprevention for Gastrointestinal Neoplasia

Paul J. Limburg, MD, MPH and Navtej Buttar, MD

INTRODUCTION

GI malignancies account for approximately 30% of all incident and 36% of all fatal cancers reported each year.[1] While early detection remains the cornerstone of prevention, chemoprevention is emerging as a complementary strategy. Within the GI tract and elsewhere, carcinogenesis is thought to proceed through a multistep process in which cellular growth becomes progressively dysregulated and ultimately results in clonal evolution and expansion.[2] Mutational (inherited or acquired) or non-mutational (epigenetic) events can lead to altered gene expression patterns.[3] Aberrant protein transcription or translation further disrupts normal cellular growth constraints. Once independent in growth signaling, cells achieve limitless replicative potential. Additional loss of usual adhesion and/or invasion controls affords the ability to breach the basement membrane.[4]

By definition, chemoprevention refers to the use of chemical compounds to prevent invasion of dysplastic epithelial cells across the basement membrane (eg, blocking carcinogenesis at a preinvasive stage). In this chapter, general concepts of GI cancer chemoprevention are reviewed, followed by discussions of candidate agents by site. Basic descriptive statistics are provided for context, and clinical trial data are emphasized where available. Due to differences in the volume of site-specific chemoprevention research conducted to date, esophageal and colorectal cancer chemoprevention are discussed in relatively greater detail than gastric, hepatobiliary, and pancreas cancer chemoprevention. Summary remarks are also provided that reflect the current state of the science in this rapidly evolving field.

GENERAL CONCEPTS

AGENT IDENTIFICATION

Data from cell culture experiments, animal model systems, and epidemiological investigations form the foundation for chemoprevention agent identification. Cell culture experiments can be used to initially screen compounds for potential effects on carcinogen synthesis, carcinogen activation, free radical scavenging, and DNA adduct formation, as well as carcinogenesis suppression at a postinitiation phase. *In vitro* studies are also useful for testing the effects of candidate agents on specific molecular targets and/or intracellular pathways. Animal model systems can be used to confirm and extend results from cell culture experiments using several different approaches. Chemical carcinogens will induce tumor formation at most GI sites, but these highly artificial constructs are of relatively limited value for chemoprevention research. Transgenic and gene-mutant animals carry specific DNA alterations and more closely approximate the human condition, at least for the subset of patients genetically predisposed to forming GI cancers. Xenograft models permit direct evaluation of anticarcinogenic properties on human tumor tissue, albeit in unnatural surroundings. Infectious organisms like *H. pylori*) can stimulate tumorigenesis in rodents that strongly mimics human disease. Lastly, surgically altered anatomy can promote inflammatory-mediated carcinogenesis in select target organs, such as the esophagus. A partial listing of candidate chemoprevention agents that appear promising based on preclinical data is shown in Table 17-1.

With respect to interpreting data from epidemiological investigations, the following factors are worthy of consideration: 1) presence or absence of a biologically plausible rationale for the proposed anticarcinogenic effect, 2) consistency of the observed risk association across studies, and 3) magnitude of the potential cancer prevention effect. Study design also affects the ability to infer potentially causal associations from observational data. Cohort, nested case-cohort, and nested case-control (prospective) studies generally provide the highest level of support, since the exposures are assessed prior to disease onset and case status is ascertained forward in time. Case-control (retrospective) studies are prone to several important biases (recall, survival, etc.); cross-sectional studies include only prevalent cases, obviating assessment of temporal relationships; and etiologic studies address population-specific, rather than person-specific, risk associations. The latter study designs are useful for hypothesis generation, but do not typically form the sole basis for moving candidate chemopreventive agents forward into clinical trials.

COHORT DEFINITION

Contrary to the traditional chemotherapy paradigm, chemopreventive interventions are intended for generally healthy patient populations. However, because most cancer prevention agents are not entirely devoid of potential toxicities, initial chemoprevention trials are often conducted among high-risk subjects, who stand to benefit the most from improved interventions. Both family cancer history and past medical history can be used to select appropriate subject cohorts for chemoprevention trials. Other factors, such as geographic location, may occasionally be useful in cohort selection as well, if residents of a specific global region are known to have increased cancer rates without defined familial, medical, or environmental associations.

Table 17-1

Promising GI Cancer Chemoprevention Agents Based on Preclinical Data

Candidate Agents	Molecular Targets	GI Cancer Site(s)	Comments
Aza-deoxycytidine, folic acid[194,195]	Promoter methylation	Colorectum	Prevent intestinal tumors and decrease aberrant crypt foci in APC Min/+ and Dnmt mice.
Perillyl alcohol, limonene[196-198]	Farnesyl transferase pathway	Hepatobiliary tract Pancreas	Inhibition of cancer development in xenograft models and decreased cell survival of cancer cell in vitro.
Genistein, erbstatin[199-201]	Tyrosine kinases	Colorectum	Decrease in azoxymethane (carcinogen)-induced aberrant crypt foci in rats.
Herceptin, VEGF, RhuMab[202]	Her2, EGFR, and VEGF	Colorectum	Inhibition of HCA-7 colon cancer cell growth in vitro and in vivo.
Anti-AP-1 retinoids, NSAIDs, Bortezomib[203,204]	AP-1 and Nf-kappa B pathway	Esophagus Colorectum	Human colorectal cell apoptosis increases with inhibition of AP-1 activation. Barrett's epithelial cell survival decreases with inhibition of Nf-kappa B activation.
1α-OH vitamin D₂, 1α-OH vitamin D₅, 1,25-(OH)2-16-ene-23-yne vitamin D₃[205-207]	Vitamin D receptor	Colorectum	Prevention of tumor formation in APC Min/+ mice. Decrease rate of DMH induced colorectal cancer. -inhibition of tumorigenesis in xenograft model of colon cancer.

continued

Table 17-1 (continued)

PROMISING GI CANCER CHEMOPREVENTION AGENTS BASED ON PRECLINICAL DATA

Candidate Agents	Molecular Targets	GI Cancer Site(s)	Comments
Troglitazone[208]	PPAR-γ	Colorectum	Decrease in azoxymethane (carcinogen)-induced aberrant crypt foci.
All-trans-RA, 9-cis RA, and others[175, 209, 210]	Retinoid acid and RXR receptors and ligands	Esophagus Colorectum Hepatobiliary tract	Apoptosis induction via tissue transglutaminase and reduced alpha-feto protein levels. Decreased esophageal cell survival. Reduction in AOM-induced aberrant crypt foci.
Celecoxib, refecoxib, NSAIDs, and triterpenoids[78, 188, 211–214]	APC, β-catenin, and Cyclo-oxygenase-2 pathway	Esophagus Colorectum Stomach Hepatobiliary tract Pancreas	Reduced tumor burden in APC Min/+ mice. Prevent esophageal adenocarcinoma and esophageal squamous cell carcinoma in rats. Decresed cell survival of gastric pancreatic and hepatic neoplastic cells.
S-adenosylmethionine decarboxylase, Difluoromethylornithine[215-217]	Polyamine biosynthesis	Esophagus Colorectum	Modify APC dependent signaling to prevent cancer. Conversion of transformed cell phenotype to normal cell phenotype.
Flavopiridol, Butyrolactone I, Olomoucine, Roscovitine[218]	Cyclin-dependent kinases	Pancreas	Growth inhibition of malignant pancreatic cells.

continued

Table 17-1 (continued)

PROMISING GI CANCER CHEMOPREVENTION AGENTS BASED ON PRECLINICAL DATA

Candidate Agents	Molecular Targets	GI Cancer Site(s)	Comments
Batimastat, Marimastat[219-221]	Matrix metalloproteinases	Colorectum Stomach Pancreas	Prevents angiogenesis in xenograft models of colon, gastric and pancreatic cancers.
Calcium, Soy isoflavin, Tea polyphenols, ursodeoxycholic acid[222-226]	Carcinogen uptake and/or activation	Colorectum Hepatobiliary tract Pancreas	Prevent hyperproliferation and tumor development in carcinogen-induced animal models of colon, pancreatic, and hepatic cancers.
Selenium, Vitamin E, Carotenoid, tea polyphenols[226]	Immune modulation ihibition of oxidative DNA damage	Esophagus Colorectum Pancreas	Decreased tumor burden in carcinogen induced colon, pancreas, and esophageal squamous cell cancers.

As shown in Table 17-2, several heritable syndromes are known to be associated with increased GI cancer risk. Of these syndromes, FAP and HNPCC are sufficiently common to form the basis for defining chemoprevention trial cohorts. Among FAP patients, APC gene mutations result in the phenotypic expression of hundreds to thousands of colorectal adenomas, usually during adolescence. Without prophylactic colectomy, FAP patients invariably develop colorectal cancer at a relatively young age (approximately 40 years).[5] Duodenal cancer risk (especially in the periampullary region) is also elevated in FAP and represents the leading cause of malignant death among patients who have undergone prophylactic colectomy.[6] HNPCC patients are predisposed to tumor formation at multiple GI sites (colorectal, gastric, small bowel, hepatobiliary tract, and pancreas), as well as in several non-GI target organs (uterus, genitourinary tract, and ovary), due to mutations in any of 5 DNA mismatch repair genes (*hMLH1, hMSH2, hPMS1, hPMS2, and hMSH6*).[7] At present, vigilant endoscopic surveillance is the only nonsurgical option for GI cancer prevention in FAP and HNPCC kindreds. While effective, this approach is intensive, invasive, and limited to a single organ system. Systemic interventions such as chemoprevention are therefore particularly attractive for patients with these genetic disorders.

Comprehensive reviews regarding the spectrum of medical conditions associated with esophageal,[8-10] gastric,[11] colorectal,[12,13] hepatobiliary,[14,15] and pancreas[16] cancers have been recently published. Patients with BE, *H. pylori* infection, prior colorectal adenomas, or idiopathic inflammatory bowel disease have well-defined risks for site-specific GI cancers and represent realistic cohorts for chemoprevention trials. BE, wherein normal squamous epithelium is replaced by specialized metaplastic columnar epithelium, results from chronic exposure to refluxed gastric contents.[17] In a subset of BE patients, histologic transformation progresses beyond metaplasia, to form LGD, HGD, and eventually adenocarcinoma. Compared to the general population, BE patients have a 30- to 60-fold increase in esophageal adenocarcinoma risk,[18] with an estimated cancer incidence rate of approximately 0.5% to 1.0% per year.[19] *H. pylori* is a gram-negative bacterium that colonizes approximately one-half of the world's population[20] and has been classified as a class I carcinogen by the International Agency for Research on Cancer.[21] Based on a recent meta-analysis of existing observational data,[22] the odds ratio for gastric cancer is 2.0 (95% CI =1.7 to 2.5) among *H. pylori*-positive vs *H. pylori*-negative patients. More strikingly, Parkin estimated that 42% of all gastric cancers may be ascribed to this infectious organism.[23]

Patients with prior colorectal adenomas are approximately 3 times more likely to develop recurrent (metachronous) neoplasia compared to average-risk patients of similar age and gender. Adenomas with the following features carry the highest risk for recurrence: ≥1 cm in diameter, ≥3 in total number, villous histology, or HGD.[24] History of colorectal cancer is also a risk factor for metachronous neoplasia, with a median time to detection of about 24 months after curative resection.[25] These patients may be particularly motivated to participate in chemoprevention trials. Idiopathic inflammatory bowel disease (including both chronic ulcerative colitis and Crohn's disease) affects approximately 400,000 patients in the United States.[26] Longstanding ulcerative colitis is associated with cumulative colorectal cancer incidence rates of 2%, 8%, and 18% after 10, 20, and 30 years of disease, respectively.[27] Data for patients with Crohn's disease are more limited, but the colorectal cancer risk seems to be similarly increased.

Table 17-2

HERITABLE SYNDROMES ASSOCIATED WITH INCREASED GASTROINTESTINAL CANCER RISK

Heritable Syndrome	Inheritance Pattern	Esophagus	Stomach	Small Bowel	Colorectum	Hepatobiliary Tract	Pancreas
Ataxia-telangiectasia	Autosomal Recessive		X				X
Basal cell nevus	Autosomal Dominant				X		
Bloom	Autosomal Recessive	X			X		
Cowden (gingival multiple hamartoma)	Autosomal Dominant				X		
FAP	Autosomal Dominant		X	X	X	X	
Familial gastric cancer	Autosomal Dominant		X				
Familial melanoma	Autosomal Dominant						X
Familial pancreatic cancer	Unknown						X
Fanconi's anemia	Autosomal Recessive	X				X	X
Hereditary breast/other cancer (BRCA2)	Autosomal Dominant				X		X
Hereditary breast/ovarian (BRCA1)	Autosomal Dominant				X		

continued

Table 17-2 (continued)

HERITABLE SYNDROMES ASSOCIATED WITH INCREASED GASTROINTESTINAL CANCER RISK

Heritable Syndrome	Inheritance Pattern	Esophagus	Stomach	Small Bowel	Colorectum	Hepatobiliary Tract	Pancreas
(HNPCC)	Autosomal Dominant		X	X	X	X	X
Li-Fraumeni	Autosomal Dominant		X				X
Multiple endocrine neoplasia I	Autosomal Dominant						X
Peutz-Jeghers	Autosomal Dominant		X	X	X		X
Tylosis (nonepidermolytic plamoplantar keratosis)	Autosomal Dominant	X					
VonHippel-Lindau disease	Autosomal Dominant						X
Werner's syndrome	Autosomal Recessive		X				
Wilm's tumor	Autosomal Dominant					X	
Xeroderma pigmentosum	Autosomal Recessive		X				

Adapted from Lindor NM, Greene MH. The concise handbook of family cancer syndromes. Mayo Familiar Cancer Program. *J Natl Cancer Inst.* 1998; 90(14):1039-71.

ENDPOINT EVALUATION

Cancer incidence and mortality remain the most definitive outcomes for judging the effects of candidate chemoprevention agents. However, these endpoints are impractical for early phase chemoprevention trials, since hundreds to thousands of subjects are typically needed to observe an adequate number of incident or fatal cancers, even within high-risk subject populations. Also, years to decades of follow-up are often required to achieve statistically meaningful results. Thus, the effects of candidate agents are commonly measured against surrogate endpoint biomarkers (SEBs) to demonstrate preliminary efficacy. Two key features of suitable SEBs are 1) level of association between the surrogate biomarker and the GI cancer outcome (ie, the degree to which the biomarker is on the causal pathway for disease), and 2) accuracy of the biomarker measurement technique. At the macroscopic level, several SEBs can be assessed by endoscopy. Length of columnar metaplasia predicts adenocarcinoma risk among BE patients[28] and can be easily measured pre- and postintervention. Colorectal adenoma size and number are both positively correlated with colorectal cancer risk[24] and have been successfully monitored in previous chemoprevention trials. Vital staining can also be used to highlight mucosal abnormalities in both the upper and lower GI tract, but data regarding the potential utility of chromoendoscopy-defined SEBs are only beginning to emerge.

To date, intraepithelial neoplasia has been the primary phenotypic SEB applied in chemoprevention trials sponsored by the National Cancer Institute.[29] Histologic grade of noninvasive neoplasia (or dysplasia) predicts GI cancer risk at multiple sites and represents a potentially modifiable target for esophageal, gastric, and colorectal cancer chemoprevention trials. In the esophagus, patients with BE-associated HGD experience a much higher adenocarcinoma incidence rate (22%) than patients with no dysplasia (2%) over a relatively short time interval.[30-33] Similarly, esophageal biopsy specimens with mild, moderate, and severe squamous dysplasia were associated relative risks for incident cancer of 2.9, 9.8, and 28.3, respectively, after extended follow-up among residents of a high-risk region in China.[34,35] In a prospective study of noninvasive gastric neoplasia, Rugge et al found that invasive cancer risk was significantly correlated with baseline histology grade over an average follow-up period of 52 months.[36] Because polyp resection convincingly decreases incident colorectal cancer,[37] large bowel adenomas are usually removed rather than monitored for signs of progression. However, cross-sectional studies have demonstrated that colorectal adenomas with LGD are less likely to contain foci of adenocarcinoma (0.3%) compared to adenomas with HGD (27%).[38]

Other tissue-based SEBs include assays related to growth regulation in general, such as proliferation and apoptosis, or specific intracellular pathways of carcinogenesis. An example of the latter group includes proteins involved in arachidonic acid metabolism. Esophageal biopsy specimens from patients with BE show a parallel increase in cyclooxygenase-2 (COX-2) expression and neoplastic progression.[39] Higher PGE2 concentration has also been observed in metaplastic BE epithelium compared to normal squamous epithelium.[40] Further, PGE2 induces proliferation in BE epithelial cells[41] and inhibition of PGE2 normalizes the proliferation rate.[40] These observations help form the basis for evaluating antireflux therapy in combination with COX-2 inhibition in BE chemoprevention trials, as discussed on page 337.

CANDIDATE CHEMOPREVENTION AGENTS BY SITE

Compounds that demonstrate chemopreventive potential in preclinical studies, epidemiological investigations, or a combination of both are further developed through a series of clinical trials designed to assess dose, bioavailability and toxicity (phase I); preliminary efficacy against molecular, imaging, or histologic SEBs (phase II); and ultimately definitive efficacy against cancer outcomes (phase III). The developmental status of candidate chemopreventive agents for esophageal, colorectal, gastric, hepatobiliary tract, and pancreas cancers is reviewed in the following sections.

ESOPHAGUS

Based on GLOBOCAN data, 412,327 incident and 337,501 fatal esophageal cancer cases were recorded worldwide in 2000.[1] High risk global regions include China, India, Northern Iran, and South Africa[10] for ESC and Scotland, the United Kingdom, the Netherlands, and the United States for EAC.[9,42] In the United States, age-adjusted incidence and mortality rates for esophageal cancer are 4.7/100,000 population and 4.4/100,000 population, respectively.[43] Incidence rates are markedly higher for men than for women (8.2 vs 1.9 per 100,000 population) and are also higher for African-Americans than for Caucasians (6.3 vs 4.7 per 100,000 population). For cases diagnosed in 1995 to 2000, the estimated 5-year survival rate was 14.3% overall (29.3% for localized disease). Candidate agents for esophageal cancer chemoprevention are discussed below, with data from randomized, controlled trials presented in Table 17-3.

Selenium

Selenium may interrupt carcinogenesis through several mechanisms, including immune modulation, decreased carcinogen activation, reduced proliferation, and increased apoptosis.[44] Cell culture and animal model studies have demonstrated few beneficial effects from selenium compounds on esophageal carcinogenesis.[44-49] In fact, selenium administration resulted in increased EAC incidence as well as tumor volume in a surgically altered rat model.[49] However, epidemiological data are more encouraging. Case-control and cohort studies have shown that selenium status (as measured in either peripheral blood samples or toenail clippings) is inversely associated with incident ESC and EAC.[50-54]

Two randomized, placebo-controlled trials have directly analyzed selenium as a potential esophageal cancer chemoprevention agent. In the US Nutritional Prevention of Cancer Study (n=1312), subjects who were treated with 200 mg/day of selenized yeast for a mean duration of 4.5 years had a nonstatistically significant reduction in esophageal cancer risk (RR=0.40; 95% CI=0.08 to 2.07) compared to placebo-treated subjects.[55] However, case numbers in both intervention arms were small (n=2 and n=5, respectively) and esophageal cancer was analyzed as a secondary endpoint in this study. Limburg et al conducted a pilot study of selenomethionine 200 mg/day (2-x-2 factorial design) among subjects from Linxian, PRC who had histologically confirmed mild or moderate squamous dysplasia at baseline. After a 10-month intervention period, selenomethionine was found to have a marginally significant effect on change in squamous dysplasia grade overall (p=0.08), although subjects who began the trial with mild dysplasia derived a statistically significant benefit (p=0.02).[56]

Two multinutrient intervention trials have also been conducted in Linxian, PRC. Asymptomatic adults enrolled in the General Population Trial (n=29,584) experienced

Table 17-3

RANDOMIZED, CONTROLLED CHEMOPREVENTION TRIALS FOR ESOPHAGEAL CANCER

Candidate Agent(s)	N[1]	Risk Cohort	Intervent. Period	Form and Dose	Endpoint	Risk Est. (95% CI)[2]	Comments
Selenium[55]	1312	Subjects enrolled in a skin cancer prevention trial	7.4 years	Selenized yeast 200 µg/day	Cancer incidence	0.40 (0.08 to 2.07)	Esophageal cancer analyzed as a secondary endpoint, without respect to histologic subtype.
Selenium, COX-2 inhibitor[56]	267	Histologically-confirmed squamous dysplasia at baseline	10 months	Selenomethionine 200 µg/day Celecoxib 200 mg bid	Change in squamous dysplasia grade	N/A[3]	Selenomethionine had marginal effect among all subjects (p=0.08) and significant effect among subjects with mild dysplasia at baseline (p=0.02); Celecoxib had no appreciable effect
Multinutrient[57]	29,584	Residents of a high-risk global region	5.25 years	Selenized yeast 50 µg/day β-carotene 15 µg/day α-tocopherol 30 mg/day	Cancer incidence Cancer mortality	1.02 (0.87 to 1.19) 0.96 (0.78 to 1.18)	Squamous cell carcinoma.
				Retinol 5000 IU/day Zinc 22.5 mg/day	Cancer incidence Cancer mortality	1.07 (0.92 to 1.25) 0.93 (0.92 to 1.25)	

continued

Table 17-3 (continued)

RANDOMIZED, CONTROLLED CHEMOPREVENTION TRIALS FOR ESOPHAGEAL CANCER

Candidate Agent(s)	N[1]	Risk Cohort	Intervent. Period	Form and Dose	Endpoint	Risk Est. (95% CI)	Comments
Multinutrient[57] (con't)	29,584	Residents of a high-risk global region	5.25 years	Ascorbic acid 120 mg/day Molybdenum 30 µg/day	Cancer incidence Cancer mortality	1.06 (0.91 to 1.24) 1.05 (0.85 to 1.29)	Squamous cell carcinoma.
				Riboflavin 3.2 mg/day Niacin 40 mg/day	Cancer incidence Cancer mortality	0.86 (0.74 to 1.01) 0.90 (0.73 to 1.11)	
Multinutrient[58]	3318	Cytologically-detected squamous dysplasia	6 years	26 vitamins and minerals (various doses)	Cancer incidence	0.94 (0.73 to 1.20)	Squamous cell carcinoma.
Multinutrient[76]	610	Residents of a high-risk global region	13.5 months	Retinol 50,000 IU/week Riboflavin 200 mg/week Zinc 50 mg/week	Spectrum of histologically-defined lesions	N/A	Prevalence of esophagitis with or without atrophy or dysplasia found to be nearly the same in the placebo group (45%) and the vitamin/zinc treated group (49%).

[1]N=number randomized; CI=confidence interval; N/A=not available

minimally reduced esophageal cancer incidence (RR=0.1.02; 95% CI=0.87 to 1.19) and mortality (RR=0.96; 95% CI=0.78 to 1.18) rates after 5.25 years of selenium (50 mg/day as selenized yeast), ß-carotene (15 mg/day), and α-tocopherol (30 mg/day).[57] In the smaller Dysplasia Trial, subjects with cytologically-detected dysplasia at baseline (n=3318) had similar risks for incident (RR=0.94; 95% CI=0.73 to 1.20) and fatal (RR=0.84; 95% CI=0.54 to 1.29) esophageal cancer regardless of whether they received daily supplementation with 26 vitamins and minerals (including sodium selenate 50 mg/day) vs placebo over the 6-year intervention period.[58]

Antioxidant Vitamins

Vitamins A, C, and E (as well as their biochemical precursors) may prevent esophageal and/or other cancers by neutralizing free radicals and blocking carcinogen formation. Retinoids are also thought to inhibit cellular proliferation and decrease angiogenesis. Alpha-tocopherol appears to stimulate immunosurveillance, induce apoptosis, and regulate cell signaling pathways, in addition to having other putative cancer prevention effects.[59-61] In animal models of esophageal cancer, supplementation with vitamin A, vitamin C, and related compounds has yielded minimal cancer protective effects (tumorigenesis was actually enhanced in Fischer 344 rats).[62-65] In contrast, vitamin E has shown chemopreventive potential in both carcinogen-treated and surgically altered rodents.[49,66] Observational studies from diverse geographic regions support inverse associations between antioxidant vitamins and esophageal cancer risk based on either dietary data[67-71] or serum/plasma levels,[72-75] although not all reports are consistent.

In the Linxian General Population Trial, antioxidant vitamins in combination with other micronutrients did not meaningfully alter the observed esophageal cancer incidence or mortality rates:

- Retinol 5000 IU and zinc 22.5 mg/day (RR=1.07; 95% CI=0.92 to 1.25 and RR=0.93; 95% CI=0.76 to 1.15, respectively)
- Ascorbic acid 120 mg and molybdenum 30 mg/day (RR=1.06; 95% CI=0.91 to 1.24 and RR=1.05; 95% CI=0.85 to 1.29, respectively)
- Selenium 50 mg, ß-carotene 15 mg, and a-tocopherol 30 mg/day (RR=1.02; 95% CI=0.87 to 1.19 and RR=0.96; 95% CI=0.78 to 1.18, respectively)

Similarly, the cadre of nutrients administered in the Linxian Dysplasia Trial, which included vitamin A 10,000 IU, vitamin C 180 mg, and vitamin E 60 IU per day, had no discernible effects with respect to either incident or fatal esophageal cancer. Another randomized trial from Huixian, PRC (n=610) found that the prevalence rates for a spectrum of histologically defined esophageal lesions (including esophagitis, atrophy, dysplasia, or cancer) were not statistically different among subjects who received retinol 50,000 IU/week (along with riboflavin 200 mg/week and zinc 50 mg/week) vs placebo after a mean intervention period of 13.5 months.[76]

NSAIDs and Selective COX-2 Inhibitors

The chemopreventive benefits afforded by traditional NSAIDs are thought to be derived primarily through COX-2 inhibition. Cell cultures from patients with either esophageal cancer or BE exhibit decreased proliferation and increased apoptosis following the application of COX-2 inhibitors.[41,77] COX-2 inhibitors have also been shown to reduce EAC risk in a surgically altered animal model of BE.[78] Inverse associations between regular use of traditional NSAIDs and esophageal cancer risk have been consistently reported in case-control and cohort studies as well. Recently, Corley et al performed a meta-analysis of existing observational data and found that any NSAID use was associated with a 43% risk reduction (OR=0.57; 95% CI=0.47 to 0.71).[79] Moreover, frequent use appeared to be more effective than intermittent use (46% vs 18% risk reduction, respectively). By histologic subtype, NSAID use was protective for both ESC (OR=0.58; 95% CI=0.43 to 0.78) and EAC (OR=0.67; 95% CI=0.51 to 0.87).[79]

In a small, uncontrolled study of BE patients (n=12), selective COX-2 inhibition with rofecoxib 25 mg/day for 10 days resulted in a statistically significant decline in cellular proliferation (p<0.005).[40] The only randomized, controlled chemoprevention trial data reported to date are from a Linxian, PCR pilot study (see page 334) wherein celecoxib 200 mg bid for 10 months had no appreciable effect on change in histologic grade of esophageal squamous dysplasia.[56] Other esophageal cancer chemoprevention trials are ongoing, including a large phase II trial of celecoxib 200 mg bid among subjects with BE.[80]

Other Candidate Agents

Prolonged acid suppression can promote the reformation of squamous mucosal islands within fields of specialized metaplastic columnar epithelium. However, proton pump inhibitors have not consistently been shown to cause regression of BE metaplasia or prevent esophageal adenocarcinoma.[19,81-84] Possible explanations are that proton pump inhibitors fail to completely suppress gastric acid secretion and also do not effectively treat duodenal-esophageal bile reflux.[85,86] Gastric acid and bile salts can activate several procarcinogenic pathways in BE.[41,78,87-90] Furthermore, using a BE organ culture system pulsed doses of acid (ie, simulating intermittent reflux) produce increased cellular proliferation.[89] Uncontrolled studies have shown that effective acid suppression therapy can favorably affect cellular proliferation among BE patients.[91] However, since bile reflux may also be important in esophageal carcinogenesis,[92] acid-suppressing agents alone are unlikely to provide substantial chemopreventive benefits.

COLORECTUM

Based on GLOBOCAN data, 944,717 incident and 492,411 fatal colorectal cancer (CRC) cases were recorded worldwide in 2000.[1] High-risk global regions include Australia, New Zealand, North America, and Northern and Western Europe.[23] In the United States, age-adjusted incidence and mortality rates for CRC are 51.8/100,000 population and 20.0/100,000 population, respectively.[43] Incidence rates are higher for men than for women (60.6 vs 44.8 per 100,000 population) and for Blacks than for Whites (61.4 vs 51.1 per 100,000 population). For cases diagnosed in 1995 to 2000, the estimated 5-year survival rate was 63.4% overall (89.9% for localized disease). Candidate agents for CRC chemoprevention are discussed below, with data from randomized, controlled trials (including at least 20 subjects and measuring at least one adenoma or cancer endpoint) presented in Table 17-4.

Fiber

Dietary fiber represents a heterogeneous class of plant-derived compounds that have potential to reduce CRC risk by 1) diluting or adsorbing intraluminal carcinogens, 2) reducing GI transit time, 3) altering bile acid metabolism, or 4) increasing the production of short-chain fatty acids. In a recent review of animal model data, Sengupta and colleagues noted that 15 of 19 experimental studies found a protective effect of fiber

Table 17-4
RANDOMIZED, CONTROLLED CHEMOPREVENTION TRIALS FOR COLORECTAL CANCER

Candidate Agent(s)	N[1]	Risk Cohort	Intervent. Period	Form and Dose	Endpoint	Risk Est. (95% CI)[2]	Comments
Fiber, antioxidant vitamins[100]	58	FAP	4 years	Wheat bran 22 gm/day Vitamin C 4 gm/day Vitamin E 400 gm/day	Rectal adenoma number	N/A[3]	No significant benefit from fiber supplement.
Fiber, antioxidant vitamins[101]	424	Prior colorectal adenoma	48 months	Wheat bran 25 gm/day ß-carotene 20 mg/day	Recurrent adenoma Recurrent adenoma	1.20 (0.80 to2.00) 1.50 (0.90 to 2.50)	
Fiber[102]	1429	Prior colorectal adenoma	34 months	Wheat bran 13.5 gm/day	Recurrent adenoma	0.88 (0.70 to 1.11)	Compared to low-fiber intervention group (2 gm/day).
Fiber[103]	201	Prior colorectal adenoma	24 months	Dietary modification: 50 gm/day	Recurrent adenoma	1.20 (0.60 to 2.20)	Combine with dietary fat reduction.
Fiber[104]	2079	Prior colorectal adenoma	3.05 years	Dietary modification: 18 gm per 1000 kcal/day	Recurrent adenoma	1.00 (0.90 to 1.12)	Combined with dietary fat reduction, increased fruit and vegetable consumption.

continued

Table 17-4 (continued)

RANDOMIZED, CONTROLLED CHEMOPREVENTION TRIALS FOR COLORECTAL CANCER

Candidate Agent(s)	N[1]	Risk Cohort	Intervent. Period	Form and Dose	Endpoint	Risk Est. (95% CI)	Comments
Fiber, Calcium[105]	665	Prior colorectal adenoma	3 years	Ispaghula husk 3.5 gm/day Elemental calcium 2000 mg/day	Recurrent adenoma Recurrent adenoma	1.67 (1.01 to 2.76) 0.66 (0.38 to 1.17)	
Antioxidant vitamins[114]	49	FAP	2 years	Vitamin C 3000 mg/day	Polyp number Polyp area	N/A	No statistically significant differences between active and placebo groups after 18 months.
Antioxidant vitamins[115]	255	Prior colorectal adenoma	18 months	Vitamin A 30,000 IU/day Vitamin C 1000 mg/day Vitamin E 70 mg/day	Recurrent adenoma	N/A	Recurrence rate lower in the vitamin group (6%) vs the placebo group (36%).
Antioxidant vitamins, selenium, calcium[117]	116	Existing colorectal polyps	3 years	Vitamin C 150 mg/day Vitamin E 75 mg/day β-carotene 15 mg/day Selenium 101 mg/day Calcium carbonate 1600 mg/day	Recurrent adenoma	0.31 (0.11 to 0.84)	
Antioxidant vitamins[118]	200	Prior colorectal adenoma	2 years	Vitamin C 400 mg/day Vitamin E 400 mg/day	Recurrent adenoma	0.86 (0.51 to 1.45)	

continued

Table 17-4 (continued)

RANDOMIZED, CONTROLLED CHEMOPREVENTION TRIALS FOR COLORECTAL CANCER

Candidate Agent(s)	N^1	Risk Cohort	Intervent. Period	Form and Dose	Endpoint	Risk Est. (95% CI)	Comments
Antioxidant vitamins[119]	864	Prior colorectal adenoma	48 months	Vitamin C 1000 mg/day Vitamin E 400 mg/day Beta-carotene 25 mg/day	Recurrent adenoma Recurrent adenoma	0.94 (0.81 to 1.08) 1.04 (0.90 to 1.21)	β-carotene risk estimate significantly reduced among nonsmokers and nondrinkers (RR= 0.56; 95% CI=0.35 to 0.89).
Antioxidant vitamins[121]	29,133	Subjects enrolled in a lung cancer prevention trial	5 to 8 years	β-carotene 20 mg/day Vitamin E 50 mg/day	Cancer incidence Cancer incidence	1.05 (0.75 to 1.47) 0.78 (0.55 to 1.09)	Subjects were all Finnish male smokers, ages 50 to 69 at baseline.
Calcium[124]	25	FAP	6 months	Calcium carbonate 1500 mg/day	Adenoma size Adenoma number	N/A	No significant difference between active and placebo groups.
Calcium[128]	930	Prior colorectal adenoma	48 months	Calcium carbonate 3000 mg/day	Recurrent adenoma	0.85 (0.74 to 0.98)	

continued

Table 17-4 (continued)

RANDOMIZED, CONTROLLED CHEMOPREVENTION TRIALS FOR COLORECTAL CANCER

Candidate Agent(s)	N^1	Risk Cohort	Intervent. Period	Form and Dose	Endpoint	Risk Est. (95% CI)	Comments
NSAIDs[227]	22	FAP	9 months	Sulindac 150 mg BID	Polyp size Polyp number	N/A	Decrease in polyp number (p=0.014) and polyp diameter (p<0.001) in active compared to placebo group.
NSAIDs[134]	41	FAP gene mutation carriers without adenomas	4 years	Sulindac 75 mg BID Sulindac 150 mg BID	Polyp incidence	N/A	No significant difference between the active and placebo groups.
NSAIDs[139]	635	Prior colorectal cancer	31 months	Aspirin 325 mg/day	Recurrent adenoma	0.65 (0.46 to 0.91)	
NSAIDs[140]	1121	Prior colorectal adenoma	36 months	Aspirin 325 mg/day Aspirin 81 mg/day	Recurrent adenoma Recurrent adenoma	0.95 (0.80 to 1.12) 0.83 (0.70 to 0.98)	
NSAIDs[138]	291	Prior colorectal adenoma	4 years	Aspirin 160 to 300 mg/day	Recurrent adenoma	0.61 (0.37 to 0.99)	Based on interim analyses after 12 months.

continued

Table 17-4 (continued)

RANDOMIZED, CONTROLLED CHEMOPREVENTION TRIALS FOR COLORECTAL CANCER

Candidate Agent(s)	N[1]	Risk Cohort	Intervent. Period	Form and Dose	Endpoint	Risk Est. (95% CI)	Comments
NSAIDs[137]	22,071	Health professionals	Up to 12 years	Aspirin 325 mg QOD	Cancer incidence	1.03 (0.83 to 1.28)	Secondary analyses; all men.
COX-2 inhibitors[141]	77	FAP	6 months	Celecoxib 100 mg BID Celecoxib 400 mg BID	Polyp burden	N/A	Significant reduction in polyp burden among subjects in the higher (p=0.001), but not the lower (p=0.09) dose group compared to placebo.
Exogenous hormones[145]	16,608	Postmenopausal women	5.6 years	Equine estrogen 0.625 mg/day Medroxyprogesterone acetate 2.5 mg/day	Cancer incidence	0.61 (0.42 to 0.87)	Colorectal cancer cases diagnosed at a more advanced stage among subjects in the active arm.

[1]N=number randomized; CI=confidence interval; N/A=not available

against tumor induction compared with controls.[93] Poorly fermentable fibers, such as wheat bran and cellulose, appeared to be more effective than soluble fibers in these systems. A meta-analysis of 16 early case-control studies by Trock et al showed that high fiber consumption was associated with a 43% decrease in CRC risk.[94] However, subsequent data from 5 cohort studies have been inconsistent[95-99] and clinical trial data have been somewhat disappointing. Among FAP patients (n=58), DeCosse et al observed marginal benefits from a 4-year intervention of wheat bran fiber at 22 gm/ day (in combination with ascorbic acid 4 gm/day and α-tocopherol 400 mg/day).[100] Wheat bran supplementation has been similarly unimpressive with respect to prevention of recurrent sporadic colorectal adenomas.[101,102] McKeown-Eyssen et al[103] and Schatzkin et al[104] also noted no appreciable effects on adenoma recurrence rates from dietary modifications to raise fiber intake, while Bonithon-Kopp et al reported that adenoma recurrence rates were actually increased by using ispaghula husks to augment fiber consumption.[105]

Antioxidant Vitamins

Mechanisms for the putative anticarcinogenic effects of antioxidant vitamins are described above. Because fecal bacteria can produce high concentrations of reactive oxygen species,[106] the rationale for CRC chemoprevention with these compounds has been particularly compelling. In carcinogen-induced animal model systems, retinoids reportedly reduce rectal aberrant foci formation, decrease cellular proliferation, and increase apoptosis.[107-109] In contrast, ascorbic acid has yielded mixed results[110,111] and α-tocopherol has demonstrated minimal effects.[112] Associations between antioxidant vitamins and CRC risk, based on either dietary intake (with or without inclusion of supplements) or blood concentrations, have been evaluated in numerous observational studies with generally favorable results, as recently reviewed.[113]

In an early clinical trial among FAP subjects (n=49), treatment with vitamin C 3 gm/day vs placebo for up to 2 years resulted in transiently reduced polyp number and polyp area, but the effects were not sustained by the end of the trial.[114] Five additional trials have been performed with recurrent sporadic adenomas as the primary endpoint. In a relatively small trial reported by Roncucci et al, subjects who were treated with vitamin A 30,000 IU/day, vitamin C 1000 mg/day, and vitamin E 70 mg/day for a mean period of 18 months had a lower adenoma recurrence rate (6%) compared to placebo-treated subjects (36%).[115] However, a subsequent follow-up study from these same investigators has revealed less striking effects from lower vitamin doses based on preliminary data analyses.[116] Hofstad et al found that a 3-year intervention using vitamin C 150 mg/day and vitamin E 75 mg/day (along with ß-carotene 15 mg/day, selenium 101 μg/day, and calcium carbonate 1600 mg/day) resulted in a 69% reduction in recurrent adenoma risk compared to placebo.[117] Conversely, the Toronto Polyp Prevention Group (n=200) and the Antioxidant Polyp Prevention Study (n=864) reported no appreciable chemopreventive benefits from vitamin C (400 mg/day and 1000 mg/ day, respectively) and vitamin E (400 mg/day in each trial).[118,119] Stratified analyses from the Antioxidant Polyp Prevention Study found that ß-carotene 25 mg/day was associated with a 44% reduction in recurrent adenoma risk (RR=0.56; 95% CI=0.35 to 0.89) among subjects who were both nonsmokers and nondrinkers.[120] Yet, secondary analyses of data from the Alpha Tocopherol, Beta Carotene Cancer Prevention (ATBC) Study of Finnish male smokers revealed no significant benefits from 5 to 8 years of ß- carotene 20 mg/day with respect to CRC incidence (RR=1.05; 95% CI=0.75 to 1.47).[121] Treatment with vitamin E 50 mg/day did result in fewer incident CRC cases in the ATBC study, but this result was not statistically significant (RR=0.78; 95% CI=0.55 to 1.09).

Calcium

Calcium binds to potentially toxic bile acids within the colorectal lumen and may also directly reduce cellular proliferation and increase apoptosis. Chemopreventive effects have been demonstrated extensively in preclinical studies.[122] A recent analysis of pooled data from 16 case-control and 8 cohort studies yielded summary risk estimates of 1.13 (95% CI=0.91 to 1.39) for colorectal adenomas and 0.86 (95% CI=0.74 to 0.98) for CRC among subjects with high vs low calcium intake.[123] Thomas et al administered calcium 1500 mg/day vs placebo for 6 months to a small number of FAP subjects (n=25). Neither size nor number of rectal adenomas was meaningfully affected in this trial, but a decline in the crypt cell production rate was reported.[124] Conversely, another FAP chemoprevention trial by Stern et al (n=31) detected no appreciable change in mucosal proliferation rate from calcium 1200 mg/day for 9 months.[125] Two phase II trials conducted among HNPCC kindreds have also demonstrated mixed results on cellular proliferation from calcium doses of 1250 to 4500 mg/day for up to 3 months.[126,127]

With respect to sporadic CRC, Hofstad et al found no appreciable benefit on adenoma growth rate after 36 months of treatment with calcium 1600 mg/day (along with vitamins C and E, selenium, and ß-carotene) vs placebo among 116 polyp-bearing subjects.[117] In the large Calcium Polyp Prevention Study (n=930), 48 months of calcium carbonate 3000 mg/day (elemental calcium 1200 mg/day) resulted in a 15% reduction in risk for recurrent adenomas (RR=0.85; 95% CI=0.74 to 0.98).[128] The European Cancer Prevention Organization Study Group also reported a potential benefit on adenoma recurrence rate at 3 years from elemental calcium 2000 mg/day among subjects with a history of prior colorectal adenomas (n=665). However, this result was not statistically significant (RR=0.66; 95% CI=0.38 to 1.17).[105] Definitive data are anticipated from the US Women's Health Initiative Clinical Trial and Observational Study (n=45,000), an ongoing study designed to evaluate the effects of calcium 1000 mg/day (along with vitamin D_3 400 IU/day) on several chronic disease endpoints, including incident CRC.[129]

NSAIDs and Selective COX-2 Inhibitors

To date, traditional NSAIDs and their derivatives have received the most attention as candidate agents for CRC chemoprevention. Mechanisms for the putative chemopreventive effects of NSAIDs and selective COX-2 inhibitors were described previously (see page 337). A variety of animal systems have been used to demonstrate the anticarcinogenic effects of COX-2 inhibitors, including APC gene mutant, COX-2 compound mutant, and tumor xenografted mice.[130,131] In addition, more than 30 epidemiological studies have described 40% to 50% CRC risk reductions among regular NSAID users compared to nonusers.[132] Recently, Rahme et al conducted a nested case-control study of older patients (≥65 years) and found that colorectal adenoma risk was reduced among regular users of either rofeco xib (OR=0.67; 95% CI=0.46-0.98) or celecoxib (OR=0.87; 95% CI=0.63 to 1.19), although the latter point estimate was not statistically significant.[133]

Multiple controlled trials have reported positive results from sulindac 300 to 400 mg/day when given for 3 to 48 months to FAP patients,[7] based on variably defined SEBs including cellular proliferation, polyp size, and polyp number. However, Giardiello, et al recently found that sulindac 150 to 300 mg/day for 48 months was not an effective primary preventive intervention (ie, suppressing polyp expression) among *APC* mutation carriers.[134] Preliminary data suggest that polymorphisms in one or more sulindac metabolizing enzymes may have contributed to this negative result.[135] NSAID chemoprevention of sporadic colorectal neoplasia has been reported in 4 randomized, controlled clinical trials.[136-140] Sandler et al investigated the effects of aspirin 325 mg/day versus placebo among subjects (n=635) with a history of curatively resected CRC.[139] After a median intervention period of 31 months, the recurrent adenoma rate was significantly lower among subjects in the aspirin arm compared to the placebo arm (17% vs 27%; p=0.004). Recurrent adenomas were also fewer in number (p=0.003) and recurred later (p=0.02) among aspirin-treated subjects. Baron et al examined 2 aspirin doses, 325 mg/day and 81 mg/day, among subjects with prior colorectal adenomas (n=1121).[140] After a mean follow-up period of 33 months, subjects in the aspirin 81 mg/day group were 17% less likely to develop recurrent adenomas (RR=0.8; 95% CI=0.7 to 1.0) compared to subjects in the placebo group. For reasons that remain incompletely defined, subjects in the aspirin 325 mg/day group had essentially the same risk for recurrent adenomas as subjects in the placebo group. Benamouzig et al reported interim data from the APACC trial, which showed a statistically significant decrease in recurrent adenoma risk (RR=0.61; 95% CI=0.37 to 0.99) after 1 year of aspirin 300 mg/day vs placebo among subjects with prior colorectal adenomas.[138] In the large US Physicians' Health Study (n=22,071), aspirin 325 mg every other day had no apparent effect on CRC incidence rates, which were analyzed as a secondary endpoint, after either 5 years (RR = 1.2; 95% CI=0.8 to 1.7) or 12 years (RR = 1.03; 95% CI = 0.83 to 1.28) of follow-up.[136,137]

In a chemoprevention trial of selective COX-2 inhibitors among FAP subjects (141), Steinbach et al found that celecoxib 400 mg BID for 6 months resulted in a reduced colorectal polyp burden (30.7%; p=0.003) compared to placebo.[141] This dose of the active agent also resulted in statistically significant duodenal polyp regression (14.5%) among subjects with >5% mucosal involvement at baseline (p=0.05 compared to placebo).[142] In a smaller (n=8), uncontrolled trial, Hallak et al detected a beneficial effect from rofecoxib 25 mg/day for 12 months on the rate of colorectal polyp formation as well.[143] At least 2 additional sporadic CRC chemoprevention trails using selective COX-2 inhibitors have been conducted. However, the overall risk-to-benefit ratio remains to be determined.

Other Candidate Agents

Estrogen compounds appear to inhibit bile acid synthesis, decrease cellular proliferation, and reduce circulating insulin-like growth factor-1 (IGF-1) concentration, all of which may contribute to CRC chemoprevention. A meta-analysis of 28 observational studies by Grodstein et al showed that ever- vs never-use of hormone replacement therapy was inversely associated with both colon (RR=0.8; 95% CI=0.7 to 0.9) and rectal (RR=0.8; 95 % CI=0.7 to 0.9) cancer risk.[144] In the Women's Health Initiative clinical trial group (n=16,608), subjects randomly assigned to receive equine estrogens 0.625 mg/day and medroxyprogesterone acetate 2.5 mg/day developed fewer incident CRCs than subjects who received placebo (43 vs 72 cases, respectively; p=0.003).[145] However, CRC cases among subjects in the active arm were diagnosed at a more advanced stage.

Ursodeoxycholic acid (UDCA), a hydrophilic epimer of chenodeoxycholate, enhances immunosurveillance and may beneficially affect cellular growth and differentiation.[146] Among a select group of subjects who had both primary biliary cirrhosis and ulcerative colitis, Pardi et al observed a statistically significant decrease in colorectal dysplasia risk (including CRC) associated with UDCA 13 to 15 mg/kg body weight/day after a median intervention period of 42 months (RR=0.26; 95% CI=0.06 to 0.92).[147]

Diflouromethylornithine (DFMO) irreversibly inhibits ornithine decarboxylase, an enzyme that appears to be functionally involved in tumor growth regulation. In the clinical trials reported to date, DFMO has shown favorable effects on tissue-based biomarkers obtained from histologically normal colorectal mucosa.[148-150] Additional studies are underway to explore the effects of DFMO on sporadic colorectal carcinogenesis.

STOMACH

Based on GLOBOCAN data, 876,341 incident and 646,567 fatal gastric cancer cases were recorded worldwide in 2000.[1] High risk global regions include China, Japan, and select areas of Eastern Europe and tropical South America.[23] In the United States, age-adjusted incidence and mortality rates for gastric cancer are 7.5/100,000 population and 4.3/100,000 population, respectively.[43] Incidence rates are higher for men than for women (10.9 vs 5.0 per 100,000 population) and for Blacks than for Whites (12.3 vs 6.3 per 100,000 population). For cases diagnosed in 1995 to 2000, the estimated 5-year survival rate was 23.3% overall (58.4% for localized disease).

Gastric adenocarcinomas account for >95% of all stomach tumors and consist of 2 histologic subtypes (intestinal and diffuse), which are thought to arise through distinct carcinogenic pathways.[151] *H. pylori* infection appears to be the most important environmental risk factor for gastric cancer subtypes.[152] However, dietary constituents also affect gastric carcinogenesis. Low fruit and vegetable consumption has been consistently linked to increased gastric cancer risk, as recently reviewed.[153] Interestingly, *H. pylori* infection has been associated with multiple micronutrient deficiencies, including ß-carotene, ascorbic acid, and α-tocopherol.[154,155] Correa, et al conducted a randomized clinical trial of *H. pylori* triple therapy (amoxicillin, metronidazole, and bismuth subsalicylate for 14 days) and/or ß-carotene 30 mg/day, ascorbic acid 1000 mg BID, or placebo among subjects with precancerous gastric lesions from a high-risk region in Colombia, South America.[156] Based on a comparison of gastric biopsy samples taken at baseline and 72 months for subjects who completed the trial (n=631), *H. pylori* eradication and nutritional supplementation both resulted in statistically significant histologic regression of the precancerous lesions. Relative risks for the active versus placebo agents ranged from 3- to 8-fold in various subset analyses. Subsequent studies have shown that COX-2 expression is increased by *H. pylori* infection,[157] suggesting a possible role for COX-2 inhibitors in gastric cancer chemoprevention as well. Indeed, administration of celecoxib to carcinogen-induced rats led to a decreased gastric cancer incidence in a recently reported experiment, although the investigators speculated that some of the observed chemopreventive benefit may have been derived through COX-independent pathways.[158]

Gastric cancer endpoints were assessed in 2 intervention trials conducted among residents of Linxian, PRC. In the Linxian General Population Trial,[57] 5.25 years of selenium 50 mg/day (as selenized yeast), ß-carotene 15 mg/day, and α-tocopherol 30 mg/day resulted in a 16% lower risk for incident gastric cancer (RR=0.84; 95% CI=0.71-1.00) and a 21% lower risk for fatal gastric cancer (RR=0.79; 95% CI=0.64 to 0.99). None of the other nutritional agent combinations was significantly associated with gastric cancer risk. In the Linxian Dysplasia Trial, daily supplementation with 26 vitamins and minerals had no discernible effect on gastric cancer incidence (RR=1.17; 95% CI=0.87 to 1.58) or mortality (RR=1.18; 95% CI=0.76 to 1.85) compared to placebo.[58] Another trial using anti-*H. pylori* therapy combined with dietary supplementation (vitamin C, vitamin E, selenium, and garlic derivatives) was initiated in 1995 among subjects from

Linqu County, PRC (n=3599),[159] but final results from this study have yet to be reported. In a small phase I, multiorgan chemoprevention trial, curcumin was found to be relatively nontoxic at doses up to 8000 mg/day for 3 months.[160] Histologic improvement of intestinal metaplasia was noted in gastric biopsy samples from 1 of 6 subjects as well. Traditional NSAIDs, soy products, and DFMO have been considered for gastric cancer chemoprevention,[161-163] but clinical trial data for these compounds are currently unavailable.

HEPATOBILIARY TRACT

Based on GLOBOCAN data, 564,336 incident and 548,554 fatal liver cancer cases were recorded worldwide in 2000.[1] High-risk global regions include Western and Central Africa, Eastern and Southeast Asia, and Melanesia.[23] In the United States, age-adjusted incidence and mortality rates for liver and bile duct cancer are 5.2/100,000 population and 4.7/100,000 population, respectively.[43] Incidence rates are higher for men than for women (8.0 vs 2.9 per 100,000 population) and for Blacks than for Whites (7.5 vs 4.0 per 100,000 population). For cases diagnosed in 1995 to 2000, the estimated 5-year survival rate was 8.3% overall (18.4% for localized disease).

HCC is the most common primary malignant tumor in the liver. Major HCC risk factors include chronic hepatitis B or hepatitis C virus infection, cirrhosis of any cause (including excess alcohol intake), previously resected HCC, and exposure to aflatoxin (a fungal toxin). Nonalcoholic fatty liver disease has also been positively associated with HCC[164] and the rapid rise of the former condition in the United States and other industrialized countries will no doubt be an important contributor to future HCC incidence rates. Relatively rare HCC risk factors include hereditary hemochromatosis, α-1-antitrypsin deficiency, primary biliary cirrhosis, Wilson's disease, and exposure to thorium dioxide (a contrast agent previously used in radiology studies). In select high-risk global regions, hepatitis B vaccination programs have resulted in reduced HCC incidence rates.[165,166] To date, other HCC primary prevention strategies have been minimally effective at best. Although dysplasia is a likely precursor lesion to HCC,[167] the degree of invasiveness involved and potential for sampling error associated with liver biopsy prohibits routine application of this SEB for chemoprevention trials. More feasible SEBs include viral load, serum protein levels (such as alpha-fetoprotein), excreted aflatoxin metabolites, and serial imaging tests.[168]

Although data from clinical trials are currently limited, several candidate HCC chemoprevention agents appear promising. Interferon-alpha therapy can eradicate hepatitis C virus and has been shown to slow the progression of fibrosis, decrease viral load, and reduce biochemical markers of inflammation.[169] Observational data further support the potential for HCC risk reduction with interferon-alpha therapy.[170] In a randomized, prospective trial among Japanese patients with HCV-related cirrhosis (n=90), interferon-alpha 6 MU 3 times per week for 12 to 24 weeks resulted in substantially fewer incident HCC cases compared to controls (2 vs 17 cases; p=0.002).[171] Lin et al reported lower HCC recurrence rates at 1 and 4 years among subjects (n=30) randomized to receive intermittent or continuous interferon-alpha for 24 months.[172] Kubo et al also observed beneficial effects on HCC recurrence from long-term interferon-alpha treatment (up to 104 months).[173] Interferon-beta 6 MU twice per week was found to have favorable effects on incident HCC after a median observation period of 25 months in a relatively small clinical trial (n=20) as well.[174]

Glycyrrhizin, which resembles cortisone in chemical structure,[175] modulates immune function, releases interferon-gamma, decreases hepatic inflammation, and possess, antioxidant properties. When given to carcinogen-induced mice, glycyrrhizin appears to reduce the HCC incidence rate and prolong the time to initial HCC occurrence.[176] In a multicenter, double-blind study from Japan, daily intravenous injection of a glycyrrhizin preparation resulted in a lower HCC incidence rate compared to controls after long-term follow-up (13% vs 25% at year 15; p<0.002).[177] Chlorophyllin is a water soluble form of chlorophyll that acts to decrease carcinogen bioavailability, including aflatoxin. In a placebo controlled trial among residents of a high-risk region in China (n=180), chlorophyllin 100 mg TID for 16 weeks resulted in decreased urinary excretion of an aflatoxin-DNA adduct.[178] Oltipraz, which induces enzymes that detoxify carcinogens, has also been shown to favorably affect aflatoxin exposure biomarkers in a Chinese clinical trial.[179] Additional candidate HCC chemoprevention agents are being actively investigated, including green tea polyphenols, antioxidant vitamins, COX-2 inhibitors, D-limonene, and ginseng among others.[180,181] Chemopreventive interventions for bile duct cancer have not been aggressively pursued to date. However, recent development of a carcinogen-induced animal model for cholangiocarcinoma[182] may stimulate further interest in this area.

PANCREAS

Based on GLOBOCAN data, 216,367 incident and 213,462 fatal pancreas cancer cases were recorded worldwide in 2000.[1] Residents of developed countries are at greater risk than residents of developing countries.[23] In the United States, age-adjusted incidence and mortality rates for pancreatic cancer are 10.7/100,000 population and 10.5/100,000 population, respectively.[43] Incidence rates are higher for men than for women (12.4 vs 9.5 per 100,000 population) and for Blacks than for Whites (13.5 vs 10.5 per 100,000 population). For cases diagnosed in 1995 to 2000, the estimated 5-year survival rate was 4.4% overall (15.2% for localized disease).

Pancreas cancer chemoprevention research has been stymied by the high case fatality rate, limited awareness of premalignant conditions, and lack of a broadly applicable screening tool. Tobacco use has been convincingly associated with incident pancreas cancer, and smokers who consume alcohol appear to be at even greater risk.[183] Emerging data further suggest that COX-2 may be overexpressed in pancreatic adenocarcinoma and intraepithelial neoplasia.[184-187] In an experimental model of pancreatic cancer induced by transplacental exposure to alcohol and the tobacco carcinogen NNK, Schuller et al found that nonselective COX inhibition afforded significant cancer preventive effects.[183] Other mechanistic data show that DNA adducts derived from exposure to polycyclic aromatic hydrocarbon and aromatic amines can be detected in pancreatic cancer tissue[188] and the level of aromatic DNA adducts has been correlated with K-*ras* mutations. Additionally, a high proportion of G to A transitions appears to be present in pancreatic tumors, suggesting that nitrosamines and/or alkylating agents may effect carcinogenesis in this target organ.[188] Furthermore, there appears to be a gradual decrease in antioxidant enzyme expression in normal pancreas, chronic pancreatitis, and pancreatic cancer.[189] Consistent with the latter observation, selenium supplementation has been noted to prevent pancreatic cancer in a carcinogen-induced hamster model.[190] However, neither ß carotene 20 mg/day nor α-tocopherol 50 mg/day had a statistically significant effect on pancreas cancer risk based on secondary analyses from the ATBC study.[191] Further insights regarding familial pancreatic cancer, as described elsewhere in this volume, may provide new opportunities for chemoprevention among these high-risk patients.

SUMMARY

The NCI's Division of Cancer Prevention began systematically reviewing nutritional and pharmaceutical compounds with potential to interrupt carcinogenesis at a preinvasive stage more than 2 decades ago.[192] Since then, significant advances have been made with respect to GI cancer chemoprevention. Most notably, celecoxib (a selective COX-2 inhibitor) has been approved by the FDA for use as an adjunct to usual measures in reducing the number of colorectal polyps among FAP patients.[193] Ongoing trials should yield informative data regarding the chemopreventive benefit and overall safety profile of COX-2 inhibitors and other candidate agents among patients with BE, prior colorectal adenomas, or other conditions associated with increased GI cancer risk. Pending further positive trial results, GI cancer chemoprevention has the potential to complement current clinical practice by allowing delayed onset of average-risk cancer screening, prolonged intervals between high-risk screening/surveillance examinations, and increased disease-free survival rates among curatively-resected cancer patients. Ongoing research into synergistic agent combinations (eg, COX-2 inhibitors and DFMO), earlier SEBs (eg, rectal aberrant crypt foci), and molecularly defined risk stratification (eg, using genetic or epigenetic characteristics to assist cohort selection) should facilitate future progress in GI cancer chemoprevention as well.

REFERENCES

1. Ferlay JF, Bray F, Pisani P, et al. *GLOBOCAN 2000: Cancer Incidence, Mortality and Prevalence Worldwide, Version 1.0. 2001, IARC Cancer Base No. 5.* Lyon: IARC Press.

2. Nowell PC. The clonal evolution of tumor cell populations. *Science.* 1976;194(4260): 23-28.

3. Chemoprevention Working Group. Prevention of cancer in the next millennium: report of the Chemoprevention Working Group to the American Association for Cancer Research. *Cancer Research.* 1999;59(19):4743-4758.

4. Hanahan D, Weinberg RA. The hallmarks of cancer. *Cell.* 2000;100(1):57-70.

5. Lindor NM, Greene MH. The concise handbook of family cancer syndromes. Mayo Familial Cancer Program. *J Natl Cancer Inst.* 1998;90(14):1039-1071.

6. Johnson JC, DiSario JA, Grady WM. Surveillance and treatment of periampullary and duodenal adenomas in familial adenomatous polyposis. *Curr Treat Options Gastroenterol.* 2004;7(2):79-89.

7. Hawk E, Lubet R, Limburg P. Chemoprevention in hereditary colorectal cancer syndromes. *Cancer.* 1999;86(11 Suppl):2551-2563.

8. Enzinger PC, Mayer RJ. Esophageal cancer. *N Engl J Med.* 2003;349(23):2241-2252.

9. el-Serag HB. The epidemic of esophageal adenocarcinoma. *Gastroenterol Clin North Am.* 2002;31(2):viii,421-440.

10. Messmann H. Squamous cell cancer of the oesophagus. *Best Pract Res Clin Gastroenterol.* 2001;15(2):249-265.

11. Plummer MS, Franceschi S, Munoz N. Epidemiology of gastric cancer. *IARC Sci Publ.* 2004;(157):311-326.

12. Sandler RS. Epidemiology and risk factors for colorectal cancer. *Gastroenterol Clin North Am.* 1996;25(4):717-735.

13. Potter JD. Colorectal cancer: molecules and populations. *J Natl Cancer Inst.* 1999; 91(11):916-932.

14. Monto A, Wright TL. The epidemiology and prevention of hepatocellular carcinoma. *Semin Oncol.* 2001;28(5):441-449.

15. Michaud DS. The epidemiology of pancreatic, gallbladder, and other biliary tract cancers. *Gastrointest Endosc.* 2002;56(6 Suppl):S195-S200.

16. Ghadirian P., Lynch HT, Krewski D. Epidemiology of pancreatic cancer: an overview. *Cancer Detect Prev.* 2003;27(2):87-93.

17. Cameron AJ, Ott BJ, Payne WS. The incidence of adenocarcinoma in columnar-lined (Barrett's) esophagus. *N Eng J Med.* 1985;313(14):857-859.

18. Cossentino MJ, Wong RK. Barrett's esophagus and risk of esophageal adenocarcinoma. *Semin Gastrointest Dis.* 2003;14(3):128-135.

19. Shaheen N, Ransohoff DF. Gastroesophageal reflux, Barrett esophagus, and esophageal cancer: scientific review. *JAMA.* 2002;287(15):1972-1981.

20. Williams MP, Pounder RE. *Helicobacter pylori*: from the benign to the malignant. *Am J Gastroenterol.* 1999;94(11 Suppl):S11-S16.

21. Moller H, Heseltine E, Vainio H. Working group report on schistosomes, liver flukes and Helicobacter pylori. *Int J Cancer.* 1995;60(5):587-589.

22. Eslick GD, Lim LL, Byles JE, et al. Association of Helicobacter pylori infection with gastric carcinoma: a meta-analysis. *Am J Gastroenterol.* 1999;94(9):2373-2379.

23. Parkin DM, Pisani P, Ferlay J. Global cancer statistics. *CA Cancer J Clin.* 1999;49(1): 1, 33-64.

24. Bond JH. Polyp guideline: diagnosis, treatment, and surveillance for patients with colorectal polyps. Practice Parameters Committee of the American College of Gastroenterology. *Am J Gastroenterol.* 2000;95(11):3053-3063.

25. Neugut AI, Lautenbach E, Abi-Rached B, et al. Incidence of adenomas after curative resection for colorectal cancer. *Am J Gastroenterol.* 1996;91(10):2096-2098.

26. Lashner BA. Colorectal cancer surveillance for patients with inflammatory bowel disease. *Gastrointest Endosc Clin N Am.* 2002;12(1):viii, 135-143.

27. Eaden JA, Abrams KR, Mayberry JF. The risk of colorectal cancer in ulcerative colitis: a meta-analysis. *Gut.* 2001;48(4):526-535.

28. Weston AP, Badr AS, Hassanein RS. Prospective multivariate analysis of clinical, endoscopic, and histological factors predictive of the development of Barrett's multifocal high-grade dysplasia or adenocarcinoma [comment]. *Am J Gastroenterol.* 1999;94(12): 3413-3419.

29. Kelloff GJ, Sigman CC, Johnson KM, et al. Perspectives on surrogate end points in the development of drugs that reduce the risk of cancer. *Cancer Epidemiol Biomarkers Prev.* 2000;9(2):127-137.

30. Weston AP, Badr AS, Hassanein RS. Prospective multivariate analysis of clinical, endoscopic, and histological factors predictive of the development of Barrett's multifocal high-grade dysplasia or adenocarcinoma [see comments]. *Am J Gastroenterol.* 1999; 94(12):3413-3419.

31. Reid BJ, Levine DS, Longton G, et al. Predictors of progression to cancer in Barrett's esophagus: baseline histology and flow cytometry identify low- and high-risk patient subsets. *Am J Gastroenterol.* 2000;95(7):1669-1676.

32. Schnell TG, Sontag SJ, Chejfec G, et al. Long-term nonsurgical management of Barrett's esophagus with high-grade dysplasia [comment]. *Gastroenterology.* 2001; 120(7):1607-1619.

33. Buttar NS, Wang KK, Sebo TJ, et al. Extent of high-grade dysplasia in Barrett's esophagus correlates with risk of adenocarcinoma [comment]. *Gastroenterology.* 2001;120(7): 1630-1639.

34. Dawsey SM, Lewin KJ, Wang GQ, et al. Squamous esophageal histology and subsequent risk of squamous cell carcinoma of the esophagus. A prospective follow-up study from Linxian, China. *Cancer.* 1994;74(6):1686-1692.

35. Wang GQ, Abnet CC, Liu FS, et al. Squamous dysplasia is the histologic precursor of invasive esophageal squamous cell carcinoma. *Gastroenterology.* 2003;124:A297.

36. Rugge M, Correa P, Dixon MF, et al. Gastric dysplasia: the Padova international classification. *Am J Surg Pathol.* 2000;24(2):167-176.

37. Winawer SJ, Zauber AG, Ho MN, et al. Prevention of colorectal cancer by colonoscopic polypectomy. The National Polyp Study Workgroup. *N Engl J Med.* 1993;329(27): 1977-1981.

38. Muto T, Bussey MN, Morson BC. The evolution of cancer of the colon and rectum. *Cancer.* 1975;36(6):2251-2270.

39. Shirvani VN, Ouatu-Lascar R, Kaur BS, et al. Cyclooxygenase 2 expression in Barrett's esophagus and adenocarcinoma: ex vivo induction by bile salts and acid exposure. *Gastroenterology.* 2000;118(3):487-496.

40. Kaur BS, Khamnehei N, Iravani M, et al. Rofecoxib inhibits cyclooxygenase 2 expression and activity and reduces cell proliferation in Barrett's esophagus. *Gastroenterology.* 2002;123(1):60-67.

41. Buttar NS, Wang KK, Anderson MA, et al. The effect of selective cyclooxygenase-2 inhibition in Barrett's esophagus epithelium: an in vitro study. *J Nat Cancer Instit.* 2002;94(6):422-429.

42. Wei JT, Shaheen N. The changing epidemiology of esophageal adenocarcinoma. *Semin Gastrointest Dis.* 2003;4(3):112-127.

43. Ries LAG, Eisner MP, Kosary CL, et al. *SEER Cancer Statistics Review, 1975-2001.* Bethesda, Md: National Cancer Institute; 2004.

44. Kim YS, Milner J. Molecular targets for selenium in cancer prevention. *Nutr Cancer.* 2001;40(1):50-54.

45. van Rensburg SJ, Hall JM, Gathercole PS. Inhibition of esophageal carcinogenesis in corn-fed rats by riboflavin, nicotinic acid, selenium, molybdenum, zinc, and magnesium. *Nutr Cancer.* 1986;8(3):163-170.

46. Bogden JD, Chung HR, Kemp FW, et al. Effect of selenium and molybdenum on methylbenzylnitrosamine-induced esophageal lesions and tissue trace metals in the rat. *J Nutr.* 1986;116(12):2432-2342.

47. Lijinsky W, Milner JA, Kovatch, FW, et al. Lack of effect of selenium on induction of tumors of esophagus and bladder in rats by two nitrosamines. *Toxicol Ind Health.* 1989;5(1):63-72.

48. Hu G, Han C, Wild CP, et al. Lack of effects of selenium on N-nitrosomethylbenzylamine-induced tumorigenesis, DNA methylation, and oncogene expression in rats and mice. *Nutr Cancer.* 1992;18(3):287-295.

49. Chen X, Mikhail SS, Ding YW, et al. Effects of vitamin E and selenium supplementation on esophageal adenocarcinogenesis in a surgical model with rats. *Carcinogenesis.* 2000;21(8):1531-1536.

50. Jaskiewicz K, Marasas WF, Rossouw JE, et al. Selenium and other mineral elements in populations at risk for esophageal cancer. *Cancer.* 1988;62(12):2635-2639.

51. Knekt P, Aromaa A, Maatela J, et al. Serum micronutrients and risk of cancers of low incidence in Finland. *Am J Epidemiol.* 1991;134(4):356-361.

52. Krishnaswamy K, Prasad MP, Krishna TP, et al. A case control study of selenium in cancer. *Indian J Med Res.* 1993;98:124-128.

53. Nayar D, Kapil U, Joshi YK, et al. Association of vitamin A, zinc, selenium and magnesium with oesophageal cancer. *Trop Gastroenterol.* 1998;19(4):148-149.

54. Mark SD, Qiao YL, Dawsey SM, et al. Prospective study of serum selenium levels and incident esophageal and gastric cancers. *J Natl Cancer Inst.* 2000;92(21):1753-1763.

55. Duffield-Lillico AJ, Reid ME, Turnbull BW, et al. Baseline characteristics and the effect of selenium supplementation on cancer incidence in a randomized clinical trial: a summary report of the Nutritional Prevention of Cancer Trial. *Cancer Epidemiol Biomarkers Prev.* 2002;11(7):630-639.

56. Limburg P, Wei W, Ahnen D, et al. Chemoprevention of esophageal squamous cancer: randomized, placebo-controlled trial in a high-risk population. *Gastroenterol.* 2002; 122:A71.

57. Blot WJ, Li JY, Taylor PR, et al. Nutrition intervention trials in Linxian, China: supplementation with specific vitamin/mineral combinations, cancer incidence, and disease-specific mortality in the general population. *J Natl Cancer Inst.* 1993;85(18): 1483-1492.

58. Li JY, Taylor PR, Li B, et al. Nutrition intervention trials in Linxian, China: multiple vitamin/mineral supplementation, cancer incidence, and disease-specific mortality among adults with esophageal dysplasia. *J Natl Cancer Inst.* 1993;85(18):1492-1498.

59. Tengerdy RP. Effect of vitamin E on immune function. In: Machlin LJ, ed. *Vitamin E: a Comprehensive Treatise.* New York, NY: Marcel Dekker; 1980:429-444.

60. Zhang D, Okada S, Yu Y, et al. Vitamin E inhibits apoptosis, DNA modification, and cancer incidence induced by iron-mediated peroxidation in Wistar rat kidney. *Cancer Res.* 1997;57(12):2410-2414.

61. Leibold, E, Schwarz LR. Inhibition of intercellular communication in rat hepatocytes by phenobarbital, 1,1,1-trichloro-2,2-bis(p-chlorophenyl)ethane (DDT) and gamma-hexachlorocyclohexane (lindane): modification by antioxidants and inhibitors of cyclooxygenase. *Carcinogenesis.* 1993;14(11):2377-2382.

62. Nauss KM, Bueche D, Newberne PM. Effect of vitamin A nutriture on experimental esophageal carcinogenesis. *J Natl Cancer Inst.* 1987;79(1):145-147.

63. Daniel EM, Stoner GD. The effects of ellagic acid and 13-cis-retinoic acid on N-nitrosobenzylmethylamine-induced esophageal tumorigenesis in rats. *Cancer Lett.* 1991; 56(2):117-124.

64. Cohen M, Bhagavan HN. Ascorbic acid and gastrointestinal cancer. *J Am Coll Nutr.* 1995;14(6):565-578.

65. Gupta A, Nines R, Rodrigo KA, et al. Effects of dietary N-(4-hydroxyphenyl)retinamide on N-nitrosomethylbenzylamine metabolism and esophageal tumorigenesis in the Fischer 344 rat. *J Natl Cancer Inst.* 2001;93(13):990-998.

66. Odeleye OE, Eskelson CD, Mufti SI, et al. Vitamin E protection against nitrosamine-induced esophageal tumor incidence in mice immunocompromised by retroviral infection. *Carcinogenesis.* 1992;13(10):1811-1816.

67. Zheng W, Sellers TA, Doyle TJ, et al. Retinol, antioxidant vitamins, and cancers of the upper digestive tract in a prospective cohort study of postmenopausal women. *Am J Epidemiol.* 1995;142(9):955-960.

68. Launoy G, Milan C, Day NE, et al. Diet and squamous-cell cancer of the oesophagus: a French multicentre case-control study. *Int J Cancer.* 1998;76(1):7-12.

69. Terry P, Lagergren J, Ye W, et al. Antioxidants and cancers of the esophagus and gastric cardia. *Int J Cancer.* 2000;87(5):750-754.

70. Siassi F, Pouransari Z, Ghadirian P. Nutrient intake and esophageal cancer in the Caspian littoral of Iran: a case-control study. *Cancer Detect Prev.* 2000;24(3):295-303.

71. Bollschweiler E, Wolfgarten E, Nowroth T, et al. Vitamin intake and risk of subtypes of esophageal cancer in Germany. *J Cancer Res Clin Oncol.* 2002;128(10):575-580.

72. Yang CS, Sun YH, Yang QP, et al. Nutritional status of the high esophageal cancer risk population in Linxian, People's Republic of China: effects of vitamin supplementation. *Natl Cancer Inst Monogr.* 1985;69:23-27.

73. Knekt P, Aromaa A, Maatela J, et al. Serum vitamin E, serum selenium and the risk of gastrointestinal cancer. *Int J Cancer.* 1988;42(6):846-850.

74. Taylor PR, Qiao YL, Abnet CC, et al. Prospective study of serum vitamin E levels and esophageal and gastric cancers. *J Natl Cancer Inst.* 2003;95(18):1414-1416.

75. Abneth CC, Qiao YL, Dawsey SM, et al. Prospective study of serum retinol, beta-carotene, beta-cryptoxanthin, and lutein/zeaxanthin and esophageal and gastric cancers in China. *Cancer Causes Control.* 2003;14(7):645-655.

76. Munoz N, Wahrendorf J, Bang LJ, et al. No effect of riboflavin, retinol, and zinc on prevalence of precancerous lesions of oesophagus. Randomised double-blind intervention study in high-risk population of China. *Lancet.* 1985;2(8447):111-114.

77. Souza RF, Shewmake K, Beer DG, et al. Selective inhibition of cyclooxygenase-2 suppresses growth and induces apoptosis in human esophageal adenocarcinoma cells. *Cancer Res.* 2000;60(20):5767-5772.

78. Buttar NS, Wang KK, Leontovich O, et al. Chemoprevention of esophageal adenocarcinoma by COX-2 inhibitors in an animal model of Barrett's esophagus. *Gastroenterology.* 2002;122(4):1101-1112.

79. Corley DA, Kerlikowske K, Verma R, et al. Protective association of aspirin/NSAIDs and esophageal cancer: a systematic review and meta-analysis. *Gastroenterology.* 2003;124(1):47-56.

80. Heath EI, Canto MI, Wu TT, et al. Chemoprevention for Barrett's esophagus trial. Design and outcome measures. *Dis Esophagus.* 2003;16(3):177-186.

81. Sampliner RE, Garewal HS, Fennerty MB, et al. Lack of impact of therapy on extent of Barrett's esophagus in 67 patients. *Dig Dis Sci.* 1990;35(1):93-96.

82. Csendes A, Braghetto I, Burdiles P, et al. Long-term results of classic antireflux surgery in 152 patients with Barrett's esophagus: clinical, radiologic, endoscopic, manometric, and acid reflux test analysis before and late after operation. *Surgery.* 1998;126(6):645-657.

83. Peters FT, Ganesh S, Kuipers EJ, et al. Endoscopic regression of Barrett's oesophagus during omeprazole treatment; a randomised double blind study. *Gut.* 1999;45(4):489-494.

84. Yau P, Watson DI, Devitt PG, et al. Laparoscopic antireflux surgery in the treatment of gastroesophageal reflux in patients with Barrett esophagus. *Arch Surg.* 2000;135(7):801-805.

85. Ouatu-Lascar R, Triadafilopoulos G. Complete elimination of reflux symptoms does not guarantee normalization of intraesophageal acid reflux in patients with Barrett's esophagus. *Am J Gastroenterol.* 1998;93(5):711-716.

86. Fass R, Sampliner RE, Malagon JB, et al. Failure of oesophageal acid control in candidates for Barrett's oesophagus reversal on a very high dose of proton pump inhibitor. *Aliment Pharmacol Ther.* 2000;14(5):597-602.

87. Fitzgerald RC, Omary MB, Triadafilopoulos G. Dynamic effects of acid on Barrett's esophagus. An ex vivo proliferation and differentiation model. *J Clin Invest.* 1996;98(9):2120-2128.

88. Zhang F, Subbaramaiah K, Altorki N, et al. Dihydroxy bile acids activate the transcription of cyclooxygenase-2. *J Bio Chem.* 1998;273(4):2424-2428.

89. Kaur BS, Ouatu-Lascar R, Omary MB, et al. Bile salts induce or blunt cell proliferation in Barrett's esophagus in an acid-dependent fashion. *Am J Physiol Gastrointest Liver Physiol.* 2000;278(6):G1000-G1009.

90. Zhang F, Altorki NK, Wu YC, et al. Duodenal reflux induces cyclooxygenase-2 in the esophageal mucosa of rats: evidence for involvement of bile acids. *Gastroenterology.* 2001;121(6):1391-1399.

91. Ouatu-Lascar R, Fitzgerald RC, Triadafilopoulos G. Differentiation and proliferation in Barrett's esophagus and the effects of acid suppression [comments]. *Gastroenterology.* 1999;117(2):327-335.

92. Triadafilopoulos G. Acid and bile reflux in Barrett's esophagus: a tale of two evils. *Gastroenterology.* 2001;121(6):1502-1506.

93. Sengupta S, Tjandra JJ, Gibson PR. Dietary fiber and colorectal neoplasia. *Dis Colon Rectum.* 2001;44(7):1016-1033.

94. Trock B, Lanza E, Greenwald P. Dietary fiber, vegetables, and colon cancer: critical review and meta-analyses of the epidemiologic evidence. *J Natl Cancer Inst.* 1990;82(8):650-661.

95. Thun MJ, Calle EE, Namboodiri MM, et al. Risk factors for fatal colon cancer in a large prospective study. *J Natl Cancer Inst.* 1992;84(19):1491-1500.

96. Platz EA, Giovannucci E, Rimm EB, et al. Dietary fiber and distal colorectal adenoma in men. *Cancer Epidemiol Biomarkers Prev.* 1997;6(9):661-670.

97. Fuchs CS, Giovannucci EL, Colditz GA, et al. Dietary fiber and the risk of colorectal cancer and adenoma in women. *N Engl J Med.* 1999;340(3):169-176.

98. Peters U, Sinha R, Chatterjee N, et al. Dietary fibre and colorectal adenoma in a colorectal cancer early detection programme. *Lancet.* 2003;361(9368):1491-1495.

99. Bingham SA, Day NE, Luben R, et al. Dietary fibre in food and protection against colorectal cancer in the European Prospective Investigation into Cancer and Nutrition (EPIC): an observational study. *Lancet.* 2003;361(9368):1496-1501.

100. DeCosse JJ, Miller HH, Lesser ML. Effect of wheat fiber and vitamins C and E on rectal polyps in patients with familial adenomatous polyposis. *J Natl Cancer Inst.* 1989;81(17):1290-1297.

101. MacLennan R, Macrae F, Bain C, et al. Randomized trial of intake of fat, fiber, and beta carotene to prevent colorectal adenomas. The Australian Polyp Prevention Project. *J Natl Cancer Inst.* 1995;87(23):1760-1766.

102. Alberts DS, Martinez ME, Roe DJ, et al. Lack of effect of a high-fiber cereal supplement on the recurrence of colorectal adenomas. Phoenix Colon Cancer Prevention Physicians' Network. *N Engl J Med.* 2000;342(16):1156-1162.

103. McKeown-Eyssen GE, Bright-See E, Bruce WR, et al. A randomized trial of a low fat high fibre diet in the recurrence of colorectal polyps. Toronto Polyp Prevention Group. *J Clin Epidemiol.* 1994;47(5):525-536.

104. Schatzkin A, Lanza E, Corle D, et al. Lack of effect of a low-fat, high-fiber diet on the recurrence of colorectal adenomas. Polyp Prevention Trial Study Group. *N Engl J Med.* 2000;342(16):1149-1155.

105. Bonithon-Kopp C, Kronborg O, Giacosa A, et al. Calcium and fibre supplementation in prevention of colorectal adenoma recurrence: a randomised intervention trial. European Cancer Prevention Organisation Study Group. *Lancet.* 2000;356(9238):1300-1306.

106. Stone WL, Papas AM. Tocopherols and the etiology of colon cancer. *J Natl Cancer Inst.* 1997; 89(14):1006-1014.

107. Pereira MA. Prevention of colon cancer and modulation of aberrant crypt foci, cell proliferation, and apoptosis by retinoids and NSAIDs. *Adv Exp Med Biol.* 1999;470:55-63.

108. Zheng Y, Kramer PM, Lubet RA, et al. Effect of retinoids on AOM-induced colon cancer in rats: modulation of cell proliferation, apoptosis and aberrant crypt foci. *Carcinogenesis.* 1999;20(2):255-260.

109. Wargovich MJ, Jimenez A, McKee K, et al. Efficacy of potential chemopreventive agents on rat colon aberrant crypt formation and progression. *Carcinogenesis.* 2000;21(6): 1149-1155.

110. Colacchio TA, Memoli VA. Chemoprevention of colorectal neoplasms. Ascorbic acid and beta-carotene. *Arch Surg.* 1986;121(12):1421-1424.

111. Shirai T, Ikawa E, Hirose M, et al. Modification by five antioxidants of 1,2-dimethylhydrazine-initiated colon carcinogenesis in F344 rats. *Carcinogenesis.* 1985;6(4):637-639.

112. Chung H, Wu D, Han SN, et al. Vitamin E supplementation does not alter azoxymethane-induced colonic aberrant crypt foci formation in young or old mice. *J Nutr.* 2003;133(2):528-532.

113. Hercberg S, Galan P, Preziosi P, et al. The potential role of antioxidant vitamins in preventing cardiovascular diseases and cancers. *Nutrition.* 1998;14(6):513-520.

114. Bussey HJ, DeCosse JJ, Deschner EE, et al. A randomized trial of ascorbic acid in polyposis coli. *Cancer.* 1982;50(7):1434-1439.

115. Roncucci L, Di Donato P, Carati L, et al. Antioxidant vitamins or lactulose for the prevention of the recurrence of colorectal adenomas. Colorectal Cancer Study Group of the University of Modena and the Health Care District 16. *Dis Colon Rectum.* 1993;36(3): 227-234.

116. Ponz de Leon M, Roncucci L. Chemoprevention of colorectal tumors: role of lactulose and of other agents. *Scand J Gastroenterol Suppl.* 1997;222:72-75.

117. Hofstad B, Almendingen K, Vatn M, et al. Growth and recurrence of colorectal polyps: a double-blind 3-year intervention with calcium and antioxidants. *Digestion.* 1998; 59(2):148-156.

118. McKeown-Eyssen G, Holloway C, Jazmaji V, et al. A randomized trial of vitamins C and E in the prevention of recurrence of colorectal polyps. *Cancer Res.* 1988;48(16): 4701-4705.

119. Greenberg ER, Baron JA, Tosteson TD, et al. A clinical trial of antioxidant vitamins to prevent colorectal adenoma. Polyp Prevention Study Group. *N Engl J Med.* 1994; 331(3):141-147.

120. Baron JA, Cole BF, Mott L, et al. Neoplastic and antineoplastic effects of beta-carotene on colorectal adenoma recurrence: results of a randomized trial. *J Natl Cancer Inst.* 2003;95(10):717-722.

121. Albanes D, Malila N, Taylor PR, et al. Effects of supplemental alpha-tocopherol and beta-carotene on colorectal cancer: results from a controlled trial (Finland). *Cancer Causes Control.* 2000;11(3):197-205.

122. Lipkin M. Preclinical and early human studies of calcium and colon cancer prevention. *Ann N Y Acad Sci.* 1999;889:120-127.

123. Bergsma-Kadijk JA, van't Veer P, Kampman E, et al. Calcium does not protect against colorectal neoplasia. *Epidemiology.* 1996;7(6):590-597.

124. Thomas MG, Thomson JP, Williamson RC. Oral calcium inhibits rectal epithelial proliferation in familial adenomatous polyposis. *Br J Surg.* 1993;80(4):499-501.

125. Stern HS, Gregoire RC, Kashtan H, et al. Long-term effects of dietary calcium on risk markers for colon cancer in patients with familial polyposis. *Surgery.* 1990;108(3):528-533.

126. Lipkin M, Newmark H. Effect of added dietary calcium on colonic epithelial-cell proliferation in subjects at high risk for familial colonic cancer. *N Engl J Med.* 1985; 313(22):1381-1384.

127. Cats A, Kleibeuker JH, van der Meer R, et al. Randomized, double-blinded, placebo-controlled intervention study with supplemental calcium in families with hereditary nonpolyposis colorectal cancer. *J Natl Cancer Inst.* 1995;87(8):598-603.

128. Baron JA, Beach M, Mandel JS, et al. Calcium supplements for the prevention of colorectal adenomas. Calcium Polyp Prevention Study Group. *N Engl J Med.* 1999; 340(2):101-107.

129. Jackson RD, LaCroix AZ, Cauley JA, et al. The Women's Health Initiative calcium-vitamin D trial: overview and baseline characteristics of participants. *Ann Epidemiol.* 2003; 13(9 Suppl):S98-S106.

130. Oshima M, Taketo MM. COX selectivity and animal models for colon cancer. *Curr Pharm Des.* 2002;8(12):1021-1034.

131. Chan TA. Cyclooxygenase inhibition and mechanisms of colorectal cancer prevention. *Curr Cancer Drug Targets.* 2003;3(6):455-463.

132. Hawk ET, Umar A, Viner JL. Colorectal cancer chemoprevention—an overview of the science. *Gastroenterology.* 2004;126(5):1423-1447.

133. Rahme E, Barkun AN, Toubouti Y, et al. The cyclooxygenase-2-selective inhibitors rofecoxib and celecoxib prevent colorectal neoplasia occurrence and recurrence. *Gastroenterology.*. 2003;125(2):404-412.

134. Giardiello FM, Yang VW, Hylind LM, et al. Primary chemoprevention of familial adenomatous polyposis with sulindac. *N Engl J Med.* 2002;346(14):1054-1059.

135. Wehbi M, Hisamuddin IM, Wyre H, et al. Prevalence of Flavin Monooxygenase 3 (FMO3) Polymorphisms in Sulindac-Mediated Primary Chemoprevention Trial in Familial Adenomatous Polyposis (FAP). Presented at: Digestive Disease Week; May 2004; New Orleans, LA.

136. Gann PH, Manson JE, Glynn RJ, et al. Low-dose aspirin and incidence of colorectal tumors in a randomized trial. *J Natl Cancer Inst.* 1993;85(15):1220-1224.

137. Sturmer T, Glynn RJ, Lee IM, et al. Aspirin use and colorectal cancer: posttrial follow-up data from the Physicians' Health Study. *Ann Intern Med.* 1998;128(9):713-720.

138. Benamouzig R, Deyra J, Martin A, et al. Daily soluble aspirin and prevention of colorectal adenoma recurrence: one-year results of the APACC trial. *Gastroenterology.* 2003; 125(2):328-336.

139. Sandler RS, Halabi S, Baron JA, et al. A randomized trial of aspirin to prevent colorectal adenomas in patients with previous colorectal cancer. *N Engl J Med.* 2003;348(10): 883-890.

140. Baron JA, Cole BF, Sandler RS, et al. A randomized trial of aspirin to prevent colorectal adenomas. *N Engl J Med.* 2003;348(10):891-899.

141. Steinbach G, Lynch PM, Phillips RK, et al. The effect of celecoxib, a cyclooxygenase-2 inhibitor, in familial adenomatous polyposis. *N Engl J Med.* 2000;342(26):1946-1952.

142. Phillips RK, Wallace MH, Lynch PM, et al. A randomised, double blind, placebo controlled study of celecoxib, a selective cyclooxygenase 2 inhibitor, on duodenal polyposis in familial adenomatous polyposis. *Gut.* 2002;50(6):857-860.

143. Hallak A, Alon-Baron L, Shamir R, et al. Rofecoxib reduces polyp recurrence in familial polyposis. *Dig Dis Sci.* 2003;48(10):1998-2002.

144. Grodstein F, Newcomb PA, Stampfer MJ. Postmenopausal hormone therapy and the risk of colorectal cancer: a review and meta-analysis. *Am J Med.* 1999;106(5):574-582.

145. Chlebowski RT, Wactawski-Wende J, Ritenbaugh C, et al. Estrogen plus progestin and colorectal cancer in postmenopausal women. *N Engl J Med.* 2004;350(10):991-1004.

146. Brasitus TA. Primary chemoprevention strategies for colorectal cancer: ursodeoxycholic acid and other agents. *Gastroenterology.* 1995;109(6):2036-2038.

147. Pardi DS, Loftus EV Jr, Kremers WK, et al. Ursodeoxycholic acid as a chemopreventive agent in patients with ulcerative colitis and primary sclerosing cholangitis. *Gastroenterology.* 2003;124(4):889-893.

148. Love RR, Jacoby R, Newton MA, et al. A randomized, placebo-controlled trial of low-dose alpha-difluoromethylornithine in individuals at risk for colorectal cancer. *Cancer Epidemiol Biomarkers Prev.* 1998;7(11):989-992.

149. Meyskens FL Jr, Gerner EW, Emerson S, et al. Effect of alpha-difluoromethylornithine on rectal mucosal levels of polyamines in a randomized, double-blinded trial for colon cancer prevention. *J Natl Cancer Inst.* 1998;90(16):1212-1218.

150. Meyskens FL Jr, Emerson SS, Pelot D, et al. Dose de-escalation chemoprevention trial of alpha-difluoromethylornithine in patients with colon polyps. *J Natl Cancer Inst.* 1994;86(15):1122-1130.

151. Tahara E. Genetic pathways of two types of gastric cancer. *IARC Sci Publ.* 2004;(157): 327-349.

152. Nardone G. Review article: molecular basis of gastric carcinogenesis. *Aliment Pharmacol Ther.* 2003;17 Suppl 2:75-81.

153. Correa P, Malcom G, Schmidt B, et al. Review article: antioxidant micronutrients and gastric cancer. *Aliment Pharmacol Ther.* 1998;12 Suppl 1:73-82.

154. Annibale B, Capurso G, Delle Fave G. Consequences of Helicobacter pylori infection on the absorption of micronutrients. *Dig Liver Dis.* 2002;34 Suppl 2:S72-77.

155. Yakoob J, Jaffri W, Abid S. Helicobacter pylori infection and micronutrient deficiencies. *World J Gastroenterol.* 2003;9(10):2137-2139.

156. Correa P, Fontham ET, Bravo JC, et al. Chemoprevention of gastric dysplasia: randomized trial of antioxidant supplements and anti-*Helicobacter pylori* therapy. *J Natl Cancer Inst.* 2000;92(23):1881-1888.

157. Scheiman JM, Greenson JK, Lee J, et al. Effect of cyclooxygenase-2 inhibition on human Helicobacter pylori gastritis: mechanisms underlying gastrointestinal safety and implications for cancer chemoprevention. *Aliment Pharmacol Ther.* 2003;17(12):1535-1543.

158. Hu PJ, Yu J, Zeng ZR, et al. Chemoprevention of gastric cancer by celecoxib in rats. *Gut.* 2004;53(2):195-200.

159. Gail MH, You WC, Chang YS, et al. Factorial trial of three interventions to reduce the progression of precancerous gastric lesions in Shandong, China: design issues and initial data. *Control Clin Trials.* 1998;19(4):352-369.

160. Cheng AL, Hsu CH, Lin JK, et al. Phase I clinical trial of curcumin, a chemopreventive agent, in patients with high-risk or pre-malignant lesions. *Anticancer Res.* 2001; 21(4B):2895-2900.

161. Nagata C, Takatsuka N, Kawakami N, et al. A prospective cohort study of soy product intake and stomach cancer death. *Br J Cancer.* 2002;87(1):31-36.

162. Takahashi Y, Mai M, Nishioka K. Alpha-difluoromethylornithine induces apoptosis as well as anti-angiogenesis in the inhibition of tumor growth and metastasis in a human gastric cancer model. *Int J Cancer.* 2000;85(2):243-247.

163. Zhou XM, Wong BC, Fan XM, et al. Non-steroidal anti-inflammatory drugs induce apoptosis in gastric cancer cells through up-regulation of bax and bak. *Carcinogenesis.* 2001;22(9):1393-1397.

164. Zafrani ES. Non-alcoholic fatty liver disease: an emerging pathological spectrum. *Virchows Arch.* 2004;444(1):3-12.

165. Chang MH, Chen CJ, Lai MS, et al. Universal hepatitis B vaccination in Taiwan and the incidence of hepatocellular carcinoma in children. Taiwan Childhood Hepatoma Study Group. *N Engl J Med.* 1997;336(26):1855-1859.

166. Huang K, Lin S. Nationwide vaccination: a success story in Taiwan. *Vaccine.* 2000;18 Suppl 1:S35-S38.

167. Kojiro M. Premalignant lesions of hepatocellular carcinoma: pathologic viewpoint. *J Hepatobiliary Pancreat Surg.* 2000;7(6):535-541.

168. Johnson PJ. The role of serum alpha-fetoprotein estimation in the diagnosis and management of hepatocellular carcinoma. *Clinics in Liver Disease.* 2001;5(1):145-159.

169. Nissen NN, Martin P. Hepatocellular carcinoma: the high-risk patient. *J Clin Gastroenterol.* 2002;35(5 Suppl 2):S79-S85.

170. Hino K, Okita K. Interferon therapy as chemoprevention of hepatocarcinogenesis in patients with chronic hepatitis C. *J Antimicrob Chemother.* 2004;53(1):19-22.

171. Nishiguchi S, Kuroki T, Nakatani S, et al. Randomised trial of effects of interferon-alpha on incidence of hepatocellular carcinoma in chronic active hepatitis C with cirrhosis. *Lancet.* 1995;346(8982):1051-1055.

172. Lin SM, Lin CJ, Hsu CW, et al. Prospective randomized controlled study of interferon-alpha in preventing hepatocellular carcinoma recurrence after medical ablation therapy for primary tumors. *Cancer.* 2004;100(2):376-382.

173. Kubo S, Nishiguchi S, Hirohashi K, et al. Effects of long-term postoperative interferon-alpha therapy on intrahepatic recurrence after resection of hepatitis C virus-related hepatocellular carcinoma. A randomized, controlled trial. *Ann Intern Med.* 2001; 134(10):963-967.

174. Ikeda K, Arase Y, Saitoh S, et al. Interferon beta prevents recurrence of hepatocellular carcinoma after complete resection or ablation of the primary tumor-A prospective randomized study of hepatitis C virus-related liver cancer. *Hepatology.* 2000;32(2):228-232.

175. Okuno, M., S. Kojima, and H. Moriwaki. Chemoprevention of hepatocellular carcinoma: concept, progress and perspectives. *J Gastroenterol Hepatol.* 2001;16(12):1329-1335.

176. Shiota G, Harada K, Ishida M, et al. Inhibition of hepatocellular carcinoma by glycyrrhizin in diethylnitrosamine-treated mice. *Carcinogenesis.* 1999;20(1):59-63.

177. Kumada H. Long-term treatment of chronic hepatitis C with glycyrrhizin [stronger neo-minophagen C (SNMC)] for preventing liver cirrhosis and hepatocellular carcinoma. *Oncology.* 2002;62 Suppl 1:94-100.

178. Egner PA, Wang JB, Zhu YR, et al. Chlorophyllin intervention reduces aflatoxin-DNA adducts in individuals at high risk for liver cancer. *Proceedings of the National Academy of Sciences of the United States of America.* 2001;98(25):14601-14606.

179. Wang JS, Shen X, He X, et al. Protective alterations in phase 1 and 2 metabolism of aflatoxin B1 by oltipraz in residents of Qidong, People's Republic of China. *J Nat Cancer Instit.* 1999;91(4):347-354.

180. Guyton KZ, Kensler TW. Prevention of liver cancer. *Curr Oncol Rep.* 2002;4(6):464-470.

181. Hu KQ. Rationale and feasibility of chemoprevention of hepatocellular carcinoma by cyclooxygenase-2 inhibitors. *J Lab Clin Med.* 2002;139(4):234-243.

182. Yeh CN, Maitra A, Lee KF, et al. Thioacetamide-induced intestinal-type cholangiocarcinoma in rat: an animal model recapitulating the multi-stage progression of human cholangiocarcinoma. *Carcinogenesis.* 2004;25(4):631-636.

183. Schuller HM, Zhang L, Weddle DL, et al. The cyclooxygenase inhibitor ibuprofen and the FLAP inhibitor MK886 inhibit pancreatic carcinogenesis induced in hamsters by transplacental exposure to ethanol and the tobacco carcinogen NNK. *J Cancer Res Clin Oncol.* 2002;128(10):525-532.

184. Molina MA, Sitja-Arnau M, Lemoine MG, et al. Increased cyclooxygenase-2 expression in human pancreatic carcinomas and cell lines: growth inhibition by nonsteroidal anti-inflammatory drugs. *Cancer Res.* 1999;59(17):4356-4362.

185. Kokawa A, Kondo H, Gotoda T, et al. Increased expression of cyclooxygenase-2 in human pancreatic neoplasms and potential for chemoprevention by cyclooxygenase inhibitors. *Cancer.* 2001;91(2):333-338.

186. Aoki T, Nagakawa Y, Tsuchida A, et al. Expression of cyclooxygenase-2 and vascular endothelial growth factor in pancreatic tumors. *Oncol Rep.* 2002;9(4):761-765.

187. Maitra A, Ashfaq R, Gunn CR, et al. Cyclooxygenase 2 expression in pancreatic adenocarcinoma and pancreatic intraepithelial neoplasia: an immunohistochemical analysis with automated cellular imaging. *Am J Clin Pathol.* 2002;118(2):194-201.

188. Li D. Molecular epidemiology of pancreatic cancer. *Cancer Journal.* 2001;7(4):259-265.

189. Cullen JJ, Mitros FA, Oberley LW. Expression of antioxidant enzymes in diseases of the human pancreas: another link between chronic pancreatitis and pancreatic cancer. *Pancreas.* 2003;26(1):23-27.

190. Kise Y, Yamamura M, Kogata M, et al. Inhibitory effect of selenium on hamster pancreatic cancer induction by N'-nitrosobis(2-oxopropyl)amine. *Int J Cancer.* 1990;46(1):95-100.

191. Rautalahti MT, Virtamo JR, Taylor PR, et al. The effects of supplementation with alpha-tocopherol and beta-carotene on the incidence and mortality of carcinoma of the pancreas in a randomized, controlled trial. *Cancer.* 1999;86(1):37-42.

192. Greenwald P. Cancer prevention clinical trials. *J Clin Oncol.* 2002;20(18 Suppl):14S-22S.

193. Temple R. *NDA21-156 and NDA 20-998/S-007.* Washington, DC: United States Food and Drug Administration; 2004.

194. Trinh BN, Long TI, Nickel AE, et al. DNA methyltransferase deficiency modifies cancer susceptibility in mice lacking DNA mismatch repair. *Mol Cell Biol.* 2002;22(9):2906-2917.

195. Kim YI, Salomon RN, Graeme-Cook F, et al. Dietary folate protects against the development of macroscopic colonic neoplasia in a dose responsive manner in rats. *Gut.* 1996;39(5):732-740.

196. Kelloff GJ, Lubet RA, Fay JR, et al. Farnesyl protein transferase inhibitors as potential cancer chemopreventives. *Cancer Epidemiol Biomarkers Prev.* 1997;6(4):267-282.

197. Guyton KZ, Kensler TW. Prevention of liver cancer. *Curr Oncol Rep.* 2002;4(6):464-470.

198. Burke YD, Stark MJ, Roach SL, et al. Inhibition of pancreatic cancer growth by the dietary isoprenoids farnesol and geraniol. *Lipids.* 1997;32(2):151-156.

199. Kelloff GJ, Fay JR, Steele VE, et al. Epidermal growth factor receptor tyrosine kinase inhibitors as potential cancer chemopreventives. *Cancer Epidemiol Biomarkers Prev.* 1996;5(8):657-666.

200. Lawrence DS, Niu J. Protein kinase inhibitors: the tyrosine-specific protein kinases. *Pharmacol Therapeut.* 1998;77(2):81-114.

201. Thiagarajan DG, Bennink MR, Bourquin LD, et al. Prevention of precancerous colonic lesions in rats by soy flakes, soy flour, genistein, and calcium. *Am J Clin Nutr.* 1998;68(6 Suppl):1394S-1399S.

202. Mann M, Sheng H, Shao J, et al. Targeting cyclooxygenase 2 and HER-2/neu pathways inhibits colorectal carcinoma growth [see comment]. *Gastroenterology.* 2001;120(7): 1713-1719.

203. Mandal M, Olson DJ, Sharma T, et al. Butyric acid induces apoptosis by up-regulating Bax expression via stimulation of the c-Jun N-terminal kinase/activation protein-1 pathway in human colon cancer cells. *Gastroenterology.* 2001;120(1):71-78.

204. Buttar NS. Effect of green tea polyphenol on signaling pathways associated with esophageal adenocarcinoma in an animal model. *Gastroenterology.* 2004;126(4)Suppl 2: A-47.

205. Huerta S, Irwin RW, Heber D, et al. 1alpha,25-(OH)(2)-D(3) and its synthetic analogue decrease tumor load in the Apc(min) Mouse. *Cancer Research.* 2002;62(3):741-746.

206. Smirnoff P, Liel Y, Gnainsky J, et al. The protective effect of estrogen against chemically induced murine colon carcinogenesis is associated with decreased CpG island methylation and increased mRNA and protein expression of the colonic vitamin D receptor. *Oncology Research.* 1999;11(6):255-264.

207. Evans SR, Schwartz AM, Shchepotin EI, et al. Growth inhibitory effects of 1,25-dihydroxyvitamin D3 and its synthetic analogue, 1alpha,25-dihydroxy-16-ene-23yne-26,27-hexafluoro-19-nor-cholecalcifero l (Ro 25-6760), on a human colon cancer xenograft. *Clinical Cancer Research.* 1998;4(11):2869-2876.

208. Aoki K, Nakajima A, Mukasa K, et al. Prevention of diabetes, hepatic injury, and colon cancer with dehydroepiandrosterone. *J Steroid Biochem Mol Biol.* 2003;85(2-5):469-472.

209. Zhang W, Rashid A, Wu H, et al. Differential expression of retinoic acid receptors and p53 protein in normal, premalignant, and malignant esophageal tissues. *J Cancer Res Clin Oncol.* 2001;127(4):237-242.

210. Zheng Y, Kramer PM, Lubet RA, et al. Effect of retinoids on AOM-induced colon cancer in rats: modulation of cell proliferation, apoptosis and aberrant crypt foci. *Carcinogenesis.* 1999;20(2):255-260.

211. Dubois RN, Abramson SB, Crofford L, et al. Cyclooxygenase in biology and disease [see comments]. *FASEB Journal.* 1998;12(12):1063-1073.

212. Jacoby RF, Seibert K, Cole CE, et al. The cyclooxygenase-2 inhibitor celecoxib is a potent preventive and therapeutic agent in the min mouse model of adenomatous polyposis. *Cancer Research.* 2000;60(18):5040-5044.

213. Li Z, Shimada Y, Kawabe A, et al. Suppression of N-nitrosomethylbenzylamine (NMBA)-induced esophageal tumorigenesis in F344 rats by JTE-522, a selective COX-2 inhibitor. *Carcinogenesis.* 2001;22(4):547-51 [erratum appears in *Carcinogenesis.* 2001;22(6):981].

214. Dannenberg AJ, Altorki NK, Boyle JO, et al. Inhibition of cyclooxygenase-2: an approach to preventing cancer of the upper aerodigestive tract. *Ann N Y Acad Sci.* 2001; 952:109-115.

215. Martinez ME, O'Brien TG, Fultz KE, et al. Pronounced reduction in adenoma recurrence associated with aspirin use and a polymorphism in the ornithine decarboxylase gene. *Proceedings of the National Academy of Sciences of the United States of America.* 2003;100(13):7859-7864.

216. Seiler N, Atanassov CL, Raul F. Polyamine metabolism as target for cancer chemoprevention (review). *Inter J Oncol.* 1998;13(5):993-1006.

217. Heath EI, Limburg PJ, Hawk ET, et al. Adenocarcinoma of the esophagus: risk factors and prevention. *Oncology (Huntingt).* 2000;14(4):507-14; discussion 518-20, 522-523.

218. Iseki H, Ko TC, Xue XY, et al. A novel strategy for inhibiting growth of human pancreatic cancer cells by blocking cyclin-dependent kinase activity. *J Gastrointest Surg.* 1998;2(1):36-43.

219. Wang X, Fu X, Brown PD, et al. Matrix metalloproteinase inhibitor BB-94 (batimastat) inhibits human colon tumor growth and spread in a patient-like orthotopic model in nude mice. *Cancer Research.* 1994;54(17):4726-4728.

220. Kimata M, Otani Y, Kubota T, et al. Matrix metalloproteinase inhibitor, marimastat, decreases peritoneal spread of gastric carcinoma in nude mice. *Jap J Cancer Res.* 2002; 93(7):834-841.

221. Mirzaie M, Herse B, Oster O, et al. The matrix metalloproteinase inhibitor batimastat inhibits the lung colonization of orthotopically implanted malignant pancreatic tumor cells in SCID mice. *Swiss Surgery.* 2002;8(4):165-170.

222. Kise Y, Yamamura M, Kogata M, et al. Inhibitory effect of selenium on hamster pancreatic cancer induction by N'-nitrosobis(2-oxopropyl)amine. *Int J Cancer.* 1990;46(1): 95-100.

223. Thiagarajan DG, Bennink MR, Bourquin LD, et al. Prevention of precancerous colonic lesions in rats by soy flakes, soy flour, genistein, and calcium. *Am J Clin Nutr.* 1998; 68(6 Suppl):1394S-1399S.

224. Xue L, Lipkin M, Newmark H, et al. Influence of dietary calcium and vitamin D on diet-induced epithelial cell hyperproliferation in mice. *J Natl Cancer Inst.* 1999;91(2): 176-181.

225. Finley JW, Davis CD, Feng Y. Selenium from high selenium broccoli protects rats from colon cancer. *J Nutr.* 2000;130(9):2384-2389.

226. Kelloff GJ, Crowell JA, Steele VE, et al. Progress in cancer chemoprevention: development of diet-derived chemopreventive agents. *J Nutr.* 2000;130(2S Suppl):467S-471S.

227. Giardiello FM, Hamilton SR, Krush AJ, et al. Treatment of colonic and rectal adenomas with sulindac in familial adenomatous polyposis. *N Engl J Med.* 1993;328(18): 1313-1316.

chapter 18

New Technologies for the Detection of Gastrointestinal Neoplasia

Linda S. Lee, MD and John M. Poneros, MD

INTRODUCTION

Cancers of the GI tract have a tremendous impact on society. Colorectal cancer is the second leading cause of cancer death in the United States and accounts for 10% of all cancer deaths. Over 57,000 deaths due to colorectal cancer were expected in the United States in 2003.[1] Although esophageal cancer is significantly less common, the incidence of esophageal adenocarcinoma in the United States has increased dramatically over the past 2 decades.[2] The prognosis for esophageal cancer is grim, with an overall 5-year survival rate of less than 10%. Both colonic and esophageal adenocarcinomas arise from premalignant lesions; any success in their early detection could significantly reduce their mortality rates.

Significant research efforts are being directed toward using the interaction of light and tissue to detect precancerous lesions of the GI tract. The interaction between light and tissue can be used to study both the chemical and physical properties of the tissue being analyzed. The principles being studied could theoretically be applied to the early surveillance of many different types of cancer.

The purpose of this chapter is to review the current status of various experimental optical technologies to detect precancerous changes in the GI tract. This review will focus on the clinical applications of these technologies for the practicing gastroenterologist.

LASER-INDUCED FLUORESCENCE SPECTROSCOPY

Laser-induced fluorescence spectroscopy is a technique that uses characteristic light emission spectra to help differentiate benign from malignant or premalignant tissue. Ultraviolet (UV) or short wavelength light from a laser or filtered lamp source is typically used to illuminate the tissue being studied. Endogenous substances in the tissue known as fluorophores absorb light of a specific wavelength and emit fluorescence light of a longer wavelength; this is known as the tissue's autofluorescence.[3-5] An overview of the light-tissue interactions discussed in this chapter is presented in Figure 18-1.

Figure 18-1. Schematic illustrating examples of light-tissue interactions.

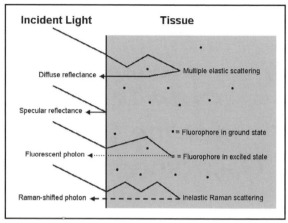

Tissue autofluorescence is dominated by the type and proportion of fluorophores it contains. Fluorophores are present in connective tissue (collagen, elastin), respiratory chain coenzymes (NADH, flavin), amino acids (tryptophan), and by-products of heme synthesis (porphyrin). Table 18-1 lists common endogenous fluorophores and their excitation and emission wavelengths. The mucosa, submucosa, and muscularis propria each have distinct fluorophore compositions; tissue autofluorescence is the sum of these layers.

Malignant and benign tissue have different emission spectra due to several specific characteristics:[4,5]

- The different distribution and concentration of fluorophores and chromophores (which absorb light without re-emission of fluorescence)
- The alteration in tissue architecture, such as mucosal thickening in epithelial tumors
- The changes in the metabolic status of tumor tissue
- The different biochemical microenvironments, such as the microbial activity that occurs in necrotic tumors which can promote porphyrin synthesis

Romer et al[6] studied the morphologic differences in fluorescence between normal colonic mucosa and adenomas, specifically which tissue components contributed to fluorescence. Fluorescence mainly arose from collagen fibers in the bowel wall and eosinophil granules in the lamina propria. Fluorescent eosinophil granules were more numerous in adenomas, and cytoplasmic fluorescence was detected in adenomas but not normal colonic epithelial cells. Determining which cellular components are responsible for the differences in polyp fluorescence will help exploit these fluorescence signatures.

The wavelength of excitation light used is critical when studying tissue autofluorescence because different wavelengths excite distinct fluorophores at varying tissue depths. The optimal excitation and emission wavelengths for various tissue types are unknown and typically determined by *ex vivo* experimentation. These results may not accurately reflect *in vivo* tissue properties due to changes in the microenvironment and metabolic state.[4]

Table 18-1

COMMON ENDOGENOUS FLUOROPHORES
AND THEIR EXCITATION AND EMISSION WAVELENGTHS

Endogenous Fluorophore	Biological Source	Wavelength of Max. Excitation (nm)	Wavelength of Max. Emission (nm)
Collagen	Connective tissue	330	390
Elastin		350	420
NADH	Respiratory chain co-enzymes	340	450
FAD, flavins		450	515
Tryptophan	Amino acids	280	350
Phenylalanine		260	280
Tyrosine		275	300
Porphyrins	Byproducts of heme synthesis	400 to 450	635, 690
Pyridoxine	Vitamin B_6 compounds	330, 340	400
Pyridoxal-5'-phosphate		330	400
Ceroid, lipofuscin	Lipopigment granules	340 to 395	430 to 460, 540 to 640

In 1990, Kapadia et al[7] reported the first use of laser-induced fluorescence spectroscopy in the GI tract. The authors examined *ex vivo* colonic tissue using a laser with an excitation wavelength of 325 nm to distinguish adenomatous polyps from hyperplastic polyps. Using linear regression analysis and a training set of 70 tissue specimens (35 normal, 35 adenomatous), a quantitative laser-induced fluorescence score was developed to discriminate adenomas from normal tissue. In the validation set, all 34 normal mucosal specimens, 16 adenomas, and 94% of hyperplastic polyps were correctly identified. These results were confirmed in the first *in vivo* study by Cothren et al[8] who compared the spectra from different specimens in the colon. They developed a spectrofluorometry system with an optical probe that could be passed through the accessory channel of a standard colonoscope and placed in direct contact with tissue. Using 460 and 680 nm excitation wavelengths, they distinguished adenomas from nonadenomas (defined as normal mucosa and hyperplastic polyps) with 97% specificity, 100% sensitivity, and 94% positive predictive value.

An *in vitro* study to determine the optimal excitation and emission wavelengths for distinguishing colonic adenomas from normal colonic tissue was performed by Richards-Kortum et al.[9] Excitation wavelengths of 330, 370, and 430 nm were studied for 11 normal mucosal specimens and 16 adenomas. Using an excitation wavelength of

370 nm, the emission wavelength of 480 nm best differentiated adenomatous from normal tissue; 96% of 26 samples were correctly identified as normal or adenomatous.

Schomacker et al[10] then specifically examined the discrimination of adenomas from hyperplastic polyps *in vivo*. During routine colonoscopy, an optical fiber probe was passed through the colonoscope and emission spectra collected from all polyps requiring resection. Similar to the study by Kapadia et al linear regression analysis was used to develop a laser-induced fluorescence score to distinguish adenomas from hyperplastic polyps.[7] For an excitation wavelength of 390 nm and using histology as the reference standard, the authors reported a slightly lower sensitivity (86%), specificity (80%), and positive predictive value (86%) compared to previous studies. They postulated that the use of a slightly longer excitation wavelength *in vivo* (390 nm vs 370 nm in the Richards-Kortum study) and the inclusion of mixed morphology polyps might explain the different results.

In the first blinded study published in 1996, Cothren's group[11] prospectively validated a diagnostic algorithm to distinguish normal colonic mucosa from hyperplastic and adenomatous polyps using fluorescence spectra. *In vivo* emission spectra were collected from 103 polypoid and 104 normal-appearing colonic mucosal sites using an optical probe passed through the colonoscope. The diagnostic algorithm was developed using emission spectra from 41 polyps and 43 normal-appearing colonic mucosal sites. This algorithm was tested in a blinded fashion using the remaining polypoid and normal colonic specimens. With an excitation wavelength of 370 nm, the sensitivity, specificity, and positive predictive value for differentiating adenomas from nonadenomas (normal mucosa and hyperplastic polyps) were 90%, 95%, and 90%, respectively. In distinguishing adenomas from hyperplastic polyps, the sensitivity and specificity were slightly lower at 90% and 82%. Table 18-2 summarizes several studies using endogenous fluorescence spectroscopy to diagnose colonic adenomas.

Laser-induced fluorescence spectroscopy has also been used to examine upper GI tract epithelia. In 1995, Panjehpour et al[12] published the first use of laser-induced fluorescence spectroscopy to identify esophageal malignancy *in vivo*. Using linear discriminate analysis, the authors developed a diagnostic algorithm that they tested on 108 normal and 26 malignant tissue specimens. At an excitation wavelength of 410 nm, the sensitivity and specificity for detecting malignant esophageal tissue was 100% and 98%. The investigators then examined the use of laser-induced fluorescence spectroscopy to detect dysplasia in BE.[13] They used the differential normalized fluorescence index to distinguish HGD from LGD or nondysplastic mucosa. For emission wavelengths of 480 and 660 nm at an excitation wavelength of 410 nm, 90% of HGD cases were correctly identified; all examples of LGD and 96% of nondysplastic BE were appropriately classified. One limitation of this study was that only 28% of LGD specimens with areas of focal HGD were correctly recognized. It should be noted that the clinical significance of focal HGD is controversial.[14,15]

Light-induced fluorescence spectroscopy has been studied as an alternative to laser excitation and appears promising.[16] Mayinger et al used violet-blue light as the excitation energy in a pilot study of 11 patients (6 with esophageal squamous cell carcinoma, 3 with gastric cancer, and 2 with gastric adenomas with severe dysplasia).[16] Biopsies were obtained after spectroscopy and used as the reference standard. The illumination and position of the probe dramatically affected the intensity of the observed spectra in this study; therefore, the spectra were normalized before comparison. After normalization, the spectra from normal and premalignant tissue were clearly different; the authors

Table 18-2

SUMMARY OF AUTOFLUORESCENCE STUDIES TO DIAGNOSE COLONIC ADENOMAS

Authors	System Studies	Excitation Wavelength (nm)	Tissues Studied	Results
Kapadia et al (1990)	Ex vivo	325	Adenoma vs hyperplastic polyp	94% accurate
Cothren et al (1990)	In vivo	460, 680	Adenoma vs hyperplastic and normal tissue	100% sensitive 97% specific 94% PPV
Richards-Kortum et al (1991)	In vitro	370	Adenoma vs normal tissue	96% accurate
Schomaker et al (1992)	In vivo	390	Adenoma vs hyperplastic polyp	86% sensitive 80% specific 86% PPV
Cothren et al (1996)	In vivo, blinded	370	Adenoma vs hyperplastic and normal tissue	90% sensitive 95% specific 90% PPV

found that esophageal squamous cell carcinoma and dysplastic gastric adenomas displayed significantly lower intensity compared to normal mucosa. In this study, interpretation of the biological significance of a spectrum was only possible after obtaining a reference spectrum from normal mucosa of the same patient. Compared to laser-induced fluorescence, light-induced fluorescence spectroscopy offers the advantage of being a less expensive technology, which would allow it to be more easily disseminated.

FLUORESCENCE SPECTROSCOPY VERSUS FLUORESCENCE SPECTROSCOPIC IMAGING

Emitted fluorescent light can be analyzed by point spectroscopy or imaging. In spectroscopy, a point measurement of fluorescence is obtained. During endoscopic GI spectroscopy, an optical fiber probe is passed through the biopsy channel of the endoscope to contact the tissue. The probe delivers excitation light, captures and transmits the emission fluorescence for analysis, and blocks scattered excitation light. During each contact and delivery of excitation light, detailed spectroscopic data are collected from a 1 to 3 mm³ volume of tissue. Conversely, fluorescence imaging analyzes a larger area of tissue. Recent prototypes involve attaching a unit with 2 light-sensitive cameras to the optical head of a fiberoptic endoscope. The images from these 2 cameras are combined into a real-time fluorescent image with normal tissue appearing a certain color and abnormal tissue a different color. The endoscopist can switch back and forth between the white-light endoscopic and real-time fluorescent imaging to image large areas of tissue rapidly. Using this system, any suspicious lesions on white-light endoscopy can be quickly examined using fluorescent imaging.[4,5] Due to the reduced signal-to-noise ratio with fluorescent imaging, the sensitivity and specificity are thought to be less than point spectroscopy.

In 1999, Wang et al[17] studied a prototype endoscopic fluorescence imaging system to diagnose colonic adenomas. Using histology as the reference standard and a fluorescence threshold of 80% of the average intensity of normal mucosa, this imaging system was 83% sensitive for identifying adenomas; all hyperplastic polyps were correctly classified as nondysplastic. White-light endoscopy was compared to combination white-light endoscopic and fluorescent imaging in differentiating nondysplastic colonic tissue (normal or hyperplastic) from adenomatous polyps in an abstract published in 2001.[18] This study demonstrated a higher sensitivity (95% vs 80%), specificity (80% vs 69%), and positive predictive value (71% vs 59%) with fluorescent imaging when examining 62 lesions.

Fluorescence spectroscopy and imaging have several limitations. Fluorescence analyzes a relatively weak signal that results from the interaction between light and tissue fluorophores and, therefore, necessitates sensitive and expensive instrumentation. In addition, fluorescence spectroscopy and imaging require that the optimal excitation and emission wavelength for each tissue be first determined through *ex vivo* experimentation, which may not accurately reflect *in vivo* results.[4] Despite these limitations, this optical technology has shown great promise and provided the earliest experience for investigators working in this field.

EXOGENOUS FLUORESCENT AGENTS

Exogenous fluorescent agents have been studied as an alternative to tissue autofluorescence in the detection of precancerous changes in the GI tract. These agents are administered before performing fluorescence spectroscopy or imaging and are used to magnify the abnormal signal from dysplastic tissue. Studies have focused on maximizing the diagnostic yield of these agents by determining the optimal dosage, method of delivery, and timing of the endoscopic procedures during which spectroscopic data are measured. Drug toxicity and imperfect localization of the drug to dysplasia are the limitations of these agents.[19,20]

One of the most studied exogenous fluorescent agents is 5-aminolevulinic acid (ALA), which is the rate-limiting precursor in heme biosynthesis. Exogenous administration of ALA promotes heme synthesis and causes an accumulation of protoporphyrin IX (PPIX), which best absorbs light at 400 nm and emits red light at 650 nm. PPIX preferentially accumulates in the mucosal epithelium of the epidermis, endometrium, urinary and GI tracts, and their malignant counterparts.[21-23] Neoplastic cells have elevated porphobilinogen deaminase levels and decreased ferrochelatase activity, which is thought to lead to excess PPIX accumulation.[24] This mechanism has been exploited by using ALA as a photosensitizer for photodynamic therapy.[25-27] The toxicity of ALA is less than other photosensitizers; phototoxicity with ALA typically lasts only 1 to 2 days. To optimize the ability to detect malignancy and premalignancy, varying the dose of ALA, mechanism of delivery (eg, intravenous vs topical spray), and the time delay between sensitization and endoscopy have been studied.[23]

In 1996, von Holstein et al[28] completed the first study using an exogenous fluorophore to perform laser-induced fluorescence spectroscopy in the GI tract. The authors injected the photosensitizer dihematoporphyrin ether (Photofrin, [Axcan Pharma Inc, Birmingham, Ala]) to help identify adenocarcinoma within Barrett's mucosa. Photofrin is an exogenous fluorophore with prolonged photosensitivity that can last for 6 to 8 weeks. It is less selectively concentrated in the GI mucosa than ALA. PPIX is typically found in highest concentration in the mucosal epithelium while Photofrin diffuses throughout the entire esophageal wall. This causes a deeper "burn" when using Photofrin to perform photodynamic therapy but also leads to a higher stricture rate.[29-31] In this preliminary study by Von Holstein et al, the investigators used both emission spectra from endogenous fluorophores (eg, autofluorescence) and Photofrin to create a fluorescence ratio to identify normal mucosa, BE, dysplasia, and adenocarcinoma. The intensity of autofluorescence at 500 nm for normal mucosa was 6.5 times higher than adenocarcinoma or severe dysplasia, while Photofrin produced a fluorescence intensity at 630 nm only 1.2 times higher in tumor compared to normal tissue. The authors concluded that autofluorescence was more useful than exogenous fluorescence with Photofrin in distinguishing normal mucosa from esophageal adenocarcinoma.

The first study using ALA-enhanced fluorescence spectroscopy to detect colonic dysplasia was published by Eker et al[32] in 1999. An oral dose of ALA of 5 mg/kg body weight was administered approximately 2 to 3 hours before colonoscopy and spectroscopy. Linear regression analysis was used to create an algorithm for classifying normal mucosa, hyperplastic polyps, and adenomas. At an excitation wavelength of 337 nm, ALA did not significantly improve the ability to differentiate between adenoma and normal or hyperplastic tissue compared to autofluorescence, but did improve discrimination using 405 and 436 nm excitation. Sensitivity was 89% with specificity of 94% at wavelength of 405 nm with similar sensitivity (86%) and specificity (100%) using 436 nm excitation.

After these initial studies using ALA-enhanced fluorescence spectroscopy, research has focused on ALA-enhanced fluorescence imaging. Mayinger et al[33] studied 22 patients with known or suspected esophageal malignancy or BE who ingested ALA at a dose of 15 mg/kg body weight. Fluorescence imaging, standard white-light endoscopy, and biopsy were performed 6 to 7 hours after ingestion. Tissue histology was used as the reference standard to determine sensitivity and specificity. While sensitivity for accurately diagnosing biopsy sites was greater with ALA-enhanced fluorescence imaging compared to white-light endoscopy (85% vs 25%), specificity was diminished (53% vs 94%) due to PPIX accumulation in inflamed mucosa. An example of ALA-enhanced fluorescence imaging is demonstrated in Figure 18-2.

In 2001, Endlicher et al[34] investigated the optimal dose and route of administration of ALA in fluorescence imaging to detect biopsy-proven low and high-grade dysplasia within BE. ALA was orally ingested at doses of 5, 10, 20, or 30 mg/kg body weight or sprayed onto Barrett's epithelium using a special spray catheter at a prior endoscopy. Imaging was performed 4 to 6 hours after systemic or 1 to 2 hours after local sensitization. At 20 and 30 mg/kg, the technique was limited by increased side effects such as nausea, vomiting, and elevated liver enzymes. The lowest dose of 5 mg/kg failed to detect dysplasia. Sensitivity and specificity for detecting dysplasia were similar for 10 mg/kg (80% and 56%) and 20 mg/kg (100% and 51%). Local sensitization with a spray

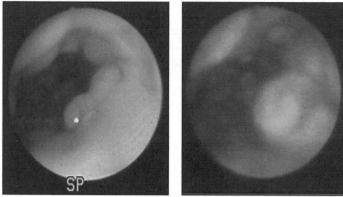

Figure 18-2. Endoscopic image of nodule with HGD and ALA-enhanced fluorescence imaging of identical nodule. (Courtesy of Norman Nishioka, MD, Boston, Mass.) *For a full-color version, see page CA-XV of the Color Atlas.*

catheter had improved specificity (69%) but reduced sensitivity (60%) and was limited by the need to perform 2 endoscopies. The overall high rate of false-positive fluorescence in this study resulted from incorrectly classifying inflammatory mucosa, ulcer margins, and bile as malignant.

Based on this work, Brand et al[35] performed the first study to use quantitative ALA-enhanced fluorescence point spectroscopy to differentiate nondysplastic from dysplastic Barrett's epithelium. Oral ALA at a dose of 10 mg/kg body weight was administered 3 hours before endoscopy. A standardized fluorescence intensity value was calculated by accounting for the contribution of autofluorescence at emission wavelengths of 635 and 750 nm. Sensitivity and specificity for distinguishing HGD from non-dysplastic Barrett's mucosa and LGD were 77% and 71%, respectively.

The use of ALA-fluorescence imaging to identify colonic dysplasia was recently studied by Messmann et al.[36] Previous studies had established that a higher dose of ALA is required to sensitize the colon compared to the esophagus.[37] Therefore, Messmann and colleagues used an oral dose of 20 mg/kg, a 3 gm ALA enema, or a spray catheter to detect dysplasia (low and high-grade) in ulcerative colitis. Endoscopy was performed 4 to 6 hours after systemic sensitization and 1 to 2 hours after local sensitization. A total of 481 biopsies were examined from 37 patients, with 42 biopsies showing dysplasia (40 with LGD, 2 with HGD). Using histology as the reference standard, sensitivity for detecting dysplasia ranged from 43% with oral ALA, 87% with enema, and up to 100% with the spray catheter. However, oral ALA had a higher specificity of 73% compared to the enema (51%) and spray catheter (62%).

Use of ALA as an exogenous fluorescent agent has shown promise in detecting dysplasia in the upper and lower GI tract, with relatively few side effects. Further studies with other exogenous fluorescent agents and improved fluorescent imaging techniques when using these agents are required.

LIGHT-SCATTERING SPECTROSCOPY

While fluorescence analyzes the biochemical properties of tissue, light-scattering spectroscopy (LSS) interrogates structural information. The wavelength of the illuminating light and the properties of the scattering particle determine the scattering pattern. Cell nuclei are predominately responsible for light scattering when tissue is analyzed, specifically the nuclear size and number. Photons are typically scattered multiple times within tissue before being emitted. LSS measures the wavelength and intensity of back-reflected light. It subtracts the diffuse background caused by multiple scattering to allow the analysis of the small amount of back-scattered light from cell nuclei. Dysplastic cells typically have an increased nuclear-to-cytoplasmic ratio and are more crowded together. LSS is a quantitative equivalent to the histologic markers for dysplasia of hyperchromasia and nuclear enlargement. One advantage of LSS compared to laser-induced fluorescence is that the signal intensity of light scattering dominates the fluorescent signal when examining biological tissue.[19,38,39]

LSS of the GI tract involves inserting an optical probe through the accessory channel of the endoscope. The tip of the probe contacts the epithelium and emits and collects the white light from about a 1 mm² area of tissue. In the first study of LSS in Barrett's epithelium with and without dysplasia, dysplastic epithelium was defined as at least 30% of the nuclei being larger than 10 μm.[40] Using this definition and histology as the gold standard, the sensitivity and specificity of LSS for correctly identifying high-grade and low-grade dysplasia was approximately 90%; all HGD samples and 87% of LGD specimens were correctly classified. The appeal of this technique is that a stronger signal is collected in real-time using white light instead of a laser source. An endoscopic imaging system using this spectroscopic technology has not been reported.

RAMAN SPECTROSCOPY

When light interacts with tissue, incident photons cause electrons in the tissue to oscillate and emit photons. If the emitted photons have the same energy as the incident photons, no energy transfer occurs and the scattering is termed elastic. Although most scattering events are elastic, some are inelastic, which refers to an energy transfer between the photon and the molecule being illuminated. The phenomenon of inelastic light scattering is termed Raman scattering. The energy transfer causes molecules to vibrate, which results in slight shifts in energy and wavelength of the emitted light relative to the excitation light. Approximately 1 photon out of 1 million will scatter at a wavelength slightly shifted from the original incident wavelength. Thus, Raman scattering is much weaker than elastic scattering, but the signal is highly specific to the molecular composition of the tissue.[19,39]

Visible, UV, or near-infrared (NIR) light may be used to induce Raman scattering, which is measured as a difference in wavelength from the excitation wavelength. When visible light is used for excitation, autofluorescence causes severe interference with the Raman signal, which is typically much weaker than the fluorescent signal. UV light is not optimal for Raman spectroscopy because it can cause tissue injury and does not penetrate tissue to the same depth as visible or NIR light. NIR light for Raman spectroscopy has the advantages of minimizing autofluorescence, penetrating more deeply to a depth of approximately 500 mm, and being nonmutagenic.[19,39]

Ex vivo studies using Raman spectroscopy to examine BE reported a sensitivity and specificity of 77% and 93%, respectively, for differentiating nondysplastic from dysplastic Barrett's epithelium.[41] Shim et al[42] then designed and built a NIR device for endoscopic *in vivo* Raman spectroscopy. In the first report using this device, the authors demonstrated the feasibility of *in vivo* measurements, but the spectral differences between normal tissue and HGD in the esophagus and colon were subtle.

In 2003, these authors used endoscopic NIR Raman spectroscopy to diagnose colonic adenomas *in vivo*.[43] They classified 19 Raman spectra from 9 polyps in 3 patients as hyperplastic or adenomatous using diagnostic algorithms. These algorithms were developed from principal component and linear discriminant analyses in a "leave-one-out" cross-validation method. In this small sample, the diagnostic algorithms were 100% sensitive and 89% specific for differentiating hyperplastic from adenomatous polyps. Raman spectroscopy is a potentially powerful tool in evaluating premalignant GI conditions but requires further study.

TRIMODAL SPECTROSCOPY

Recently, a group of investigators combined several spectroscopic techniques in an attempt to increase the accuracy of detecting dysplasia within BE.[44] Georgakoudi et al used a combination of fluorescence, reflectance, and light-scattering spectroscopies to analyze the biochemical, architectural, and morphologic characteristics of Barrett's epithelium, with and without dysplasia. The simultaneous use of all 3 techniques was named "trimodal spectroscopy." The combination of fluorescence and reflectance spectroscopies was applied to remove the distortions introduced into the measured tissue fluorescence spectrum by scattering and absorption. Undistorted fluorescence was then used to analyze the tissue biochemistry, and reflectance and light-scattering spectroscopies were used to analyze the tissue architecture and epithelial cell nuclei.

Data were collected from 40 sites in 16 patients with known BE undergoing standard surveillance endoscopy. Principal component and logistic regression analyses were used to correlate the spectral features and histopathologic diagnosis. In this data set, Trimodal spectroscopy classified HGD vs LGD and nondysplastic BE with 100% sensitivity and 100% specificity. HGD and LGD vs nondysplastic BE was identified with 100% sensitivity and 93% specificity. It should be noted that this study was not conducted in real time and used "leave-one-out" cross-validation to establish the classification algorithms. Nonetheless, Trimodal spectroscopy carries great promise for the detection of dysplastic epithelial changes by combining information regarding the biochemical and architectural characteristics of tissue.

OPTICAL COHERENCE TOMOGRAPHY

Optical coherence tomography (OCT) is a novel imaging technique that provides high resolution, 2-dimensional cross-sectional imaging of the GI tract. OCT is analogous to B mode ultrasound imaging but uses light rather than sound waves. The use of light rather than sound leads to differences in the depth of penetration and resolution of images. With the use of light, tissue resolution is increased by nearly 10 times from ~110 mm to ~10 mm but the depth of imaging is sacrificed.[45-47]

During OCT imaging, backscattered light provides information on the spatial organization of the tissue. OCT measures the echo time delay and magnitude of the backscattered light signal from microstructures within the tissue. Echo time delay refers to the time difference between the signal leaving from and returning to the detector. Because light travels too quickly for the electronic detection of its echo time delay, OCT uses a technique called interferometry to measure the delay. Light from a low coherence light source is split evenly into 2 separate pathways, with one beam directed to the tissue being imaged and the other beam delivered to a reference arm. At the end of the reference arm is a mirror that oscillates at a known distance away from the detector. Each beam of light is reflected from both the tissue and the reference mirror and recombined at the detector. The interference created by these 2 recombined light beams is then measured. Interference only occurs when the path lengths of both light beams are matched to within the coherence length of the light source. The axial resolution of an OCT image is determined by the coherence length of the light source used and is approximately 10 mm in the infrared OCT systems. The lateral or transverse resolution is determined by the spatial width of the light source and is approximately 30 mm. As the position of the mirror is moved, information is collected from different tissue levels. By scanning the optical beam across the tissue surface, a 2-dimensional picture is created.[48,49]

Several *in vitro* studies have demonstrated the feasibility of OCT imaging in the GI tract.[45,49-51] However, the clinical value of *in vitro* studies is limited because the optical properties of nonliving tissue are different from *in vivo* tissue. *In vitro* OCT images have shown esophageal squamous epithelium to be a highly scattering layer while the lamina propria demonstrated much less backscatter.[45,50] *In vivo* OCT images have shown the opposite, displaying a highly scattering lamina propria and a less scattering squamous epithelium.[52-53]

Multiple studies have demonstrated the characteristic findings for normal and abnormal GI tissue using OCT.[52-58] In 1997 Sergeev et al[54] published the first *in vivo* OCT images of normal esophageal epithelium. They imaged 4 patients and demonstrated 5 esophageal wall layers composed of mucosa, lamina propria, muscularis mucosa, submucosa, and muscularis propria. Using the same OCT system, Jäckle et al[53,55] presented data from 48 patients, including 9 esophageal images, and confirmed their findings. Bouma et al[52] studied 32 patients using a linear scanning device that produces cross-sectional images similar to those of Jäckle et al. By comparing *ex vivo* measurements of layer thickness by OCT and histology in the same specimen of normal esophagus, they were able to define precisely which OCT image layers corresponded to each esophageal wall component. In a recent *ex vivo* study using a Ti:Sapphire laser as the light source, Cilesiz et al[59] clearly visualized the muscularis propria as well as lymphoid follicles.

The OCT system used by Sivak et al[56] differs from other endoscopic OCT systems in that it acquires images with a radial scanning device similar to high-frequency ultrasound. A series by Sivak et al included 72 OCT images from 38 patients taken from the upper and lower GI tract. Zuccaro et al[57] acquired 477 images of the esophagus and stomach in 69 patients, and Li et al[58] published a descriptive study of 8 patients using both linear- and radial-scanning OCT catheter probes and spectroscopic OCT.

BE is characterized by the development of specialized intestinal metaplasia above the esophago-gastric junction. The hallmark histologic feature of specialized intestinal metaplasia is the presence of goblet cells. Visualization of individual goblet cells is beyond the resolution of currently available endoscopic OCT devices. However, OCT images of Barrett's epithelium have shown distinct morphologic features that enable the differentiation of Barrett's epithelium from other tissue types. Pitris et al and Bouma et al[45,52] identified several of these OCT features: loss of the layered esophageal structure, abnormal and disorganized glands, and increased architectural disorder and heterogeneity. The deeper structures including the lamina propria, muscularis mucosa, and submucosa were

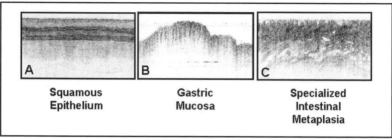

Figure 18-3. OCT images of upper GI tract tissues. (A) Squamous epithelium typically shows a 5-layered appearance. (B) Gastric mucosa demonstrates a "pit-and-crypt" morphology. (C) Barrett's epithelium, or specialized intestinal metaplasia, reveals an inhomogeneous tissue contrast, an irregular mucosal surface and submucosal glands. (Courtesy of Brett Bouma, PhD and Gary Tearney, MD, PhD, Boston, Mass.)

not visualized due to the strong backscattering from the metaplastic epithelium. Figure 18-3 demonstrates OCT images of normal esophageal squamous epithelium, gastric mucosa, and specialized intestinal metaplasia.

In 2001, Poneros et al[60] developed and prospectively validated the first objective OCT image criteria for diagnosing BE. These criteria were developed by examining 166 OCT-correlated biopsy specimens that served as the training set. The presence of 2 or more of the following OCT findings was considered diagnostic for Barrett's epithelium: absence of normal esophageal layering, disorganized architecture, and the presence of submucosal glands that look like areas of low reflectance below the tissue surface or invaginations through the epithelium. An experienced blinded observer used these criteria to analyze 122 OCT images prospectively in the validation set. Using histology as the standard, the OCT criteria were 97% sensitive and 92% specific for Barrett's mucosa with or without dysplasia.

This same group studied the use of OCT in identifying dysplasia in Barrett's mucosa.[61] Because the degree of light reflectivity depends on nuclear size, OCT may be able to characterize dysplasia within Barrett's epithelium by quantifying the OCT signal as a function of depth (eg, higher degrees of dysplasia characterized by larger nuclei would be expected to cause more light scattering). This alteration in the light reflection characteristics of dysplastic tissue may be more reliable than morphologic criteria in identifying dysplasia.

In order to differentiate specialized intestinal metaplasia from dysplasia, the authors used 2 parameters that are calculated from the OCT images: slope reflectivity and layer ratio. In a preliminary retrospective study of 11 images of LGD, 4 of HGD, and 23 of nondysplastic Barrett's epithelium, sensitivity for HGD was 100% with a specificity of 82% to 85%.

Another group also recently published a study in abstract form using OCT to diagnose dysplastic Barrett's epithelium.[62] Isenberg et al used morphologic rather than quantitative criteria to identify dysplasia. Four endoscopists independently reviewed 152 images from 23 patients and rated them from 1 (dysplasia absent) to 5 (dysplasia present). A 2 or higher was considered positive for dysplasia. A pathologist blinded to the OCT images reviewed the corresponding biopsies. OCT was 69% sensitive and 71% specific with a positive predictive value of 36% and a negative predictive value of 91%.

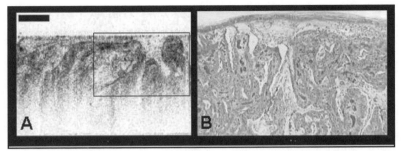

Figure 18-4. (A) OCT image of esophageal adenocarcinoma. Scale bar 500 μm. (B) Corresponding histopathology (H&E, orig. mag x 40). (Courtesy of Brett Bouma, PhD and Gary Tearney, MD, PhD, Boston, Mass.) *For a full-color version, see page CA-XVI of the Color Atlas.*

The authors concluded that the high negative predictive value suggested that OCT could be used to target biopsies to areas of higher suspicion for dysplasia in Barrett's epithelium.

OCT images of malignant GI tissue have been published by several groups. Jäckle et al[55] studied 6 patients with esophageal adenocarcinoma arising from Barrett's mucosa. They described a complete loss of layering and increased heterogeneity in esophageal adenocarcinoma when imaged by OCT. Bouma et al[52] confirmed these results in two patients and described a cellular stroma with large pockets of mucin. Figure 18-4 demonstrates an OCT image of esophageal adenocarcinoma and its corresponding histology. Because of the limited depth of penetration with OCT, the role of OCT in staging esophageal tumors is unclear. EUS accurately stages most endoscopically apparent tumors. However, superficial esophageal squamous cell carcinomas in which the tumor echogenicity does not differ significantly from the surrounding normal squamous mucosa are poorly staged by EUS. OCT may be useful in this instance but experience with OCT in esophageal squamous carcinoma is limited. Jäckle et al[53] and Pitris et al[45] each reported one case of squamous carcinoma identified by loss of normal esophageal layering using OCT.

Gastric tissue is very distinct and easily distinguishable from esophageal epithelium by OCT.[52-54,56-58] Instead of horizontal layering, gastric tissue displays a characteristic vertical "pit-and-crypt" architecture (see Figure 18-3). The depth of penetration in the stomach with OCT is the lowest in the GI tract, measuring approximately 0.7 mm. Studies are lacking regarding the OCT findings in gastric dysplasia or gastritis.

In the lower GI tract, colonic mucosa is readily identified by OCT due to its narrow and ordered crypts. Jäckle et al[53] reported that adenomas contain dark round areas that represent expansion of adenomatous glands. In colonic adenocarcinoma, similar to esophageal adenocarcinoma, there is a loss of the mucosal architecture with an uneven surface and dilated and disorganized crypts.[45,53] Mucosal inflammation is seen as areas of high backscattering on OCT,[49] and destruction of normal mucosa with ulcerative lesions are seen in ulcerative colitis.[45]

OCT images of colonic adenomas were examined in a recent study by Pfau et al.[63] During routine colonoscopy, OCT images were obtained from 44 polyps (30 adenomas, 14 hyperplastic polyps) and nearby normal-appearing mucosa in 24 patients. Real-time subjective assessments of the degree of organization and light scattering were performed by the endoscopists who rated the images from 0 (least organization or scattering) to 5 (most organization or scattering). Digital imaging analysis was performed to quantify the degree of light scattering, and histology was used as the reference standard. Adenomas were significantly more disorganized, with less light scattering compared to hyperplastic polyps; normal colonic mucosal specimens were similar to hyperplastic polyps. The authors concluded that OCT could differentiate adenomatous from hyperplastic polyps and normal tissue based upon the degree of tissue organization and light scattering.

OCT images of the biliary tree obtained during ERCP were published in 2002.[64] OCT images of normal bile duct, cholangiocarcinoma, and a malignant biliary stricture due to metastatic colon cancer were acquired from 5 patients. If proven sensitive for cholangiocarcinoma, OCT would be particularly useful in this disease given the frequent difficulty in obtaining diagnostic tissue.

OCT is an exciting technology that allows real-time tomographic visualization of tissue structures at a higher resolution than any other currently available endoscopic modality. During OCT, an optical probe is passed down the accessory channel of the endoscope without the need for a conducting medium. Endoscopic OCT is an evolving technology with several current limitations, which include the length of time required to obtain images, a shallow depth of visualization, and the inability to visualize subcellular structures. "High resolution OCT" imaging that is comparable to histology is closer to becoming a reality, with the development of ultrashort pulse laser technology. Drexler et al[65] published OCT images taken with a Ti:Sapphire laser system that achieves a longitudinal resolution of ~1 μm and transverse resolution of 3 μm *in vitro*. Subcellular structures such as nuclei are readily seen at these resolutions. As currently configured, this system is limited in that it is not catheter-based or readily portable, and safety data regarding its interrogating light beam lacking. However, once these limitations are overcome, high resolution OCT could provide a significant advancement in endoscopic optical imaging of the GI tract. Figure 18-5 demonstrates an OCT image of an African frog tadpole (Xenopus laevis) using this system.

MOLECULAR BEACONS

Recently exciting work has been published on the use of optically-based, enzyme-activatable fluorescent sensors for the *in vivo* detection of protease activity. Proteolytic enzymes have been shown to play an essential role during tumor progression, specifically during high cell turnover, invasion, and angiogenesis.[66] Cathepsin B, a cysteine protease, has been demonstrated to be up-regulated in areas of inflammation, necrosis, angiogenesis, and during the focal invasion of colorectal carcinomas and dysplastic adenomas.[67-69] Fluorescent sensors that operate in the NIR region have been developed to allow noninvasive detection and monitoring of enzyme activity.[70,71] These targeted NIR fluorochromes have an advantage over other reporters such as isotopes in that they can be "silenced" and "activated" by the enzymes they are used to identify. In their native state, the enzymes are essentially nonfluorescent but upon enzymatic cleavage, they become fluorescent in the NIR.

In 2002, a group of investigators reported their work using a fluorescent molecular "beacon" to assess cathepsin B protease activity in adenomatous polyps.[72] The authors used a mouse model, which is heterozygous for the germ-line mutation of the mouse homologue of the human APC gene. These animals develop multiple adenomas in the small and large bowel that simulate adenomatous polyps in humans.[73]

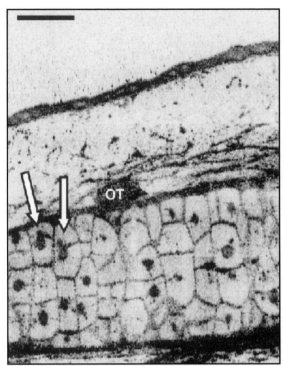

Figure 18-5. In vitro OCT image of Xenopus laevis. Scale bar represents 100 μm. The olfactory tract (OT) and mitosis of 2 cell pairs (arrows) are shown. (Reprinted with permission from Drexler W, et al. *Optics Letters.* 1999; 24:1221-3.)

Using a control set of mice injected with a nonactivatable fluorochrome, indocyanine green, the authors demonstrated that cathepsin B expression was ubiquitous in adenomatous polyps and highest in larger polyps with higher degrees of dysplasia. Immunohistochemistry and fluorescence confocal microscopy were used to examine the resected murine colonic mucosa. Adenomas as small as 50 mm in diameter could be readily identified with the aid of the fluorescent beacon. To quantify the fluorescence signal the authors calculated a target (adenoma)-to-background (mucosa) contrast (TBC contrast). A value of 100 represented a 100% higher fluorescence signal of the adenoma compared with the colonic mucosa. Contrast in the large adenomas (TBC=220% + 97%) was thought to be caused by the higher amount of converting enzyme per lesion. Adenomas in the mice that received indocyanine green showed a significantly lower TBC contrast compared to those that received the cathepsin B sensing probe (TBC= 34% ± 4% vs 119 ± 71%, p <0.01).

In humans cathepsin B-positive tumor cells have been observed in 67% of adenomas and 100% of adenomas with HGD or adenocarcinoma.[74] Optically visible activatable fluorescent beacons could provide an important technology to screen patients for late stage adenomas. This technology could eventually be adapted to conventional endoscopy or even external NIR imaging of the bowel.

CONCLUSION

The optical techniques outlined in this chapter offer an exciting, potentially powerful means of detecting premalignancy in the GI tract. The technologies being investigated to detect early GI malignancies could be transferable to other organs. The ultimate goal of "optical biopsy" refers to the establishment of a tissue diagnosis based on *in situ* optical measurements without the need for tissue removal. Laser-induced and ALA-induced fluorescence have demonstrated high sensitivity and specificity for detecting colonic adenomas as well as dysplastic BE. The issue of improving fluorescence imaging technology to visualize larger areas of tissue more rapidly without sacrificing diagnostic accuracy remains to be solved. Determining the optimal excitation and emission wavelengths as well as the optimal dosage and route of administration of ALA-enhanced fluorescence requires further study. Light-scattering spectroscopy holds promise but is limited by the inability to survey large tissue surfaces. Raman spectroscopy offers a powerful method to visualize molecular activity, but is limited by a weak signal-to-noise ratio. By combining fluorescence, reflectance, and light-scattering spectroscopic techniques, "Trimodal spectroscopy" accurately classified nondysplastic and dysplastic Barrett's epithelium. This suggests that combining various spectroscopic techniques may be more powerful than each technique alone. OCT offers the highest resolution endoscopic tomographic imaging currently available. It has been shown to be a highly sensitive and specific means of identifying BE and appears capable of grading dysplasia in Barrett's epithelium. Molecular beacons have not yet been investigated in humans but may offer another potent method to target dysplastic and malignant cells based on the presence of proteolytic activity. These experimental technologies offer an exciting glimpse into the future of endoscopic diagnostic capabilities and the ever closer goal of performing an "optical biopsy."

REFERENCES

1. Jemal A, Murray T, Samuels A, Ghafoor A, Ward E, Thun MJ. Cancer statistics. *Cancer J Clinic.* 2003;53:5-26.
2. Blot WJ, Devesa SS, Kneller RW, Fraumeni JF Jr. Rising incidence of adenocarcinoma of the esophagus and gastric cardia. *JAMA.* 1991;265:1287-1289.
3. Bohorfoush AG. Tissue spectroscopy for gastrointestinal disease. *Endoscopy.* 1996; 28:372-380.
4. Stepp H, Sroka R, Baumgartner R. Fluorescence endoscopy of gastrointestinal disease: basic principles, techniques, and clinical experience. *Endoscopy.* 1998;30:379-386.
5. DaCosta RS, Wilson BC, Marcon NE. Light-induced fluorescence endoscopy of the gastrointestinal tract. *Gastrointest Endosc Clin N Am.* 2000;10:37-69.
6. Romer TJ, Fitzmaurice M, Cothren RM, et al. Laser-induced fluorescence microscopy of normal colon and dysplasia in colonic adenomas: implications for spectroscopic diagnosis. *Am J Gastroent.* 1995;90(1):81-87.
7. Kapadia CR, Cutruzzola FW, O'Brien KM, et al. Laser-induced fluorescence spectroscopy of human colonic mucosa. *Gastroenterology.* 1990;99:150-157.
8. Cothren RM, Richards-Kortum R, Sivak MV, et al. Gastrointestinal tissue diagnosis by laser-induced fluorescence spectroscopy at endoscopy. *Endoscopy.* 1990;36(2):105-111.
9. Richards-Kortum R, Rava RP, Petra RE, et al. Spectroscopic diagnosis of colonic dysplasia. *Photochemistry and Photobiology.* 1991;53(6):777-786.

10. Schomacker KT, Frisoli JK, Compton CC, et al. Ultraviolet laser-induced fluorescence of colonic polyps. *Gastroenterology.* 1992;102:1155-1160.

11. Cothren RM, Sivak MV, Van Dam J, et al. Detection of dysplasia at colonoscopy using laser-induced fluorescence: a blinded study. *Gastrointest Endosc.* 1996;44(2):168-176.

12. Panjehpour M, Overholt BF, Schmidhammer JL, Farris C, Buckley PF, Vo-Dinh T. Spectroscopic diagnosis of esophageal cancer: new classification model, improved measurement system. *Gastrointest Endosc.* 1995;41(6):577-581.

13. Panjehpour M, Overholt BF, Vo-Dinh T, Haggit RC, Edwards DH, Buckley FP. Endoscopic fluorescence detection of high-grade dysplasia in Barrett's esophagus. *Gastroenterology.* 1996;111:93-101.

14. Buttar NS, Wang KK, Sebo TJ, et al. Extent of high-grade dysplasia in Barrett's esophagus correlates with risk of adenocarcinoma. *Gastroenterology.* 2001;120:1630-1639.

15. Dar MS, Goldblum JR, Rice TW, Falk GW. Can extent of high grade dysplasia in Barrett's esophagus predict the presence of adenocarcinoma at esophagectomy? *Gut.* 2003;52(4):486-489.

16. Mayinger B, Horner P, Jordan M, et al. Light-induced autofluorescence spectroscopy for tissue diagnosis of GI lesions. *Gastrointestinal Endoscopy.* 2000;52(3):395-400.

17. Wang TD, Crawford JM, Feld MS, et al. In vivo identification of colonic dysplasia using fluorescence endoscopic imaging. *Gastrointest Endosc.* 1999;49(4):447-455.

18. Song WK, Wilson BC, Marcon NE. Diagnostic potential of light-induced fluorescence endoscopy in the colon. *Am J Gastroent.* 2001;96:S167.

19. Dacosta RS, Wilson BC, Marcon NE. New optical technologies for earlier endoscopic diagnosis of premalignant gastrointestinal lesions. *J Gastroentol Hepatol.* 2002; 17(Suppl):S85-S104.

20. Marcon NE, Wilson BC. The value of fluorescence techniques in gastrointestinal endoscopy—better than the endoscopist's eye? II: the North American experience. *Endoscopy.* 1998;30:419-421.

21. Loh CS, MacRobert AJ, Buonaccorsi G, Krasner N, Bown SG. Mucosal ablation using photodynamic therapy for the treatment of dysplasia: an experimental study in the normal rat stomach. *Gut.* 1996;38:71-78.

22. van den Boogert J, Houtsmuller AB, de Rooij FWM, et al. Kinetics, localization, and mechanism of 5-aminolevulinic acid-induced porphyrin accumulation in normal and Barrett's-like rat esophagus. *Lasers Surg Med.* 1999;24:3-13.

23. Messmann H. 5-aminolevulinic acid-induced protoporphyrin IX for the detection of gastrointestinal dysplasia. *Gastrointest Endoscop Clin N Am.* 2000;10(3):497-512.

24. Hinnen P, de Rooij FW, Velthuysen ML, et al. Biochemical basis of 5-aminolevulinic acid-induced protoporphyrin IX accumulation: a study in patients with (pre)malignant lesions of the esophagus. *Br J Cancer.* 1998;78:679.

25. Kennedy JC, Pottier RH. Endogenous protoporphyrin IX, a clinically useful photo-sensitizer for photodynamic therapy. *J Photochem Photobiol B.* 1992;14:275-292.

26. Barr H, Shepherd NA, Dix A, et al. Eradication of high-grade dysplasia in columnar-lined (Barrett's) esophagus by photodynamic therapy with endogenously generated protoporphyrin IX. *Lancet.* 1996;348:584-585.

27. Gossner L, Stolte M, Sroka R, et al. Photodynamic ablation of high-grade dysplasia and early cancer in Barrett's esophagus by means of 5-aminolevulinic acid. *Gastroenterology.* 1998;114:448-455.

28. von Holstein CS, Nilsson AMK, Andersson-Engels S, et al. Detection of adenocarcinoma in Barrett's esophagus by means of laser induced fluorescence. *Gut.* 1996;39(5):711-716.

29. Nishioka NS. Drug, light and oxygen: a dynamic combination in the clinic. *Gastroenterology.* 1998;114:604-606.

30. Overholt BF, Panjehpour M, Haydek JM. Photodynamic therapy for Barrett's esophagus: follow-up of 100 patients. *Gastrointest Endosc.* 1999;49:1-7.

31. Overholt BF, Panjehpour M. Photodynamic therapy for Barrett's esophagus. *Gastrointest Endoscop Clin N Am.* 1997;7:207-220.

32. Eker C, Montan S, Jaramillo E, et al. Clinical spectral characterization of colonic mucosal lesions using autofluorescence and delta aminolevulinic acid sensitization. *Gut.* 1999;44(4):511-518.

33. Mayinger B, Neidhardt S, Reh H, Martus P, Hahn EG. Fluorescence induced with 5-aminolevulinic acid for the endoscopic detection and follow-up of esophageal lesions. *Gastrointest Endosc.* 2000;54:572-578.

34. Endlicher E, Kneuchel R, Hauser T, et al. Endoscopic fluorescence detection of low and high grade dysplasia in Barrett's esophagus using systemic or local 5-aminolevulinic acid sensitization. *Gut.* 2001;48(3):314-319.

35. Brand S, Wang TD, Schomacker KT, et al. Detection of high-grade dysplasia in Barrett's esophagus by spectroscopy measurement of 5-aminolevulinic acid-induced protoporphyrin IX fluorescence. *Gastrointest Endosc.* 2002;56(4):479-487.

36. Messmann H, Endlicher E, Freunek G, Rummele P, Scholmerich J, Knuchel R. Fluorescence endoscopy for the detection of low and high grade dysplasia in ulcerative colitis using systemic or local 5-aminolevulinic acid sensitization. *Gut.* 2003;52(7): 1003-1007.

37. Regula J, MacRobert AJ, Gorchein A, et al. Photosensitization and photodynamic therapy of esophageal, duodenal, and colorectal tumors using 5-aminolevulinic acid induced protoporphyrin IX—a pilot study. *Gut.* 1995;36:67-75.

38. Backman V, Wallace MB, Perlman LT, et al. Detection of preinvasive cancer cells. *Nature.* 2000;406:35-36.

39. Rollins AM, Sivak MV. Potential new endoscopic techniques for the earlier diagnosis of pre-malignancy. *Best Pract Res Clin Gastroenterol.* 2001;15(2):227-247.

40. Wallace MB, Perelman LT, Backman V, et al. Endoscopic detection of dysplasia in patients with Barrett's esophagus using light-scattering spectroscopy. *Gastroenterology.* 2000;119:677-682.

41. Shim MG, Wilson BC. The effects of ex vivo handling procedures on the near-infrared Raman spectra of normal mammalian tissues. *Photochem Photobiol.* 1996;63:662-671.

42. Shim MG, Song LM WK, Marcon NE, Wilson BC. In vivo near-infrared Raman spectroscopy: demonstration of feasibility during clinical gastrointestinal endoscopy. *Photochem Photobiol.* 2000;72(1):146-150.

43. Molckovsky A, Song LM, Shim MG, Marcon NE, Wilson BC. Diagnostic potential of near-infrared Raman spectroscopy in the colon: differentiating adenomatous from hyperplastic polyps. *Gastrointest Endosc.* 2003;57(3):396-402.

44. Georgakoudi I, Jacobson BC, Van Dam J, et al. Fluorescence, reflectance, and light-scattering spectroscopy for evaluating dysplasia in patient's with Barrett's esophagus. *Gastroenterology.* 2001;120:1620-1629.

45. Pitris C, Jesser C, Boppart SA, et al. Feasibility of optical coherence tomography for high-resolution imaging of human gastrointestinal tract malignancies. *J Gastroenterol.* 2000;35:87-92.

46. Brand S, Poneros JM, Bouma BE, et al. Optical coherence tomography in the gastrointestinal tract. *Endoscopy.* 2000;32(10):796-803.

47. Wallace MB, Van Dam J. Enhanced gastrointestinal diagnosis: light-scattering spectroscopy and optical coherence tomography. *Gastrointest Endosc Clin N Am.* 2000; 10(1):71-80.

48. Tearney GJ, Brezinski ME, Bouma BE, et al. In vivo endoscopic optical biopsy with optical coherence tomography. *Science.* 1997;276(5321):2037-2039.

49. Tearney GJ, Brezinski ME, Southern JF, et al. Optical biopsy in human gastrointestinal tissue using optical coherence tomography. *Am J Gastroenterol.* 1997;92(10):1800.

50. Kobayashi K, Izatt JA, Kulkarni MD, Willis J, Sivak MV. High-resolution cross-sectional imaging of the gastrointestinal tract using optical coherence tomography: preliminary results. *Gastrointest Endosc.* 1998;47:515-523.

51. Tearney GJ, Brezinski ME, Southern JF, et al. Optical biopsy in human pancreatobiliary tissue using optical coherence tomography. *Dig Dis Sci.* 1998;43(6):1193-1199.

52. Bouma BE, Tearney GJ, Compton CC, Nishioka NS. High resolution of the human esophagus and stomach in vivo using optical coherence tomography. *Gastrointest Endosc.* 2000;51:467-474.

53. Jäckle S, Gladkova N, Feldchtein F, et al. In vivo endoscopic optical coherence tomography of the human gastrointestinal tract—toward optical biopsy. *Endoscopy.* 2000; 32(10):743-749.

54. Sergeev AM, Gelikonov VM, Gelikonov GV, et al. In vivo endoscopic OCT imaging of precancer and cancer states of human mucosa. *Optics Express.* 1997;1:432-440.

55. Jäckle S, Gladkova N, Feldchtein F, et al. In vivo endoscopic optical coherence tomography of esophagitis, Barrett's esophagus, and adenocarcinoma of the esophagus. *Endoscopy.* 2000;32(1):750-755.

56. Sivak MV Jr, Kobayashi K, Izatt JA, et al. High-resolution endoscopic imaging of the GI tract using optical coherence tomography. *Gastrointest Endosc.* 2000;51:474-479.

57. Zuccaro G, Gladkova N, Vargo J, et al. Optical coherence tomography of the esophagus and stomach in health and disease. *Am J Gastroenterol.* 2001;96(9):2633-2639.

58. Li XD, Boppart SA, Van Dam J, et al. Optical coherence tomography: advanced technology for the endoscopic imaging of Barrett's esophagus. *Endoscopy.* 2000;32(12):921-930.

59. Cilesiz I, Fockens P, Kerindongo R, et al. Comparative optical coherence tomography imaging of human esophagus: how accurate is localization of the muscularis mucosae? *Gastrointest Endosc.* 2002;56:852-857.

60. Poneros JM, Brand S, Bouma BE, et al. Diagnosis of specialized intestinal metaplasia by optical coherence tomography. *Gastroenterol.* 2001;120:7-12.

61. Poneros JM, Tearney GJ, Bouma BE, Lauwers GY, Nishioka NS. Diagnosis of dysplasia in Barrett's esophagus using optical coherence tomography. *Gastrointest Endosc.* 2001;53:AB 113.

62. Isenberg G, Sivak MV, Chak A, et al. Accuracy of endoscopic optical coherence tomography in the detection of dysplasia in Barrett's esophagus. *Gastrointest Endosc.* 2003; AB77.

63. Pfau PR, Sivak MV, Jr., Chak A, et al. Criteria for the diagnosis of dysplasia by endoscopic optical coherence tomography. *Gastrointest Endosc.* 2003;58:196-202.

64. Poneros JM, Tearney GJ, Shiskov M, et al. Optical coherence tomography of the biliary tree during ERCP. *Gastrointest Endosc.* 2002;55:84-88.

65. Drexler W, Morgner U, Kaertner FX, Pitris C, Boppart SA, Li XD, et al. In vitro ultrahigh resolution of optical coherence tomography. *Optics Letters.* 1999;24:1221-1223.

66. Koblinski JE, Ahram M, Sloane BF. Unraveling the role of proteases in cancer. *Clinica Chimica Acta.* 2000;291:113-135.

67. Emmert-Buck MR, Roth MJ, Zhuang Z, et al. Increased gelatinase A (MMP-2) and cathepsin B activity in invasive tumor regions of human colon cancer samples. *Am J Pathol.* 1994;145(6):1285-1290.

68. Hazen LG, Bleeker FE, Lauritzen B, et al. Comparative localization of cathepsin B protein and activity in colorectal cancer. *J Histochem Cytochem.* 2000;48(10):1421-1430.

69. Herszenyi L, Plebani M, Carraro P, et al. The role of cysteine and serine proteases in colorectal carcinoma. *Cancer.* 1999;86(7):1135-1142.

70. Weissleder R, Tung CH, Mahmood U, Bogdanov A Jr. In vivo imaging of tumors with protease-activated near-infrared fluorescent probes. *Nat Biotechnology.* 1999;17:375-378.

71. Mahmood U, Tung C, Bogdanov A, Weissleder R. Near infrared optical imaging system to detect tumor protease activity. *Radiology.* 1999;213:866-870.

72. Marten K, Bremer C, Khazaie K, et al. Detection of dysplastic intestinal adenomas using enzyme-sensing molecular beacons in mice. *Gastroenterology.* 2002;122(2):406-414.

73. Moser AR, Pitot HC, Dove WF. A dominant mutation that predisposes to multiple intestinal neoplasia in the mouse. *Science.* 1990;247(4940):322-324.

74. Khan A, Krishna M, Baker SP, Banner BF. Cathepsin B and tumor-associated laminin expression in the progression of colorectal adenoma to carcinoma. *Modern Pathology.* 1998;11(8):704-708.

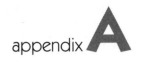

Esophageal Cancer Staging

DEFINITION OF TNM

PRIMARY TUMOR (T)

TX   Primary tumor cannot be assessed

T0   No evidence of primary tumor

Tis   Carcinoma *in situ*

T1   Tumor invades lamina propria or submucosa

T2   Tumor invades muscularis propria

T3   Tumor invades adventitia

T4   Tumor invades adjacent structures

REGIONAL LYMPH NODES (N)

NX   Regional lymph nodes cannot be assessed

N0   No regional lymph node metastasis

N1   Regional lymph node metastasis

DISTANT METASTASIS (M)

MX   Distant metastasis cannot be assessed

M0   No distant metastasis

M1   Distant metastasis

Tumors of the Lower Thoracic Esophagus

M1a   Metastasis in celiac lymph nodes

M1b   Other distant metastasis

Tumors of the Midthoracic Esophagus

M1a   Not applicable

M1b   Nonregional lymph nodes and/or other distant metastasis

Tumors of the Upper Thoracic Esophagus

M1a   Metastasis in cervical nodes

M1b   Other distant metastasis

STAGE GROUPING

Stage 0	Tis	N0	M0
Stage I	T1	N0	M0
Stage IIA	T2	N0	M0
	T3	N0	M0
Stage IIB	T1	N1	M0
	T2	N1	M0
Stage III	T3	N1	M0
	T4	Any N	M0
Stage IV	Any T	Any N	M1
Stage IVA	Any T	Any N	M1a
Stage IVB	Any T	Any N	M1b

Gastric Cancer Staging

DEFINITION OF TNM

PRIMARY TUMOR (T)

TX   Primary tumor cannot be assessed

T0   No evidence of primary tumor

Tis   Carcinoma *in situ*: intraepitheal tumor without invasion of the lamina propria

T1   Tumor invades lamina propria or submucosa

T2   Tumor invades muscularis propria or subserosa*

T2a   Tumor invades muscularis propria

T2b   Tumor invades subserosa

T3   Tumor penetrates serosa (visceral peritoneum) without invasion of adjacent structures**, ***

T4   Tumor invades adjacent structures**,***

Note. A tumor may penetrate the muscularis propria with extension into the gastrocolic or gastrohepatic ligaments, or into the greater or lesser omentum, without perforation of the visceral peritoneum covering these structures. In this case, the tumor is classified as T2. If there is perforation of the visceral peritoneum covering the gastric ligaments or the omentum, the tumor should be classified as T3.

**Note*. The adjacent structures of the stomach include the spleen, transverse colon, liver, diaphragm, pancreas, abdominal wall, adrenal gland, kidney, small intestine, and retroperitorneum.

****Note*. Intramural extension to the duodenum or esophagus is classified by the depth of the greatest invasion in any of these sites, including the stomach.

REGIONAL LYMPH NODES (N)

NX   Regional lymph node(s) cannot be assessed

N0   No regional lymph node metastasis*

N1   Metastasis in 1 to 6 regional lymph nodes

N2   Metastasis in 7 to 15 regional lymph nodes

N3   Metastais in more than 15 regional lymph nodes

*Note: A designation of pN0 should be used if all examined lymph nodes are negative, regardless of the total number removed and examined.

DISTANT METASTASIS (M)

MX   Distant metastasis cannot be assessed

M0   No distant metastasis

M1   Distant metastasis

STAGE GROUPING

Stage 0	Tis	N0	M0
Stage IA	T1	N0	M0
Stage IB	T1	N1	M0
	T2a	N0	M0
	T2b	N0	M0
Stage II	T1	N2	M0
	T2a	N1	M0
	T2b	N1	M0
	T3	N0	M0
Stage IIIA	T2a	N2	M0
	T2b	N2	M0
	T3	N1	M0
	T4	N0	M0
Stage IIIB	T3	N2	M0
Stage IV	T4	N1-3	M0
	T1	N3	M0
	T2	N3	M0
	T3	N3	M0
	Any T	Any N	M1

Pancreas Cancer Staging

DEFINITION OF TNM

PRIMARY TUMOR (T)

TX Primary tumor cannot be assessed

T0 No evidence of primary tumor

Tis Carcinoma *in situ**

T1 Tumor limited to the pancreas, 2 cm or less in greatest dimension

T2 Tumor limited to the pancreas, more than 2 cm in greatest dimension

T3 Tumor extends beyond the pancreas but without involvement of the celiac axis or the superior mesenteric artery

T4 Tumor involves the celiac axis or the superior mesenteric artery (unresectable primary tumor)

*Note: This includes the "PainInIII" classification N3 "metastasis"

REGIONAL LYMPH NODES (N)

NX Regional lymph node(s) cannot be assessed

N0 No regional lymph node metastasis

N1 Regional lymph node metastasis

DISTANT METASTASIS (M)

MX Distant metastasis cannot be assessed

M0 No distant metastasis

M1 Distant metastasis

STAGE GROUPING

Stage 0	Tis	N0	M0
Stage IA	T1	N0	M0
Stage IB	T2	N1	M0
Stage IIA	T3	N2	M0
Stage IIB	T1	N1	M0
	T2	N1	M0
	T3	N1	M0
Stage III	T4	Any N	M0
Stage IV	Any T	Any N	M1

Used with the permission of the American Joint Committee on Cancer (AJCC7), Chicago, Illinois. The original source for this material is the *AJCC Cancer Staging Manual,* 6th edition (2002). Springer-Verlag: New York, Inc., New York, New York.

Colon and Rectum Cancer Staging

DEFINITION OF TNM

The same classification is used for both clinical and pathologic staging.

PRIMARY TUMOR (T)

TX   Primary tumor cannot be assessed

T0   No evidence of primary tumor

Tis   Carcinoma *in situ*: intraepitheal or invasion of the lamina propria*

T1   Tumor invades submucosa

T2   Tumor invades muscularis propria

T3   Tumor invades through the muscularis propria into the subserosa, or into nonperitonealized pericolic or perirectal tissues

T4   Tumor directly invades other organs or structures, and/or perforates visceral peritoneum**,***

*Note: Tis includes cancer cells confined within the gladular basement membrane (intraepithelial) or lamina propria (intramucosal) with no extension through the muscularis mucosae into the submucosa.

**Note: Direct invasion in T4 includes invasion of other segments of the colorectum by way of the serosa; for example, invasion of the sigmoid colon by a carcinoma of the cecum.

***Note: Tumor that is adherent to other organs or structures, macroscopically, is classified as T4. However, if no tumor is present in the adhesion, microscopically, the classification should be pT3. The V and L substaging should be used to identify the presence or absence of vascular or lymphatic invasion.

REGIONAL LYMPH NODES (N)

NX   Regional lymph node(s) cannot be assessed

N0   No regional lymph node metastasis

N1   Metastasis in 1 to 3 regional lymph nodes

N2   Metastasis in 4 or more regional lymph nodes

Note: A tumor nodule in the pericolorectal adipose tissue of a primary carcinoma without histologic evidence of residual lymph node in the nodule is classified in the pN category as a regional lymph node metastasis if the nodule has the form and smooth contour of a lymph node. If the nodule has an irregular contour, it should be classified in the T category and also coded as V1 (microscopic venous invasion) or as V2 (if it was grossly evident), because there is a strong likelihood that it represents venous invasion.

DISTANT METASTASIS (M)

MX   Distant metastasis cannot be assessed

M0   No distant metastasis

M1   Distant metastasis

STAGE GROUPING

Stage	T	N	M	Dukes*	MAC*
0	Tis	N0	M0	-	-
I	T1	N0	M0	A	A
	T2	N0	M0	A	B1
IIA	T3	N0	M0	B	B2
IIB	T4	N0	M0	B	B3
IIIA	T1-T2	N1	M0	C	C1
IIIB	T3-T4	N1	M0	C	C2/C3
IIIC	Any T	N2	M0	C	C1/C2/C3
IV	Any T	Any N	M1	-	D

*Dukes B is a composite of better (T3 N0 M0) and worse (T4 N0 M0) prognostic groups, as is Dukes C (Any TN1 M0 and Any T N2 M0). MAC is the modified Astler-Coller classification.

Note: The y prefix is to be used for those cancers that are classified after pretreatment, whereas the r prefix is to be used for those cancers that have recurred.

Used with the permission of the American Joint Committee on Cancer (AJCC7), Chicago, Illinois. The original source for this material is the *AJCC Cancer Staging Manual,* 6th edition (2002). Springer-Verlag: New York, Inc., New York, New York.

Index

WAIT
...There's More!